TECHNOLOGY
for DIAGNOSTIC
SONOGRAPHY

WAYNE R. HEDRICK, Ph.D., FACR

Professor, Medical Radiation Biophysics,
Northeast Ohio Medical University, Rootstown, Ohio,
Aultman Hospital, Canton, Ohio

ELSEVIER

ELSEVIER
MOSBY

3251 Riverport Lane
St. Louis, Missouri 63043

Technology for Diagnostic Sonography   ISBN: 978-0-323-08198-6

Notices

Knowledge and best practice in this field are constantly changing. As new research and experience broaden our understanding, changes in research methods, professional practices, or medical treatment may become necessary.

Practitioners and researchers must always rely on their own experience and knowledge in evaluating and using any information, methods, compounds, or experiments described herein. In using such information or methods they should be mindful of their own safety and the safety of others, including parties for whom they have a professional responsibility.

With respect to any drug or pharmaceutical products identified, readers are advised to check the most current information provided (i) on procedures featured or (ii) by the manufacturer of each product to be administered, to verify the recommended dose or formula, the method and duration of administration, and contraindications. It is the responsibility of practitioners, relying on their own experience and knowledge of their patients, to make diagnoses, to determine dosages and the best treatment for each individual patient, and to take all appropriate safety precautions.

To the fullest extent of the law, neither the Publisher nor the authors, contributors, or editors, assume any liability for any injury and/or damage to persons or property as a matter of products liability, negligence or otherwise, or from any use or operation of any methods, products, instructions, or ideas contained in the material herein.

Previous editions copyrighted

Library of Congress Cataloging-in-Publication Data
Hedrick, Wayne R.
   Technology for diagnostic sonography / Wayne R. Hedrick.
      p. ; cm.
   ISBN 978-0-323-08198-6 (pbk. : alk. paper)
   I. Title.
   [DNLM: 1. Ultrasonography–methods. 2. Ultrasonics. 3. Ultrasonography–instrumentation.
WN 208]

616.07'543–dc23

                                                                    2011043781

Publisher: Jeanne Olson
Managing Editor: Linda Woodard
Publishing Services Manager: Catherine Jackson
Project Manager: Sara Alsup
Design Direction: Paula Catalano

PREFACE

What an exciting time for diagnostic medical sonography! Although the fundamental principles were established over 30 years ago, technological innovations continue to improve image quality and performance capabilities. The images of today bear little resemblance to those of the 1970s.

Technology for Diagnostic Sonography and its companion volume, *Study Guide and Laboratory Exercises*, are designed to help the student acquire the theoretical knowledge that is the basis for ultrasound scanning, as well as the practical application of that knowledge. Structured in eighteen chapters, which are designed to be read in sequence, this text provides comprehensive coverage of physics principles, ultrasound transducers, pulse echo instrumentation, Doppler instrumentation, clinical safety, and quality control. It includes the latest information on real-time imaging techniques, plus an extensive discussion of image artifacts. The intended audience is the beginning sonographer, who, with effort, can master this subject matter. No other imaging modality is as dependent on operator interaction. To achieve the optimal images for the benefit of every patient, the sonographer must have thorough understanding of sonography physics and instrumentation. Sonography offers challenges but also a sense of accomplishment to its practitioners.

FEATURES

- **A focus on essential physics and instrumentation** provides the fundamental technical content.
- **Examples** make the connection between theory and practical applications.

- **The latest information on equipment and scanning methods** ensures an understanding of how to competently and safely use ultrasound instrumentation.
- **Comprehensive discussion of image artifacts** with illustrative examples helps you recognize artifacts and respond appropriately to their presence.
- **Detailed description of performance testing with tissue mimicking phantoms** allows assessment of the proper operation of B-mode scanners.
- **Practical guidance on the clinical use of mechanical index and thermal index** enables practice of the ALARA principle when scanning patients.
- **Key terms** in each chapter focus your study on important information.
- **Summaries of essential principles and equations** reinforce the most important concepts.
- **Glossary** of common sonography terms that includes definitions for all the key terms in the book.

FOR THE READER

The companion Evolve website includes a randomized practice quiz feature that includes over 600 questions that cover all topics in the book. The user chooses the topic and number of questions in each quiz. Feedback is included for each question.

FOR THE INSTRUCTOR

The following instructor resources are available on Evolve.
- A test bank, available in Examview or Word, which includes over 400 questions.
- PowerPoint slides, designed to be lecture ready.

ACKNOWLEDGMENTS

During many hours of discussion Bruce K. Daniels, RDCS; Eileen M. Nemec, RDCS' Jo Ann Lamb, RDMS, RVT, RT (R) (M); Paul Wagner, BS, RDCS; RDMS, RVT; and Paul A. Cardullo, MS, BSN, RVT, provided insight to the practical clinical applications of sonography principles.

For assistance in the acquisition of sonographic images the author thanks Linda Metzger, RT(R), RDMS, RVT, and Yvette Ramos, RDMS, RVT.

Jeanne Olson's editorial direction created a new approach for teaching sonography physics and instrumentation. Linda Woodard was able to balance two manuscripts simultaneously while contributing her editorial expertise.

TABLE OF CONTENTS

Properties of Sound Waves

Chapter Objectives

To describe ultrasound transmission in tissue, which includes type of wave, frequency, particle density, and energy flow
To define common descriptors of waves
To identify the properties of the medium that affect sound transmission
To state the relationship between acoustic velocity, wavelength, and frequency

Key Terms

Acoustic velocity
Amplitude
Bulk modulus
Compressibility
Compression
Cycle

Density
Elasticity
Frequency
Intensity
Longitudinal waves
Period

Propagation
Rarefaction
Transducer
Transverse waves
Wavelength

SOUND

Sound is mechanical energy that is transmitted through a medium (e.g., air, water, iron, or tissue) by forces acting on molecules. The induced molecular motion is periodic, whereby the molecules oscillate back and forth about their unperturbed positions. These fluctuations cause variations in molecular density and pressure (greater than and lower than the natural state) along the path of the sound wave. As vibrating molecules interact with their neighbors, the periodic changes in pressure and molecular density are conveyed from one location to another. The term propagation describes this transmission of mechanical energy to distant regions remote from the sound source.

Compression and Rarefaction

Consider the diaphragm in an audio speaker as a sound source. The motion of the diaphragm can be visualized as a piston. When the diaphragm moves forward, the air molecules (or particles) immediately in front are pushed together, producing a region of increased air density characterized by a small zone of increased pressure. The term compression describes the formation of the high-pressure region (Fig. 1-1). When the diaphragm vibrates back, a zone of decreased molecular density results. The term rarefaction describes the creation of this low-pressure region.

The vibration of the diaphragm alternately compresses the air on a forward thrust and rarefies the air on a backward thrust. The regions of compression and rarefaction are transmitted through the medium by molecular interactions. The originally affected molecules collide with adjacent molecules to propagate the action of the diaphragm. Thus the transmission of mechanical energy through the medium creates regions of varying particle density and pressure. Compression zones alternate with

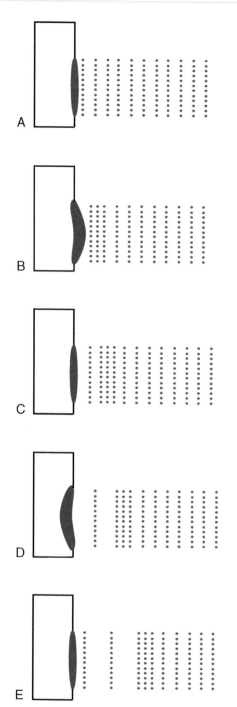

Figure 1-1 Oscillation of air molecules produced by a speaker. However, the collective action of the molecules is complex. **A,** Undisturbed medium (no movement of diaphragm). **B,** Diaphragm moving outward, compressing the medium. **C,** Diaphragm returning to its original position as a region of compression advances. **D,** Diaphragm moving inward, creating rarefaction in the medium. **E,** Diaphragm returning to its original position as the regions of compression and rarefaction advance.

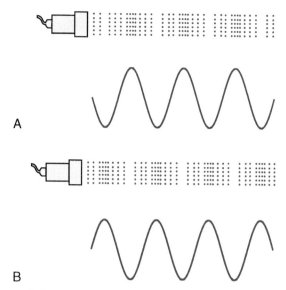

Figure 1-2 Particle density along the path of propagation varies with time. Regions of high and low density alternate, as shown by the sinusoidal curves. **A,** Initial observation. **B,** After a short time the regions of high and low density are displaced to the right.

rarefaction zones. Between adjacent compression zones, particle density decreases from a maximum in the compression zone to a minimum in the rarefaction zone; then it increases back to a maximum at the succeeding compression zone. If the action of sound propagation is suspended in time, a plot of particle density as a function of

distance exhibits a sinusoidal wave pattern (Fig 1-2, *A*). At a later instant in time, the sinusoidal wave pattern of particle density is maintained (Fig. 1-2, *B*), but the compression and rarefaction zones have shifted to new locations along the direction of propagation. This is described as linear propagation, since molecular density follows a sine-wave variation along the transmission path (a plot of molecular density with distance at an instant in time is a sine wave). Molecular density is not constant at a particular position but oscillates with a certain time dependence imposed by the action of the sound source. The rate of change from high density to low density depends on how fast the sound source vibrates (how rapidly the diaphragm moves in and out).

The molecules are displaced from and vibrate about their customary positions (a distance of only several microns) as the sound wave passes through the medium. A micron is equal to 10^{-6} meter. The motion of the molecules at a particular location is also sinusoidal and is dictated by the vibrational rate of the sound source (Fig. 1-3). Molecules do not travel from one end of the medium to the other; there is no flow of particles. Rather, the effect is transmitted over long distances because of neighbor-to-neighbor interactions. Sound transmission cannot occur in a vacuum because no molecules are available to transfer the mechanical vibrations.

Sound transmission is usually portrayed diagrammatically by showing the compression zones. A compression zone is often considered the leading portion of the sound wave and hence is called the wavefront. Wavefronts are helpful in illustrating the direction in which sound travels (perpendicular to the compression zone) and the region over which sound transmission takes place (the ultrasonic field).

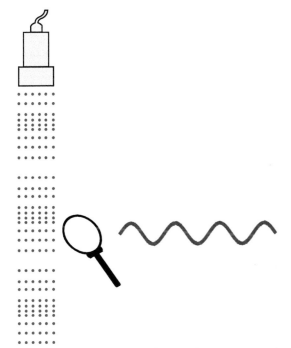

Figure 1-3 Molecular motion as a function of time at a point within the ultrasonic field. As the sound wave propagates through the medium, individual molecules vibrate back and forth over a small distance.

Amplitude is the magnitude of a physical entity from the neutral value to the maximum extent in an oscillation. The term can be applied to acoustic pressure, particle density, particle displacement, or particle velocity in the medium. It has other applications, such as to characterize the magnitude of a voltage pulse delivered to or induced within the crystal of the transducer. Since the motion of the molecules (particles) is repetitive, the term cycle is used to describe any sequence of changes in molecular motion (particle displacement, density of molecules, pressure, or particle velocity) that recurs at regular intervals.

The frequency of a wave is the number of vibrations (back-and-forth movements) that a molecule makes per second or the number of times the cycle is repeated each second. For comparative purposes, higher frequency means that the cyclic motion is executed at a faster rate and more cycles are completed in the 1-second interval than at lower frequency. Sound waves are those pressure changes that the human ear can detect. They oscillate at frequencies of 20 to 20,000 cycles per second, also referred to as hertz (Hz). Cycle is not a standard of measurement but is used as a descriptor to clarify the concept of frequency. Often frequency is expressed in units of inverse time only ($1/s$ or s^{-1}). Ultrasound is defined as mechanical waves with higher frequency than humans can hear; frequencies greater than 20,000 Hz or 20 kilohertz (kHz). *Infrasound* refers to mechanical waves with frequencies lower than humans can hear: frequencies less than 20 Hz. Sound, ultrasound, and infrasound have similar properties; thus these terms are often used interchangeably in the description of physical interactions.

Longitudinal and Transverse Sound Waves

Waves are divided into two basic types: longitudinal and transverse. Longitudinal waves are those in which particle motion is along the direction of the wave energy propagation; that is, the molecules vibrate back and forth in the same direction as the wave is traveling (Fig. 1-4). Sound waves in liquids and tissue are longitudinal.

Transverse waves are those in which the motion of the particles is perpendicular to the direction of propagation of the wave energy (Fig. 1-5). The wave motion that occurs when a stone is thrown into a pool of water is an example of a transverse wave. The water molecules vibrate up and down, like a cork floating on the water, as the wave moves away from the point of origin across the surface of the water. Bone is an example of biological tissue that can exhibit transverse waves, which are sometimes referred to as shear waves.

Wave Descriptors

Wavelength is the distance of one complete wave cycle, as illustrated by the variation in particle density along the propagation path (Fig. 1-6). Wavelength is measured between two successive zones of equivalent density (i.e., two compression zones or two rarefaction zones) and is

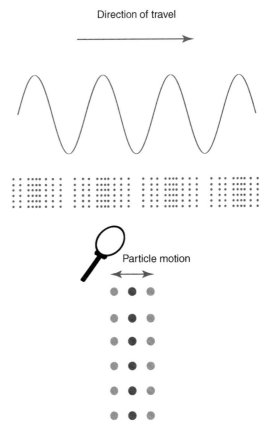

Figure 1-4 Longitudinal wave. Molecular (particle) motion is along the direction of propagation.

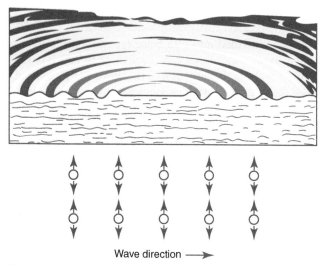

Figure 1-5 Transverse wave. The direction of travel of the wave is radially outward from the source, as when a stone is dropped into a calm pond. Molecular (particle) motion is perpendicular to the direction of propagation.

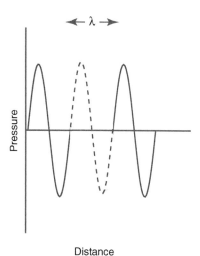

Figure 1-6 Particle density as function of distance of wave travel. The wavelength is equal to the distance between successive maxima or minima. It is also defined as the distance needed to complete one wave cycle (dotted line).

expressed in units of a meter (m), centimeter (cm), or millimeter (mm).

The frequency of a wave (f) is the number of cycles (pressure oscillations) occurring at a given point in one unit of time (usually 1 second). When the particle density at a point is plotted as a function of time, the period of the wave (τ) is defined as the time necessary for one complete cycle or the time between two successive compression zones or rarefaction zones. The frequency is equal to the reciprocal of the period ($1/\tau$).

The following equation defines the relationship between period and frequency:

1-1
$$f = \frac{1}{\tau}$$

Example 1-1

Calculate the period of a wave whose frequency is 4,000,000 Hz, or 4×10^6 cycles per second, or 4 MHz.

$$\tau = \frac{1}{f}$$

$$\tau = \frac{1}{4{,}000{,}000 \ 1/s}$$

$$\tau = 2.5 \times 10^{-7} \ s = 0.25 \ \mu s$$

Example 1-2

Calculate the frequency of a wave whose period is 5×10^{-7} second.

$$f = \frac{1}{\tau}$$

$$f = \frac{1}{5 \times 10^{-7} \ s}$$

$$f = 2.0 \times 10^6 \ 1/s = 2 \ MHz$$

Examples 1-1 and 1-2 illustrate the inverse relationship between frequency and period. When the period is doubled (from 2.5×10^{-7} s to 5.0×10^{-7} s), the frequency is halved (from 4 MHz to 2 MHz).

To facilitate communication of the very large and very small numbers encountered in ultrasound physics, engineering prefixes are used. These prefixes correspond to various multiples of powers of 10, as shown in Table 1-1. When a physical parameter is expressed in scientific notation that includes some standard unit (i.e., meter, second, hertz, watt, etc.), the prefix replaces the power of 10 and becomes a modifier of the unit. For example, 4×10^6 Hz becomes 4 MHz.

The speed at which a wave propagates through the medium (rate of transfer of the mechanical vibrations) is called the acoustic velocity (c). In physics, velocity is usually considered a vector quantity; magnitude and direction are assigned. In ultrasound physics, the term *velocity* traditionally refers to magnitude only (a scalar quantity). The velocity of sound is determined by the rate at which the

Table 1-1	Unit Prefixes Representing Powers of 10	
Factor	**Prefix**	**Symbol**
10^9	giga	G
10^6	mega	M
10^3	kilo	k
10^{-2}	centi	c
10^{-3}	milli	m
10^{-6}	micro	μ
10^{-9}	nano	n
10^{-12}	pico	p

wave energy is transmitted through the medium, which depends on the physical density (mass per unit volume) and compressibility of the medium. Note that the acoustic velocity is not the same as the particle velocity, which is the speed at which the particles move when acted on by mechanical force.

The rate at which the wave transmits energy over a small area is the intensity, expressed in units of watts per centimeter squared (W/cm^2) or milliwatts per centimeter squared (mW/cm^2). As sound intensity is increased, the molecular density and acoustic pressure in the compression zone are also increased; this is accompanied by longer particle oscillation length and faster particle velocity. Intensity does not affect frequency, wavelength, or acoustic velocity during linear propagation. In a stereo system, the volume control adjusts the loudness of the sound output but does not alter the pitch (frequency). As volume is increased, the diaphragm moves over a greater distance, but the time for an in-and-out oscillation is unchanged.

At high intensity, as in tissue harmonic imaging, propagation is no longer linear. Nonlinear propagation alters particle velocity during rarefaction compared with that during compression, and the sinusoidal wave becomes distorted. However, the change in waveform proceeds in a predictable manner (introduction of harmonics) and can be used to image tissue where nonlinear propagation occurs.

SOUND-PROPAGATION MEDIA

Sound waves are mechanical in nature, but they are not restricted to transmission through air. Mechanical pressure waves, however, require an elastic deformable medium for propagation, which can be gas, liquid, or solid. A solid is deformable because increased pressure applied to it causes a change in its shape. Elasticity is demonstrated by a return to the original shape when the pressure is lowered to its initial value. The amount of this distortion depends on the strength of the force and the elastic properties of the object. The latter is determined by molecular interactions. An ultrasound wave traveling through soft tissue causes elastic deformations by the separation and compression of neighboring molecules.

Density is the mass of a medium per unit volume. If all other physical properties of the medium are maintained unchanged, an increase in density will impede the rate of sound propagation through the medium. As the density increases, more mass is contained within a given volume. For particles with increasingly larger mass, more force is required to produce molecular motion; and once the molecules are moving, more force is required to stop them. This is true for the rhythmic starting and stopping required to produce sound transmission. Thus, on the basis of density alone, we would expect sound to have a greater velocity in air (low density) than in bone (high density). However, this is not the case; therefore other factors must influence acoustic velocity.

Another physical characteristic of a medium, compressibility, affects the velocity of sound through the medium. Compressibility indicates the fractional decrease in volume when pressure is applied to the material. The easier a medium is to reduce in volume, the higher is its compressibility.

The parameter relating the elastic properties of a medium to the velocity of sound through it is usually expressed as the reciprocal of the compressibility, termed the bulk modulus (B). The bulk modulus is often defined as the negative ratio of stress and strain. Stress is the force per unit area (or pressure) applied to an object. Strain is the fractional change in volume of the object. The negative sign is required, since a positive pressure causes a decrease in volume. Large values for the bulk modulus indicate that a material is resistant to change in its volume when force is applied (low compressibility). Acoustic velocity is directly proportional to the square root of the bulk modulus.

A dense material (e.g., bone or some other solid) is very difficult to reduce in volume when pressure is applied to it. This low compressibility predicts the high velocity of sound in bone. By contrast, air is easily reduced in volume because the gas molecules are far apart and can be easily brought closer together (compressibility is high). The velocity of sound in air is low. Based on differences in both density and compressibility, the velocity of sound in bone (4080 m/s) is much greater than that in air (330 m/s).

Quantitatively, the velocity of sound in a medium (c) is directly proportional to the square root of the bulk modulus and inversely proportional to the square root of the density of the medium (ρ). By combining the bulk modulus and density into one equation, the acoustic velocity for a particular medium can be determined:

$$1\text{-}2 \qquad c = \sqrt{\frac{B}{\rho}}$$

If the density can be increased without affecting the bulk modulus, then Equation 1-2 predicts that the speed of sound will decrease. The compressibility and density of a particular substance are interdependent; a change in density is often coupled with a larger and opposing change in compressibility. Because compressibility varies more rapidly, it becomes the dominant factor in the determination of acoustic velocity. The overall effect is commonly summarized by the statement that as the density of a medium increases, the velocity of sound through it increases. Exceptions can be cited; but for materials of interest to the sonographer (air, lung, fat, soft tissue, plastic, bone), this statement is generally true. The acoustic velocities for common materials are shown in Table 1-2.

For liquids in general, density and compressibility offset each other; consequently different liquids tend to transmit ultrasound at nearly the same velocity. In the transmission of sound, soft tissue behaves similarly to liquid; the acoustic velocities for various tissue types do not vary by more than a few percent.

Table 1-2	Sound Speed in Different Media
Material	**Acoustic Velocity (m/s)**
Air	330
Water	1480
Lung	600
Liver	1555
Muscle	1600
Aqueous humor	1510
Lens of eye	1620
Bone	4080
Fat	1460
Blood	1575
Soft tissue (average)	1540

Because their compressibility is low, more dense media (most solids) usually have greater velocities than do less dense media (liquids or gases). This is one of the reasons (the other will soon become evident) why, in old western movies, cowboys would put their heads to the ground or to a railroad track to hear the sound of stampeding buffalo or that of an approaching train. *Sound travels faster in media that are denser than air because of their reduced compressibility.*

The average velocity of ultrasound in tissue is 1540 m/s or 154,000 cm/s or 1.54 mm/μs. A slight dependence on the temperature of the medium and on sound frequency is exhibited; the velocity of ultrasound waves in water at 20° C is 1480 m/s, but it rises to 1570 m/s in water that is 37° C. For a few degrees' shift in temperature, the change in velocity through water is small. Thus fluctuations in room temperature are not a problem with respect to sonography, because the body maintains a nearly constant temperature.

The dependence of velocity or other physical parameter on frequency is called dispersion. The change in velocity with frequency is small (less than 0.5%) over the frequency range used in diagnostic ultrasound, which is 2 to 20 MHz. The velocity of sound in different materials (e.g., blood versus soft tissue) has varying frequency dependence, but these small differences have little importance in clinical imaging.

ACOUSTIC VELOCITY EQUATION

The acoustic velocity (c) remains constant for a particular medium. Acoustic velocity equals the product of frequency (f) and the wavelength (λ). Stated mathematically:

1-3 $$c = f\lambda$$

This is the first essential equation of sonography. Because the acoustic velocity is constant for a particular medium, increasing the frequency causes the wavelength to decrease.

Example 1-3

Using Equation 1-3, we can determine the wavelength in tissue for an ultrasound source with a 2.5-MHz frequency as follows:

$$c = f\lambda$$
$$\lambda = \frac{c}{f}$$
$$\lambda = \frac{1540 \text{ m/s}}{2.5 \times 10^6 \text{ 1/s}}$$
$$\lambda = 6.2 \times 10^{-4} \text{ m} = 0.62 \text{ mm}$$

If the frequency is increased to 5 MHz, the wavelength decreases to 0.31 mm, or half the value of 0.62 mm at 2.5 MHz, because the frequency has doubled.

In going from a medium with one acoustic velocity to a medium with another, the frequency of the sound beam remains constant. This means that a change in the wavelength of the sound beam must accompany the velocity shift, as expressed by Equation 1-3.

Example 1-4

The wavelength of an ultrasonic beam in tissue generated by a 2.5-MHz transducer is 0.62 mm in tissue, as demonstrated in Example 1-3. If the sound beam is then transmitted into bone, the wavelength becomes

$$\lambda = \frac{4080 \text{ m/s}}{2.5 \times 10^6 \text{ 1/s}}$$
$$\lambda = 1.6 \times 10^{-3} \text{ m}$$
$$\lambda = 1.6 \text{ mm}$$

The wavelength of the ultrasound wave as a function of frequency can be determined for any medium for which the acoustic velocity is known. In medical imaging the medium of interest is soft tissue, where an acoustic velocity of 1540 m/s is assumed. Equation 1-3 can be simplified by substituting the velocity of soft tissue:

1-4 $$\lambda \text{ (soft tissue)} = \frac{1.54 \text{ mm}}{f \text{ (MHz)}}$$

Dividing 1.54 by the frequency expressed in megahertz yields the wavelength in millimeters.

Example 1-5

Using Equation 1-4, we can calculate the wavelength in tissue for an ultrasound source with a 5-MHz frequency as follows:

$$\lambda \text{ (soft tissue)} = \frac{1.54 \text{ mm}}{5 \text{ (MHz)}}$$
$$\lambda \text{ (soft tissue)} = 0.31 \text{ mm}$$

Table 1-3 lists the wavelengths and periods of an ultrasound waves in soft tissue as the frequency is varied.

Table 1-3	Frequency, Wavelength, and Period for Ultrasound Waves in Soft Tissue

Frequency (MHz)	Wavelength (mm)	Period (μs)
1.0	1.54	1.00
2.5	0.62	0.40
3.5	0.44	0.29
5.0	0.31	0.20
7.5	0.21	0.13
10	0.15	0.10
15	0.10	0.07
20	0.08	0.05

SOUND TRANSMISSION

In sonography a single device, called the transducer, functions as the sound source and the detector of echoes. The transducer may operate in continuous- or pulsed-wave output mode depending on the application. Continuous-wave (CW) transmission continuously emits a constant frequency with a constant peak-pressure amplitude sound wave from the source (Fig. 1-7). Pulsed-wave (PW) transmission is a short-duration burst of sound (a few cycles in length) emitted from the sound source (Fig. 1-8). In the latter case the transducer must be turned on and off very rapidly (sound generation is less than 1 microsecond).

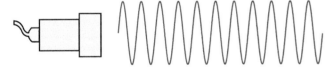

Figure 1-7 Continuous-wave output.

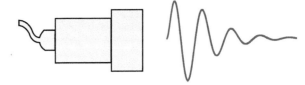

Figure 1-8 Pulsed-wave output.

SUMMARY

Sound waves in tissue are longitudinal mechanical waves. The vibrating sound source alternately compresses and rarefies the molecules in close proximity to the source and then transmits this action to more distant regions. Waves and propagation media have certain characteristics that describe them. Table 1-4 lists the common descriptors introduced in this chapter. Acoustic velocity in a medium remains constant as frequency is varied. The first essential equation of sonography reveals the interdependence of the wave properties of acoustic velocity, frequency, and wavelength. Sound transmission by an ultrasound transducer may be in the form of continuous- or pulsed-wave output.

Table 1-4	List of Physical Descriptors	
Descriptor	**Symbol**	**Units**
Bulk modulus	B	$kg/(m\text{-}s^2)$
Density	ρ	kg/m^3, g/cm^3
Frequency	f	1/s, Hz, kHz, MHz
Period	τ	s, μs
Acoustic velocity	c	m/s, cm/s, mm/μs
Wavelength	λ	m, cm, mm, μm
Intensity	I	mW/cm^2, W/cm^2

Interactions

2

Chapter Objectives

To describe the types of interactions that take place in tissue
To recognize the importance of the acoustic impedance mismatch at the interface in specular reflection
To state the conditions under which refraction occurs
To understand the frequency dependence of absorption in tissue
To explain the principle of echo ranging

Key Terms

Absorption
Acoustic impedance
Attenuation
Diffraction
Diffuse reflection
Divergence

Echo ranging
Interference
Rayl
Reflection coefficient
Reflectivity
Refraction

Scattering
Snell's law
Specular reflection
Transmission coefficient

TYPES OF INTERACTIONS

The recorded image in sonography, unlike that in radiography, is typically based on reflected rather than transmitted energy. The single device that generates the ultrasound wave and subsequently detects the reflected energy is the transducer. An ultrasound wave directed into the body interacts with tissues in accordance with the characteristics of the targeted tissues. The outcome of these interactions is detected in the form of reflected ultrasound waves (echoes). The types of interactions that occur in tissue are similar to the wave behavior observed with light: reflection, refraction, scattering, divergence, diffraction, interference, and absorption. The progression of interactions that collectively reduce the intensity (loudness of audible sound) of the beam is called attenuation. In practice, reflection at the boundary between two media is often treated separately from attenuation; in other words, all interactions that decrease the intensity as the beam is transmitted through a single, specified medium are included in the attenuation process.

Specular Reflection

A major interaction of interest for diagnostic ultrasound is specular reflection. If a sound beam is directed at right angle (called normal incidence) to a smooth interface (e.g., the boundary between different tissue types) much larger than the wavelength of the wave, it will be partially reflected toward the sound source (Fig. 2-1). This interaction is responsible for the major organ outlines seen in diagnostic ultrasound. The skull, diaphragm, and pericardium are also examples of specular reflectors. The sonogram of the fetal head in Fig. 2-2 illustrates the strong echoes obtained from the skull.

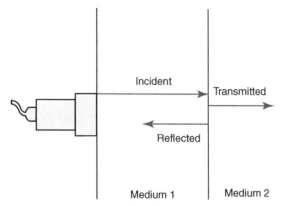

Figure 2-1 Reflection caused by a sound wave striking a large smooth interface at normal incidence. The interface is much larger than the wavelength and acts as a specular reflector. The acoustic impedances of the media that compose the interface determine the relative intensities of the transmitted and reflected waves.

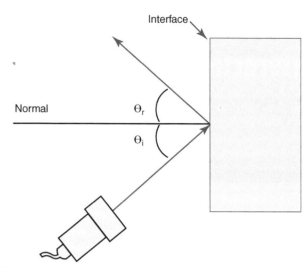

Figure 2-3 Reflection caused by a sound wave striking a specular reflector at an angle. The resulting angle of reflection (θ_r) equals the angle of incidence (θ_i).

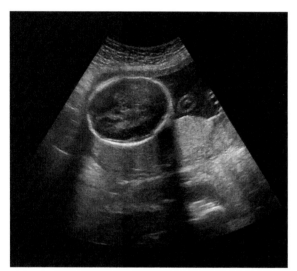

Figure 2-2 Sonogram of the fetal head showing strong echoes from the skull.

At other than normal incidence, the angle of reflection of a sound beam is equal to the angle of incidence (Fig. 2-3). These angles are defined relative to a line drawn perpendicular to the surface of the interface (normal). To obtain maximum detection of the reflected echo, the transducer (which sends and receives) must be oriented so that the generated sound beam strikes the interface close to perpendicularly and the reflected wave travels along a similar path back to transducer.

What conditions result in a reflection of energy? A useful analogy would be throwing a baseball against a brick wall; not much energy will be transferred to the wall. Conservation of energy would permit the ball to transfer all its energy to the wall and simply stop at the surface of the wall, but conservation of momentum prevents this from occurring because of the differences in mass. Only a small portion of the energy is transferred to the wall. Most is retained by the baseball, which returns with almost the same velocity as when it struck the wall.

Similarly, if a Mack truck rams into a Volkswagen, very little energy will be transferred to the Volkswagen. The truck will continue at almost the same velocity as it originally had. Most of its energy will be retained, although a great deal of damage will be done to the Volkswagen. Energy cannot be transmitted readily from large objects to small ones or from small objects to large ones. If massive transfers of kinetic energy are required, collisions between objects of equal mass must occur. For example, to slow down a baseball, the maximum amount of energy transfer will result if it collides with another baseball. To transfer energy from a Mack truck by the maximum amount, it would have to collide with another Mack truck. Vibrating molecules behave in a similar manner. As long as they are transmitting energy to identically sized molecules, maximum transfer will occur. If there is a difference in the masses of the molecules, less energy will be transferred and the energy that is not transferred will be reflected.

Acoustic Impedance

In ultrasound the quantity analogous to momentum is acoustic impedance. Here we are looking not at individual molecules but at their concerted action, thereby applying the concept of mass per unit volume (density). Whereas in classic mechanics momentum is equal to mass times velocity, in ultrasound density replaces the mass and is then multiplied by the velocity. The velocity in this case is the speed of sound in the medium. The product of density (ρ) and the acoustic velocity (c) is called the acoustic impedance (Z):

2-1 $$Z = \rho c$$

This quantity is a measure of the resistance to sound passing through the medium. It is similar to electrical resistance, which is the degree of difficulty experienced by electrons in flowing through a specific type of material. Acoustic impedance is expressed in units of kilograms per square meter per second (kg/m²-s), which is given a special name: the rayl.

Example 2-1

What is the acoustic impedance of soft tissue (which has a density of 1060 kg/m³)? Assume that the velocity of sound in soft tissue is 1540 m/s.

$$Z = \rho c = (1060 \text{ kg/m}^3)(1540 \text{ m/s})$$
$$Z = 1.63 \times 10^6 \text{ kg/(m}^2\text{-s) or 1.63 Mrayls}$$

High-density materials generally give rise to high-velocity sound waves and therefore high acoustic impedances. Similarly, low-density materials, such as gases, have low acoustic impedances. Table 2-1 lists the acoustic impedances for several materials of interest.

Impedance Mismatch

When a diver enters a pool, the ripple pattern expands outward and is reflected from the concrete wall of the pool. Very little wave energy is transferred from the water to the concrete wall. Now consider what would happen if the walls were made of Jell-O instead of concrete. The reflected wave in the water would be less intense and the walls would vibrate. Energy is transferred from the

Table 2-1	Properties of Different Media		
Material	**Density (kg/m³)**	**Velocity (m/s)**	**Acoustic Impedance (megarayls)**
Air	1.2	330	0.0004
Water (20° C)	1000	1480	1.48
Mercury	13,600	1450	20
Soft tissue			
Average*	1060	1540	1.63
Liver	1060	1550	1.64
Muscle	1080	1580	1.7
Fat	952	1459	1.38
Brain	994	1560	1.55
Kidney	1038	1560	1.62
Spleen	1045	1570	1.64
Blood	1057	1575	1.62
Bone	1912	4080	7.8
Lung	400	650	0.26
PZT	7650	3791	29
Lens	1142	1620	1.85
Aqueous humor	1000	1500	1.5
Vitreous humor	1000	1520	1.52
Lucite	1180	2680	3.16
Polystyrene	1060	2350	2.49
Castor oil	969	1477	1.43

PZT, lead zirconate titanate.
*Average tissue (e.g., abdomen).

water to the Jell-O because the composition and acoustic impedance of the two materials are similar.

If the acoustic impedance is the same in one medium as in another, sound is readily transmitted from one to the other. A difference in acoustic impedances causes some portion of the sound to be reflected at the interface. It is primarily the change in acoustic impedance at a biological interface (an impedance mismatch) that allows visualization of soft tissue structures with an ultrasonic beam.

Watching late-night western movies teaches that one does not listen for the sound of an oncoming train or a herd of buffalo in a normal standing position. Every youngster learned from old westerns that you put your ear to the rail or to the ground. The late John Wayne most likely would not have said, "Put your ear to the ground because that way you will eliminate the acoustic impedance mismatch and thus get a better sound transfer," but he should have, for that is the case.

Thus we have the second reason for placing one's ear on a solid surface. The transfer of sound from rail to air and then from air to ear is very inefficient; but with direct contact, the transmission from rail to air is eliminated and vibrations pass readily across a solid-solid interface.

Another analogy that might be used, and which would be quite correct, is the transmission of light. Light transmitted from one medium to another having different indices of refraction causes the major portion of the energy to be reflected rather than transmitted. This phenomenon can be observed in looking at sunlight reflected from a shallow pool of water. The reflection occurs at the air-water boundary because of the different indices of refraction (similar to acoustic impedance). The amount of reflection is a function of the surface only. One receives the same amount of reflected light standing over a pool of water as over the deepest part of the Pacific Ocean. *Sound is reflected at the interface regardless of the thickness of the material from which it is reflected.*

Reflection Coefficient

For perpendicular incidence, the reflection coefficient for intensity, which equals the ratio of the reflected intensity (I_r) to the incident intensity (I_i), is given by:

$$2\text{-}2 \qquad \alpha_R = \frac{I_r}{I_i} = \left(\frac{Z_2 - Z_1}{Z_2 + Z_1}\right)^2$$

where α_R is the reflection coefficient, Z_2 the acoustic impedance of medium number 2 (distal to the boundary), and Z_1 the acoustic impedance of medium number 1 (proximal to the boundary). This is the second essential equation of sonography. Multiplying the right-hand side of Equation 2-2 by 100 gives the percentage reflection.

Transmission Coefficient

The transmission coefficient (α_T), the ratio of the transmitted intensity (I_t) to the incident intensity (I_i), is calculated directly by the formula

2-3 $$\alpha_T = \frac{I_t}{I_i} = \frac{4Z_2 Z_1}{(Z_2 + Z_1)^2}$$

Alternatively, if the reflection coefficient is known, then the transmission coefficient can be determined by subtracting the reflection coefficient from unity. Multiplying the right-hand side of Equation 2-3 by 100 gives the percentage transmission through the interface.

For specular reflection, the equations for the transmission and reflection of ultrasound intensity are independent of frequency. That is, frequency does not affect the fraction of intensity transmitted and reflected at the interface.

Interface Composition

The order of the acoustic impedance for two materials that compose the interface has no effect on the reflected intensity; the difference between them squared gives the same number. *Thus the same percentage of reflection occurs at the interface, whether sound is going from a high acoustic impedance to a low acoustic impedance or vice versa.* If the difference in acoustic impedance is small, the magnitude of the reflected wave is small. Because the same device transmits and receives the sound waves, maximum intensity of the detected echo occurs when the sound beam strikes the interface with near normal incidence. If the acoustic impedance difference is large, as in bone compared with soft tissue, a large fraction of sound will be reflected; little of the transmitted beam will penetrate structures behind the bone, and much will return to the detector. This is one of the reasons why bone is usually avoided during an ultrasound examination. To visualize the liver, which is largely positioned under the ribs, one must direct the ultrasound beam either through the intercostal spaces (between the ribs) or under the ribs and back up at the liver.

Example 2-2

Calculate the percentage reflection (%R) for a bone-tissue interface using the acoustic impedance values in megarayls listed in Table 2-1:

$$\%R = \left(\frac{Z_B - Z_T}{Z_B + Z_T}\right)^2 \times 100$$

$$\%R = \left(\frac{7.8 - 1.63}{7.8 + 1.63}\right)^2 \times 100$$

$$\%R = 43\%$$

where Z_B is the acoustic impedance in bone and Z_T the acoustic impedance in tissue.

Example 2-3

Calculate the percentage transmission (%T) for a soft tissue-bone interface using the acoustic impedance values listed in Table 2-1:

$$\%T = \frac{4Z_B Z_T}{(Z_B + Z_T)^2} \times 100$$

$$\%T = \frac{4\,(7.8)\,(1.63)}{(7.8 + 1.63)^2} \times 100$$

$$\%T = 57\%$$

Note that the result for fraction reflected at the soft tissue-bone interface determined in Example 2-2, which yielded fraction reflected, can be used to calculate the fraction transmitted (T) at this interface:

$$T = 1 - 0.43 = 0.57$$

Table 2-2 lists the percentage reflections at interfaces of varying composition. The acoustic impedances used to calculate these values were obtained from Table 2-1. Note that the thickness of the medium and frequency are not considered in the calculations; only the impedance mismatch at the interface is of concern.

The acoustic impedance difference is also large for an air-tissue interface, which causes most of the incident beam to be reflected. Even if the air layer between a transducer and the patient is extremely thin, nearly total reflection occurs at the air-tissue interface. The ultrasound beam is not transmitted to structures distal to the air bubble, and the sonogram is void of information from this region (Fig. 2-4). During scanning, coupling gel is used to eliminate air gaps. The gel also serves to reduce friction between the transducer and the skin.

Remember: When the heart or other thoracic structures are being studied, the lungs must be avoided because of the large amount of reflection that occurs at the multiple air interfaces within them. Acoustic impedance differences at fat-soft tissue interfaces produce relatively strong echoes ($\sim 1\%$ of the incident intensity) and are primarily responsible for the organ outlines seen in imaging.

Table 2-2	Percentage Reflection at Different Interfaces
Interface	**Percent Reflection**
Soft tissue-air	99.9
Soft tissue-lung	52
Soft tissue-bone	43
Aqueous humor-lens	1.1
Fat-liver	0.79
Soft tissue-fat	0.69
Soft tissue-muscle	0.04

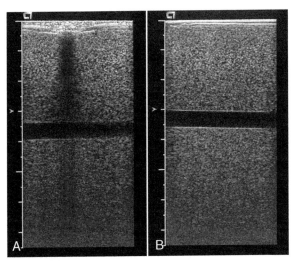

Figure 2-4 Sonogram of a tissue-mimicking phantom with **(A)** and without **(B)** an air bubble present between the transducer and the phantom surface. Note that information is lost distal to the air bubble. The ultrasound energy is reflected by the air-transducer interface and does not enter the phantom.

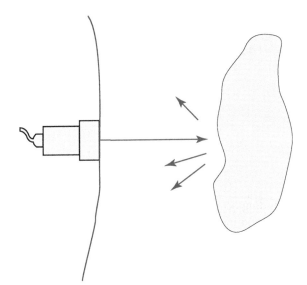

Figure 2-5 Diffuse reflection. When a sound beam is incident on an irregular interface *(light blue area)*, it is reflected in multiple directions.

Diffuse Reflection

The large smooth surface of a specular reflector acts as a mirror to form a well-defined redirected beam (echo). A large rough-surfaced interface deflects the ultrasound beam in multiple directions (Fig. 2-5). Since the interface is not entirely flat, the sound beam strikes the interface with various angles of incidence, which gives rise to differing angles of reflection. This is called diffuse reflection. The loss of coherence in the reflected beam weakens the echo returning to the transducer. Diffuse reflection is relatively independent of the orientation of the interface.

Before the bathroom mirror becomes fogged when you take a shower, it provides a true representation of objects placed in front of it. After you shower, the buildup of water on its surface causes it to act as a diffuse reflector and

the images of objects are less well defined. Water particles roughen the mirror's surface, reducing the coherence of reflected light.

Scattering

Another extremely important interaction between ultrasound and tissue is scattering, or nonspecular reflection, which is responsible for providing the internal texture of organs in the image. The scattering occurs because the interfaces are small, with physical dimensions approximately the size of the wavelength or smaller. Each interface acts as a new separate sound source, and sound is reflected in all directions independent of the direction of the incoming sound wave (Fig. 2-6). The magnitude of scattered ultrasound intensity is much weaker than for specular reflection and depends on the number of scatterers per volume, the size of the scatterers, acoustic impedance, and frequency.

Fluid regions such as cysts, urine in the bladder, and amniotic fluid lack scattering centers and produce weak ultrasound signals compared with surrounding tissue (dark areas in the image, which are called hypoechoic). Areas with increased ultrasound signals compared with the surrounding tissue are called hyperechoic. The sonogram of the fetus in Figure 2-7 illustrates low- and high-signal variations throughout the scanned tissues.

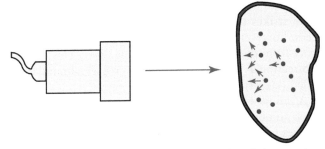

Figure 2-6 Scattering. Sound energy is emitted in all directions from small reflectors (approximately the size of the wavelength or smaller). The strength of the scattered waves is relatively independent of the incident beam's direction.

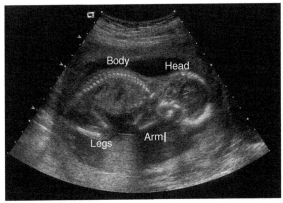

Figure 2-7 Sonogram of a fetus. Amniotic fluid is hypoechoic and bone is hyperechoic. Soft tissue structures have intermediate signal levels.

Scattering by small particles in which the linear dimensions are much smaller than the wavelength is called Rayleigh scattering. Red blood cells act as Rayleigh scatterers in Doppler ultrasound. *Rayleigh scatterers have a strong frequency dependence (f^2 to f^6).*

Reflectivity

Many factors influence the fraction of incident intensity that is reflected at an interface toward the transducer: the acoustic impedance mismatch, the angle of incidence, the size of the structure compared with the wavelength, the shape of the structure, and the texture of the surface of the interface. The combination of these factors is described by the term reflectivity.

Differences in reflectivity are partially responsible for the patient-to-patient variations observed by sonographers as they perform particular types of examinations. Ultrasound imaging systems are capable of detecting extremely small changes in reflectivity, on the order of one in a million.

Refraction

If the ultrasound beam strikes an interface between two media at an incident angle of 0 degrees (normal incidence), a fraction of the incident intensity is reflected back to the first medium and the rest is transmitted into the second medium without a change in direction. If the beam strikes the interface at an angle other than 0 degrees, however, the transmitted part is refracted or bent away from the straight-line path (Fig. 2-8). This change in direction as the ultrasound beam crosses a boundary is called refraction.

A similar effect caused by the refraction of light is seen when an object under water is viewed from above. If one reaches for the object through the water, the spatial inaccuracy becomes immediately apparent. Refraction may

contribute to the misregistration of an object depicted in the sonographic image.

Snell's Law

Refraction of sound waves obeys Snell's law, which relates the angle of transmission to the relative velocities of sound in the two media. (Note that this relationship is not based on acoustic impedance.) Snell's law, the third essential equation of sonography, is given by

$$2\text{-}4 \qquad \frac{c_i}{c_t} = \frac{\sin \theta_i}{\sin \theta_t}$$

where θ_i is the angle of incidence, θ_t the angle of transmission, c_i the velocity of sound in the incident medium, and c_t the velocity of sound in the transmitted medium. In Snell's law the angles θ_i and θ_t are defined with respect to a line drawn perpendicular to the interface.

Example 2-4

Calculate the transmitted angle if an ultrasound beam is directed at an interface composed of soft tissue and fat. The angle of incidence (θ_i) is 10 degrees. Assume that the sound beam is moving from soft tissue ($c_t = 1540$ m/s) into fat ($c_f = 1460$ m/s).

$$\frac{c_i}{c_t} = \frac{\sin \theta_i}{\sin \theta_t}$$

$$\frac{1540 \text{ m/s}}{1460 \text{ m/s}} = \frac{\sin 10°}{\sin \theta_t}$$

$$\sin \theta_t = 0.165$$
$$\theta_t = 9.5 \text{ degrees}$$

This bending occurs because the portion of the wavefront in the second medium travels at a different velocity from that in the first medium (Fig. 2-9). Note that the acoustic velocity in medium 2 is less than that in medium 1 (the spacing between successive wavefronts is smaller). The wavefront is continuous across the interface, but the portion of the wavefront in medium 2 is moving at a slower velocity than the rest and lags behind.

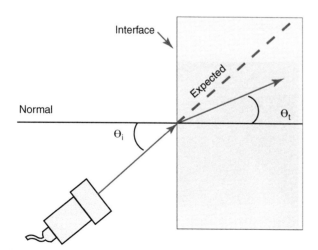

Figure 2-8 Refraction. The velocity of a sound beam in the incident medium is greater than that in the transmitted medium, causing the beam to be bent toward the normal ($\theta_i > \theta_t$).

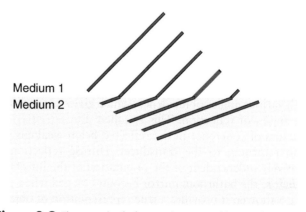

Figure 2-9 The principle of refraction demonstrated by wavefronts striking an interface between two media having different velocities.

To illustrate this shift in wavefronts, imagine successive rows of four-wheel-drive vehicles traveling through the Sahara Desert. As the vehicles cross a boundary between flat, smooth terrain and sandy terrain, their velocity is reduced. Assume that the vehicles on the left side of the row enter the sandy terrain first. If these drivers stubbornly maintain their alignment, the advance of their vehicles will be slowed compared with that of the drivers who have not yet encountered the sandy terrain. For the vehicles to continue to advance so that the row remains perpendicular to their direction of travel, the drivers in the sandy terrain must turn slightly to the right (the line of vehicles bends in the new terrain).

Three situations regarding Snell's law should be considered:

- Case 1 refraction: The velocity in the first medium is greater than that in the second medium. The angle of transmittance bends toward the normal from the expected straight-line path (Fig. 2-8). For example, this occurs at a bone-tissue interface.
- Case 2 refraction: The velocity in the first medium is less than that in the second medium. The angle of transmittance is bent away from the normal (Fig. 2-10). For example, this occurs at a tissue-bone interface.
- Case 3 refraction: This is a special extension of case 2 refraction. If the velocity in the incident medium is less than that in the transmitted medium and the angle of incidence is beyond the so-called critical angle, the refracted beam travels along the boundary and no energy enters the second medium. This is called total reflection and occurs at an incident angle of greater than 22 degrees when the interface is composed of tissue and bone.

If the velocity of sound is the same in the two media, no refraction (bending) occurs, although the acoustic impedances may be different. Nor does refraction occur at normal incidence, regardless of the relative velocities in the two media.

For refraction, the angle of reflection of a sound beam is equal to the angle of incidence, but the angle of transmission does not equal the angle of incidence. The sound wave is reflected with higher intensity compared with normal incidence (the reflection coefficient increases as the angle of incidence is increased).

For nonperpendicular incidence, the equation for intensity reflection coefficient is modified as follows:

$$2\text{-}5 \qquad \alpha_R = \frac{I_r}{I_i} = \left(\frac{Z_2 \cos\theta_i - Z_1 \cos\theta_t}{Z_2 \cos\theta_i + Z_1 \cos\theta_t} \right)^2$$

This equation reduces to the more customary form shown by Equation 2-2 if θ_i and θ_t are equal to 0 degrees.

Divergence and Diffraction

If not impeded, sound waves will spread out in all directions (called divergence) as the waves moves farther from the sound source (Fig. 2-11). The rate of divergence increases as the size (diameter) of the sound source decreases. Diffraction occurs after the beam with planar wavefronts passes through a small aperture on the order of one wavelength. Because the wave is blocked everywhere but in the area of the aperture, the aperture acts as a small sound source and the beam diverges rapidly. This is demonstrated in Fig. 2-12.

Interference

Sound waves demonstrate interference phenomena or the superposition of waves (algebraic summation). As an example of interference, consider the ripple patterns produced

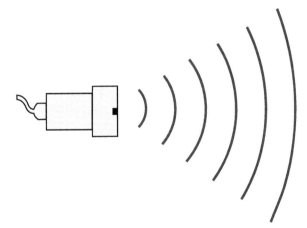

Figure 2-11 Divergence of a sound beam from a small source, shown as the blackened portion of the transducer face.

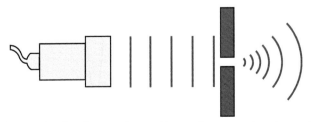

Figure 2-12 Diffraction of a sound beam after passing through a small aperture.

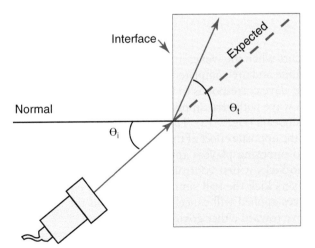

Figure 2-10 Case 2 refraction. The velocity of a sound beam in the incident medium is less than that in the transmitted medium, causing the beam to be bent away from the normal ($\theta_i < \theta_t$).

in the water when three swimmers dive into a pool one after the other from three different diving boards located alongside the pool. If the entries are separated in time, each diver will produce a characteristic ripple pattern. If all three divers enter the water simultaneously, the resulting complex ripple pattern, consisting of large and small water disturbances, is a combination of the three individual patterns.

If waves of the same frequency are in phase, they undergo constructive interference. Waves are in phase if crossing and inflection points are matched along the distance or time axis (Fig. 2-13). Constructive interference results in an increased amplitude.

If waves of the same frequency are out of phase, they undergo destructive interference; that is, a decrease in amplitude results because the peaks are not matched in the same position (Fig. 2-14). Completely destructive interference

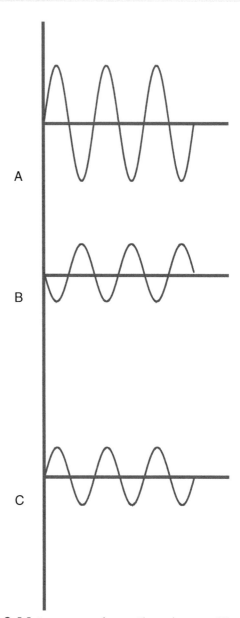

Figure 2-14 Destructive interference. The resultant wave **(C)** is the sum of waves **(A)** and **(B)** and is reduced in amplitude because the waves are out of phase.

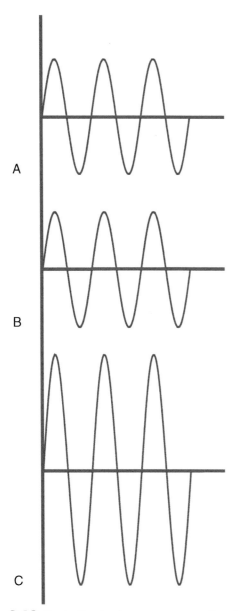

Figure 2-13 Constructive interference or superposition (algebraic summation) of waves. The resultant wave **(C)** is the sum of waves **(A)** and **(B)**.

occurs when the waves are of the same frequency and amplitude and are completely out of phase (i.e., the trough of one wave corresponds to the peak of the other). The result is a wave with zero amplitude; hence the summation wave disappears (Fig. 2-15). The effect of one wave is countered by the opposite effect of the other wave. For example, when two opposing players approach a soccer ball, the player who kicks it first controls the direction of travel. If both players kick the ball simultaneously with equal force, the forces applied will cancel each other and the ball will not move toward either goal.

Every combination, from completely constructive to completely destructive interference, can occur, resulting in a complex wave summation. Figure 2-16 shows the result when waves with differing frequencies create

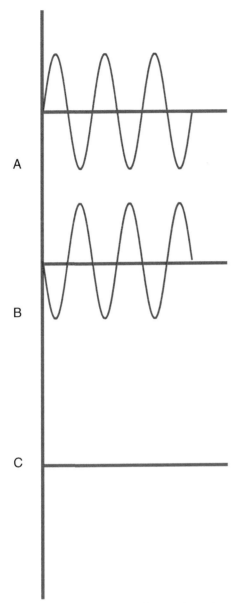

Figure 2-15 Complete destructive interference. The resultant wave **(C)** is zero because waves **(A)** and **(B)** are completely out of phase and have the same amplitude.

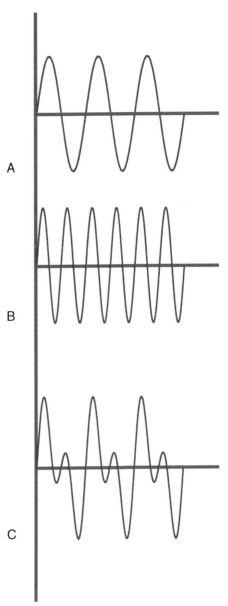

Figure 2-16 Wave interference. Note that **(B)** has a slightly different frequency from **(A)**. Thus **(C)** is the summation of these two waves.

interference. Interference plays an important role throughout sonography, including pulse transmission, electronic focusing, and the measurement of Doppler velocity.

Absorption

Absorption is the only process whereby sound energy is dissipated in a medium, primarily in the form of heat. Once energy is transferred from ultrasound to the medium, it cannot be recovered and intensity is reduced. All other modes of interaction (reflection, refraction, scattering, and divergence) decrease the intensity of the ultrasonic beam by redirecting its energy.

The absorption of an ultrasonic beam is related to the viscosity and relaxation time of the medium, but it is strongly dependent on the frequency of the wave. The relaxation time describes the rate at which molecules return to their original positions after being displaced by a force. If a substance has a short relaxation time, the molecules return to their original positions before the next wave compression arrives. If it has a long relaxation time, however, the molecules may be moving back toward their original positions as the wave crest (compression) strikes them. More energy is required to stop and then reverse the direction of the molecules, and this produces more heat (absorption).

The ability of molecules to move past one another characterizes the viscosity of a medium; high viscosity provides great resistance to molecular flow. For instance, a low-viscosity fluid (water) flows more freely than a viscous one (maple syrup). The frictional forces must be overcome by vibrating molecules; thus more heat is produced in the viscous maple syrup.

The frequency also affects absorption in relation to both the viscosity and the relaxation time. If the frequency is increased, the molecules must move more often, thereby generating more heat from the drag caused by friction (viscosity). Also, as the frequency is increased, less time is available for the molecules to recover during the relaxation process. Molecules remain in motion, and more energy is necessary to stop and redirect them, again producing more absorption. *The rate of absorption is directly related to the frequency.* If the frequency doubles, the rate of absorption also doubles.

Consider the mechanical action of rubbing one's hands together. The movement produces heat. If the hands are rubbed together more rapidly (higher frequency), increased warming occurs. If lotion is placed between the palms so that the resistance is decreased (lower viscosity), less heat will be generated.

The peak amplitude of acoustic pressure, particle density, particle displacement, and particle velocity all decrease as the wave propagates through a homogeneous medium. In Figure 2-17 the absorption of the pulsed ultrasonic beam follows an exponential function as the pulsed wave penetrates the tissue. Absorption is enhanced if the frequency is increased (Fig. 2-18).

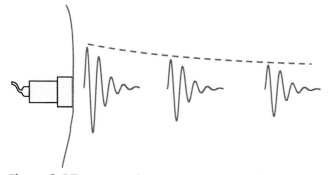

Figure 2-17 Attenuation of acoustic pressure as a sound beam penetrates the medium. The dashed curve demonstrates an exponential decrease in the peak acoustic pressure.

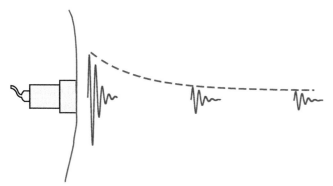

Figure 2-18 Attenuation of acoustic pressure as a high-frequency sound beam penetrates the medium. The dashed curve demonstrates an exponential decrease in the peak acoustic pressure. Compared with Figure 2-17, the frequency is increased; consequently the rate of absorption is more rapid.

Attenuation

Attenuation includes the effects of both scattering and absorption in the reduction of intensity as the ultrasound wave propagates through a medium. Attenuation of intensity is described by an exponential function dependent on the distance traveled, the composition of the medium, and the frequency. Values for the fractional intensity remaining after transmission through different media (1 cm in thickness) at a frequency of 1 MHz are listed in Table 2-3. Ultrasound readily passes through blood, whereas bone and lung are strong attenuators.

As frequency is increased, reduction of the ultrasound intensity with distance becomes more pronounced. This has a practical consequence in medical imaging. The ultrasound beam and returning echoes that form the image must travel through tissue. *The depth of penetration becomes less as frequency is increased, and the ability to observe deep-lying structures is forfeited* (Fig. 2-19).

ECHO RANGING

A system that can generate an ultrasonic pulsed wave and detect the reflected echo after a measured time permits the distance to an interface (i.e., the depth of the interface) to be determined. This technique is called echo ranging, a concept that formed the basis of sonar developed during World War II.

In diagnostic ultrasound, reflections of the sound beam from interfaces along the ultrasonic path are of primary interest. A pulsed ultrasound wave is transmitted into the body, strikes an interface (acoustic mismatch between two media), and is partially reflected to the transducer as determined by the reflection coefficient. The echoes arising from the various acoustic impedance mismatches along the path result in ultrasonic detection of reflectors within the body.

If the velocity of ultrasound in the medium (c) and the elapsed time (t) from the original transmitted pulse to the detection of the return echo are known, then the depth of the interface (z) is determined by the fourth essential equation of sonography:

2-6
$$z = \frac{ct}{2}$$

Table 2-3	Loss of Intensity by Attenuation in Different Media	
Material	**Relative Intensity* (1 cm at 1 MHz)**
Blood	0.96
Fat	0.87
Soft tissue	0.83-0.89
Skull	0.01
Lung	0.0001
Water	0.9995

*Note: A value of 1 corresponds to no reduction in intensity.

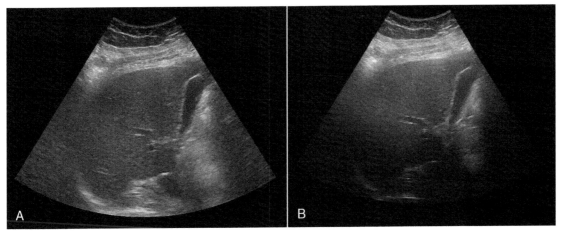

Figure 2-19 Effect of frequency on penetration. **A,** Scan of the liver acquired with a center frequency of 2.8 MHz. **B,** The depth of penetration for 5 MHz center frequency is reduced for the same patient.

where the factor 2 takes into account the fact that the distance between the sound source and the reflector must be traversed twice, once by the transmit pulse and once by the echo.

The following calculation demonstrates the time necessary to travel distances that are of clinical interest. The average velocity of ultrasound in tissue is 1540 m/s. For an interface exactly 1 cm away, the total time for the sound wave to travel out to the interface and back to the transducer is calculated by solving for time (t) in Equation 2-6:

$$t = \frac{2(0.01 \text{ m})}{1540 \text{ m/s}}$$

$$t = \frac{2 \times 10^{-2} \text{ m}}{1.54 \times 10^{3} \text{ m/s}}$$

$$t = 13 \times 10^{-6} \text{ s}$$
$$t = 13 \text{ μs}$$

Only 13 μs are required for the transmitted sound beam to travel 1 cm from the transducer and for the echo to return 1 cm in tissue (Fig. 2-20). An essential principle of sonography is that a time between transmitted pulse and detected echo is 13 μs for each centimeter in depth for soft tissue.

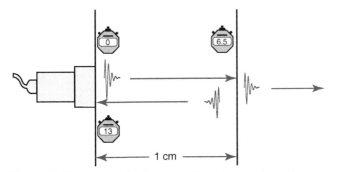

Figure 2-20 Principle of echo ranging. The distance to the interface can be determined by measuring the time between the transmitted pulse and the received echo. Constant velocity in the medium must be assumed. The time after the transmitted pulse until reception of the echo is 13 μs for a reflector 1 cm away from the transducer.

Example 2-5

A pulsed ultrasound wave is transmitted through soft tissue toward an interface composed of soft tissue and bone. The elapsed time between the transmitted pulse and the detected echo is 74 μs. What is the depth of the interface?

$$z \text{ (depth)} = \frac{t}{13 \text{ μs/cm}}$$

$$z \text{ (depth)} = \frac{74 \text{ μs}}{13 \text{ μs/cm}}$$

$$z = 5.7 \text{ cm}$$

The distance to an interface is measured by the elapsed time; in other words, the time of travel to and from the interface at a constant velocity is governed by the distance of travel. As the depth to the interface increases, the elapsed time increases. For an interface 10 cm away, 130 μs between the transmitted pulse and the returning echo are required.

For echo ranging to delineate the position of an interface correctly, certain conditions must hold: (1) the ultrasound wave must travel directly to the interface and back to the transducer along a straight-line path and (2) the velocity of sound must remain constant along the path of travel.

SUMMARY

Knowledge of the physics of ultrasound is essential to the successful clinical application of diagnostic ultrasonographic techniques. The interactions of sound waves with tissues (reflection, refraction, scattering, interference, absorption, and attenuation) influence the collection and interpretation of scan data. Specular reflectors and scatterers are the principal contributors of echoes in sonography. The technique of echo ranging determines the spatial position (depth) of the reflector. Three essential equations of sonography (reflection coefficient, Snell's law, and echo ranging) were introduced.

Intensity and Power

3

Chapter Objectives

To name the device used to measure intensity
To state common intensity descriptors
To define relative intensity measurements in decibels
To identify factors that determine the loss of intensity in tissue

Key terms

Decibel (dB)
Free-field conditions
Hydrophone
Intensity

Power
Pulse average (PA)
Spatial average (SA)
Spatial peak (SP)

Temporal average (TA)
Temporal peak (TP)

MEASUREMENT OF INTENSITY

The intensity of an ultrasonic beam is the physical parameter that describes the rate at which the energy is transmitted by the wave over a small area. Traditionally, acoustic intensity is expressed in mixed units of watts per centimeter squared (W/cm^2) or milliwatts per centimeter squared (mW/cm^2)—a combination of meter kilogram second (MKS) and centimeter gram second (CGS) system units. In other areas of physics this is considered bad form. One watt is the unit for the rate of energy generation, or flow, and is equal to one joule per second.

For ultrasound, increasing intensity means that the distribution of particles within a compression zone becomes more dense, peak acoustic pressure is higher, length of particle oscillation increases, and maximum particle velocity is greater. The intensity of an ultrasound beam is reduced as the beam propagates through tissue. The transmitted intensity and the rate of intensity loss influence the ability of a scanner to observe deep-lying as well as weakly reflecting structures. *The frequency, wavelength, and acoustic velocity of an ultrasonic beam are not affected by a change in intensity.* However, for high-intensity applications such as tissue harmonic imaging, propagation is nonlinear and the sinusoidal wave becomes distorted.

The study of potential biological effects is linked to intensity. Since the particle velocity and length of displacement are dictated by intensity, a high-intensity ultrasound wave is more disruptive to living systems than a low-intensity ultrasound wave. The clinical safety of ultrasound is examined in Chapter 17.

The instantaneous intensity (I) is determined from the measurement of acoustic pressure (p) where the acoustic velocity (c) and the density (ρ) of the medium are known.

3-1
$$I = \frac{p^2}{\rho c}$$

This is the fifth essential equation of sonography. Pressure is the force exerted on a small area and is expressed in newtons per meter squared (Nt/m^2), named pascal (Pa) in the MKS system. One atmosphere (atmospheric pressure at sea level) equals 10^5 pascals. Frequently, the pulsed-wave ultrasound is characterized by a peak negative pressure. The peak negative pressure is also called the peak rarefactional pressure (Fig. 3-1). Ultrasound instruments produce peak pressure amplitudes ranging from 0.5 to 5.5 megapascals (more than 50 times greater than atmospheric pressure).

Unfortunately, state-of-the-art experimental techniques await a good method whereby the intensity (or pressure from which intensity is calculated) is measured at a particular point within tissue (classified as an in situ measurement). Typically the transducer is characterized by using free-field conditions, in which the pressure is measured in water without reflectors or other disturbances to the ultrasonic field. Pressure, and thus the corresponding intensity in water, is converted to intensity in tissue by applying correction (derating) factors for attenuation.

Measurements of acoustic pressure are performed with a hydrophone placed in the ultrasonic field. The physical dimension of the hydrophone is typically 0.5 to 1 mm in diameter; thus, to minimize spatial averaging, a very small area is sampled by the device. The ultrasound wave incident on the hydrophone induces a voltage that is directly proportional to the acoustic pressure. Because the pressure is not constant but fluctuates as the wave passes a point in space, a time-varying waveform of the voltage is obtained. The spatial variation in intensity is mapped by moving the hydrophone to different locations in the field.

Free-field measurements do not assess the attenuation by tissue, focusing by anatomic structures, production of standing waves, or effect of reflecting boundaries. Nevertheless, free-field testing does provide measurable physical entities that characterize the ultrasound beam and allow comparisons between devices.

INTENSITY DESCRIPTORS

Because of the pulsing and scanning techniques employed, diagnostic ultrasound equipment produces complex spatial and time-varying acoustic fields. Quantification of these patterns is impractical and difficult to correlate with the bioeffect potential of the ultrasound beam. Thus, characterization of the ultrasonic field is accomplished by a few select parameters, usually related to energy, such as acoustic power, intensity, or peak negative pressure. The spatial and temporal dependence of the intensity complicates this descriptive process. Several shorthand methods have been developed to specify intensity.

Temporal Dependence

As the transducer emits pulses, it causes large fluctuations of intensity in the region through which the pulses move. Each pulse consists of multiple cycles that produce intensity variations within the pulse itself: the maximum intensity designated temporal peak (TP); the intensity averaged over the duration of a single pulse, designated pulse average (PA): and the intensity averaged over the longer interval of the pulse repetition period, designated temporal average (TA). For a given pulse sequence, TP has the highest value, followed by PA and finally by TA (Fig. 3-2).

Often the time-averaged intensity over one cycle is of interest. At any point through which an ultrasound beam passes, the pressure oscillates between high and low values. The greatest deviation from average pressure during a cycle is the peak-pressure amplitude (p_o). Since the pressure is fluctuating as a function of time, the instantaneous intensity is also oscillating between high and low values. By averaging the instantaneous intensity over one cycle, it is possible to find the time-averaged intensity (I_c):

$$3\text{-}2 \qquad I_c = \frac{p_o^2}{2\,\rho c}$$

The intensity for continuous-wave output usually refers to a time-averaged intensity. The temporal-average intensity I(TA) is related to the pulse-average intensity I(PA) by the duty factor (DF), the fraction of time the transducer is actively generating ultrasound energy:

$$3\text{-}3 \qquad I(TA) = DF \times I(PA)$$

For example, if the pulse duration is 1 μs and the time between pulses is 1 ms, the duty factor is 0.001. The PA intensity is 1000 times greater than the TA intensity. A determination of the TP intensity from the PA intensity

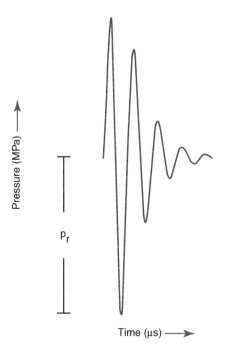

Figure 3-1 Pressure variation as a function of time at a point in the ultrasonic field. The peak rarefactional pressure is designated p_r.

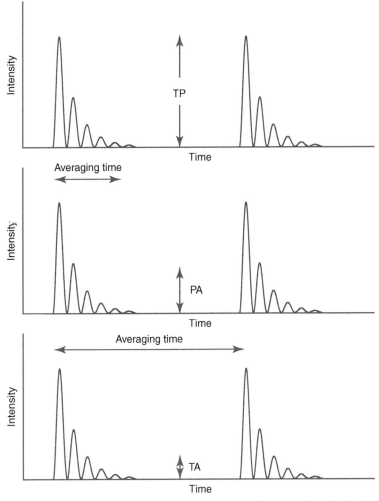

Figure 3-2 Specification of intensity with respect to time. Top graph, Temporal peak (TP). Middle graph, Pulse average (PA). Bottom graph, Temporal average (TA).

requires knowledge of the pulse shape. The ratio TP/PA is typically in the range of 2 to 10.

The relationship between intensity peak and intensity averaging is an important concept. The following analogy may help illustrate it: Suppose that a row of sand castles had been built along the seashore, as in Figure 3-3. Each castle corresponds to a single pulse. The height of the tallest point of a castle represents the temporal peak. If a castle is flattened so that the sand is spread evenly over its base, the level of the sand will be lower than the original peak. This corresponds to the pulse average. If the sand is distributed over the area between castles, it will be even lower than the original height of the peak. This represents the temporal average.

Spatial Dependence

The additional factor of space must now be considered in the shorthand description of intensity. Once more, the peak or average value with respect to the variable (in this case space) is used. The TP intensity, PA intensity, or TA intensity is mapped as a function of position within the

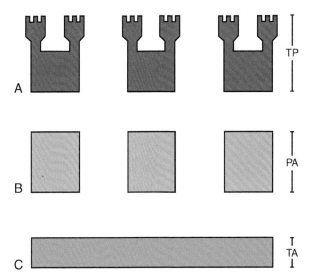

Figure 3-3 Temporal averaging. **A,** The highest points on the sand castles (turrets) correspond to the temporal peak (TP). **B,** Sand making up the turrets has been flattened and distributed across the base of each castle. This corresponds to the pulse average (PA). **C,** The sand has been flattened to cover the area between the castles. This corresponds to the temporal average (TA).

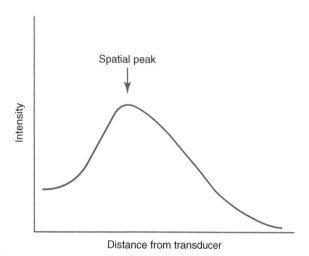

Figure 3-4 Axial intensity profile for a focused transducer. The intensity is maximal at a particular distance from the face of the transducer, which is the spatial peak intensity.

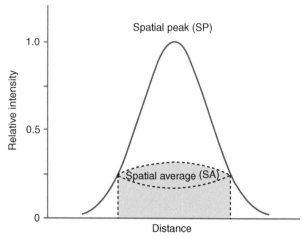

Figure 3-5 Relationship of spatial peak (SP) and spatial average (SA) intensities. The curve represents the intensity profile across the width of the beam. The SA intensity is found by averaging the intensity over the beam's cross-sectional area.

ultrasonic field. The variation in intensity along the axis of propagation for a focused transducer is illustrated in Figure 3-4. The maximum intensity of all measured values within the sound field is designated as the spatial peak (SP). Thus three combinations are possible, depending on which temporal intensity is mapped:

- I(SPTP): Spatial peak, temporal peak intensity
- I(SPPA): Spatial peak, pulse average intensity
- I(SPTA): Spatial peak, temporal average intensity

The designation of spatial peak is not clearly defined. In some applications it refers to the maximum intensity in a plane perpendicular to the beam's axis at a particular distance from the transducer. More commonly, however, it denotes the maximum intensity throughout the ultrasonic field, which usually occurs along the beam's axis. The focusing of the transducer is the most important determinant of spatial peak.

Spatial averaging (SA) over the cross-sectional area of the beam of one of the temporal intensities is also specified (Fig. 3-5). Again, three combinations are possible:

- I(SATP): Spatial average, temporal peak intensity
- I(SAPA): Spatial average, pulse average intensity
- I(SATA): Spatial average, temporal average intensity

POWER

The power is a measure of the total energy transmitted per unit time summed over the entire cross-sectional area of the beam (expressed in milliwatts or joules per second). The I(SATA) is approximated by the ratio of the power to the scan cross-sectional area.

ATTENUATION

Attenuation of an ultrasound beam causes a decrease in intensity as the beam traverses a medium. Interactions of ultrasound with tissue (reflection, scattering, divergence, and absorption) contribute to the overall attenuation of the

beam. Only absorption results in energy transfer to the tissue; the other interactions redirect ultrasonic energy.

The peak amplitude pressure decreases as the ultrasound wave propagates through a homogeneous medium. *The rate of attenuation depends on the medium and frequency of the ultrasound wave.* To a first approximation, the rate of attenuation increases linearly with frequency.

DECIBEL

Absolute determination of power and intensity of ultrasound is difficult. This is particularly true of pulsed beams, for which both temporal and spatial properties must be considered. Additionally, intensity measurements are not performed in tissue.

Although no standard reference intensity for ultrasound has been established, a useful method for determining the intensity is to make relative measurements that compare the value at one point with a reference intensity at another point. The following analogy may help to illustrate the concept: Johnny owns 25 marbles and Tommy owns 50. To find out how much Johnny's marbles weigh in ounces, we place them on a scale. If we are interested only in the relative weight of Johnny's marbles, we say they are "half as heavy as Tommy's." The absolute weight in ounces is not known, but the relative weight can be described with respect to a standard (Tommy's marbles).

Measurements of relative intensity are usually made and given in decibels (dB). The intensity variation or level expressed in decibels is the sixth essential equation of sonography:

$$3\text{-}4 \qquad \text{Level (dB)} = 10 \log\left(\frac{I}{I_{ref}}\right)$$

where I is the intensity at the point of interest and I_{ref} is the initial or reference intensity.

Example 3-1

Assume that the intensity at a particular point is reduced to half the transmitted intensity. Convert this relative intensity measurements to decibels.

$$I_1 = 0.5\, I_t$$

$$\text{Level (dB)} = 10\, \log\left(\frac{0.5\, I_t}{I_t}\right)$$

$$\text{Level (dB)} = 10\, \log 0.5$$

$$\text{Level (dB)} = (10)(-0.301)$$

$$\text{Level (dB)} = -3.01$$

This is the mathematical basis for the rule of thumb that each factor of 2 results in a loss of 3 dB in intensity.

Equation 3-4 defines decibel using the ratio of the intensities at two different points. Another equation using the ratio of the amplitudes (usually pressure) may be employed to calculate intensity changes in decibels. Recall that the square of the amplitude is proportional to the intensity. Consequently,

$$3\text{-}5 \qquad \text{Level (dB)} = 20\, \log\left(\frac{A_o}{A_{max}}\right)$$

where A_{max} is the initial peak amplitude of the beam and A_o is the peak amplitude at the point of interest. Table 3-1 lists several examples of intensity ratio, amplitude ratio, and the corresponding level in decibels. A reduction in amplitude by a factor of 2 results in a 6-dB intensity loss. This reduction is equivalent to a reduction of intensity by a factor of 4.

One advantage of decibels is that they enable a wide range of intensity and power levels to be expressed in a compact form. Decibels are not restricted to the parameters of power and intensity, however. They can also be used to describe relative measurements of pressure, noise level, percentage reflection, and many other quantities. In Equation 3-4, I_{ref} and I are replaced by the reference value and the value for the parameter of interest respectively.

Consider an ultrasonic field in which the intensity is one-half the surface intensity at 1 cm and continues to decrease to 1/10,000 of the surface intensity at a depth of

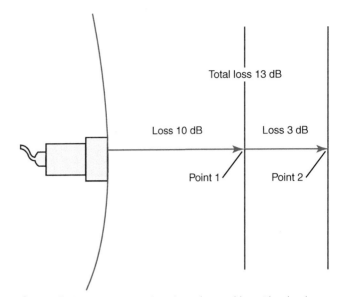

Figure 3-6 Intensity losses along the path are additive. Thus the change in intensity from the transducer to the point 2 in medium is −13 dB.

14 cm. The intensity ratio of each point to the surface requires a numerical range of 2 to 10,000. Since the decibel notation is logarithmic, a range of only −3 dB to −40 dB units is needed to express this same relationship. The negative sign indicates that the intensity of the beam has decreased from the reference point to the point of interest.

Another advantage of the decibel notation is that decibel changes along the beam path are additive. Consider the situation illustrated in Figure 3-6, in which the intensity at point 1 is one-tenth the original intensity and the intensity at point 2 is half the intensity at point 1, or 1/20 the original. By using the decibel methodology, the change in decibels can be found by adding dB change from transducer to point 1 (−10 dB) with the dB the change from point 1 to point 2 (−3 dB) to yield a total loss of 13 dB from the transducer to point 2. The sum of the decibel changes between points along the path is equal to the decibel change for the entire path.

PENETRATION

High-frequency sound waves are attenuated more rapidly than low-frequency sound waves. Thus the ability to penetrate tissue is reduced at higher frequencies. In addition, a reflector positioned at progressively greater depths generates progressively lower-intensity returning echoes. Intensity attenuation factors for human tissues are usually stated at a frequency of 1 MHz (Table 3-2). The attenuation rate at frequencies above 1 MHz is estimated by assuming that the attenuation rate is directly proportional to the frequency. For example, the attenuation rate at 4 MHz for fat is calculated by multiplying 4 MHz by 0.6 dB/(cm-MHz). The result is 2.4 dB/cm for fat when the frequency is 4 MHz.

The attenuation (neglecting reflection) of an ultrasound beam propagating through soft tissue ranges from 0.5 to

Table 3-1	Intensity Ratio and Amplitude Ratio versus Decibels	
I/I_o	A/A_o	dB
10,000	100	40
400	20	26
100	10	20
4	2	6
1	1	0
0.25	0.5	−6
0.01	0.1	−20
0.0025	0.05	−26
0.0001	0.01	−40

Table 3-2	Attenuation Rates for Different Media	
Material	**Attenuation Rate (dB/cm-MHz)**	
Blood	0.18	
Fat	0.6	
Soft tissue	0.5-0.8	
Skull	20	
Lung	40	
Water	0.0022	

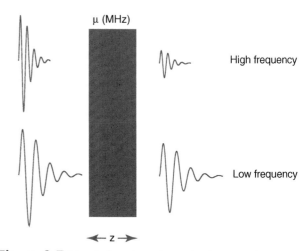

Figure 3-7 Intensity loss depends on the tissue via the attenuation coefficient (μ), the frequency of the sound wave, and the path length (z). High-frequency sound waves undergo more rapid attenuation for the same medium and path length.

1 dB/(cm-MHz). As an approximation, the attenuation rate is often assumed to be 0.5 dB/(cm-MHz), while the actual value is closer to 0.7 dB/(cm-MHz). For clinical safety, a value of 0.3 dB/(cm-MHz) is often specified to calculate a conservative estimate of the intensity at depth. For a 2-MHz ultrasound beam, approximately 30% of the energy is absorbed after 1 cm of travel in soft tissue. As a comparison, a 7.5-MHz ultrasound beam loses more than 75% of the energy after 1 cm of travel in soft tissue. *The decreased in intensity level expressed in decibels is directly proportional to both the depth of penetration and the frequency of the ultrasound beam.*

The intensity of the detected echo is often compared with the intensity of the transmitted ultrasound wave. If the relative intensity of the returning echo is 50 dB less than that of the transmitted wave, Equation 3-4 demonstrates that the echo intensity (I_e) will be a small fraction (1/100,000) of the transmitted intensity (I_t):

$$-50 = 10 \log \left(\frac{I_e}{I_t} \right)$$

$$-5 = \log \left(\frac{I_e}{I_t} \right)$$

$$\left(\frac{I_e}{I_t} \right) = \text{Antilog} \, (-5)$$

$$\left(\frac{I_e}{I_t} \right) = 0.00001$$

INTENSITY LOSS

The intensity loss in decibels caused by attenuation as the ultrasound beam passes through a medium is calculated by the seventh essential equation of sonography:

3-6   Intensity loss (dB) = μfz

where μ is the intensity attenuation coefficient expressed in dB/(cm-MHz), f is the frequency of the ultrasound wave expressed in MHz, and z is the distance traveled in the medium expressed in cm (Fig. 3-7). The intensity attenuation coefficient is tissue-specific and accounts for differences in the attenuation rate for various tissue types. *Rapid*

attenuation is indicated by high values of the intensity attenuation coefficient. The intensity loss expressed in decibels is directly proportional to both the depth of penetration and the frequency of the ultrasound beam. This can be seen more clearly by citing an example.

Example 3-2

Calculate the intensity loss in decibels for a 2.5-MHz ultrasound beam after it traverses 6 cm of soft tissue. Assume $\mu = 0.7$ dB/cm-MHz.

Intensity loss (dB) = μfz
Intensity loss (dB) = (0.7 dB/cm – MHz) (2.5 MHz) (6 cm)
Intensity loss (dB) = 10.5 dB

A loss of intensity relative to the reference intensity in the decibel equation is denoted by a negative sign. The negative sign is not included in Equation 3-6 because attenuation always causes decreased intensity as the ultrasound beam penetrates a medium. The descriptor "loss" and the negative sign would be redundant. However, if the result is used in Equation 3-4 to calculate an absolute intensity expressed in W/cm², dB intensity loss by attenuation must include the negative sign.

ECHO INTENSITY

In ultrasound imaging, the transducer sends out a pulsed wave and subsequently detects the returning echo. Intensity loss occurs by attenuation of the transmitted wave going out to the interface and also by attenuation of the reflected wave coming back toward the transducer from the interface. The rate of attenuation depends on tissue type and frequency. The intensity of the detected echo from an interface is diminished by increasing the distance of travel.

Figure 3-8 depicts the ultrasound beam striking an interface composed of soft tissue and bone at a depth of

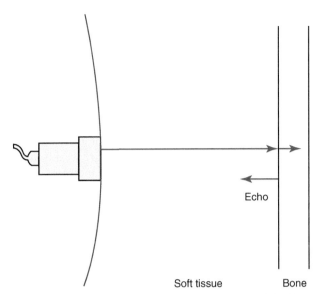

Figure 3-8 An echo is created at an interface composed of soft tissue and bone after the sound wave penetrates 6 cm of soft tissue.

$$\text{Loss (dB)} = 10 \log \left(\frac{100}{\%R} \right)$$

$$\text{Loss (dB)} = 10 \log \left(\frac{100}{43} \right)$$

$$\text{Loss (dB)} = 3.7 \text{ dB}$$

The total loss from attenuation through soft tissue and reflection at the tissue-bone interface is

$$\text{Loss (dB)} = 21 \text{ dB} + 3.7 \text{ dB} = 24.7 \text{ dB}$$

In general, absorption is a major contributor to the overall intensity loss. Structures with the same reflectivity are not always depicted with the same signal level because of differences in path length (effect of attenuation). The presence of a cyst (low attenuation) or gallstone (high attenuation) along the beam path alters the displayed signal level distal to these structures (Figs. 3-9 and 3-10).

6 cm. An echo is created at the interface, which returns toward the transducer. What is the change in intensity of a sound beam after undergoing various interactions, specifically attenuation and reflection? From Example 3-2, the intensity loss in decibels for a 2.5-MHz ultrasound beam after traversing 6 cm of soft tissue is 10.5 dB. Since the echo must repeat the path back to the transducer, the total intensity loss is twice this amount (21 dB). Remember that the dB losses along the path are additive. Additionally, intensity is reduced by reflection at the soft tissue-bone interface.

We will now consider the combined effect of attenuation and reflection on the intensity of a detected echo. *Attenuation* refers to all processes that act to reduce ultrasound intensity in a homogeneous medium. Reflection at the boundary also contributes to intensity loss. Losses from attenuation and reflection must be expressed in the same units, usually decibels. To convert percentage reflection into decibels, we modify Equation 3-4 by the percentage reflection:

3-7 $$\text{Loss (dB)} = 10 \log \left(\frac{100}{\%R} \right)$$

The following example illustrates the total effect of attenuation and reflection on the intensity of the detected echo.

Example 3-3

Calculate the relative intensity in decibels for an echo generated at a bone-tissue interface that is 6 cm deep in soft tissue. The transducer operates at a frequency of 2.5 MHz. Include the contribution of reflection at the interface.

Attenuation loss is 21 dB. Considering reflection at this soft tissue-bone interface the percentage reflection of 43%, must be converted into decibels:

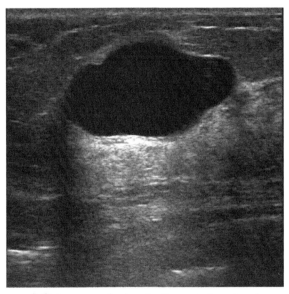

Figure 3-9 Sonogram of a breast with a cyst. Acoustic enhancement occurs distal to the liquid-filled structure, which has a low rate of attenuation.

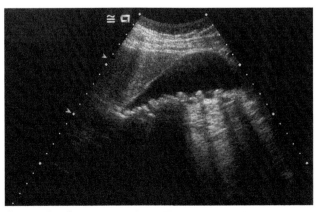

Figure 3-10 Sonogram of a gallbladder with gallstones. Acoustic shadowing occurs distal to the strongly attenuating structures.

Once the total attenuation from all sources (i.e., attenuation and reflection) in decibels is found, the intensity ratio can be calculated. For a loss of 30 dB, Equation 3-4 demonstrates that the original intensity is reduced by a factor of 1000.

The intensity ratio can be used to calculate the actual intensity value for I or I_{max} if one of them is known. For example, if I_{max} is 10 mW/cm^2, the intensity at the point of interest (I) will be 0.01 mW/cm^2.

Example 3-4

Calculate the intensity in watts per square centimeter for the detected echo in Example 3-3. The transmitted intensity is 5 W/cm^2 (I_{max}).

$$\text{Level (dB)} = -24.7 \text{ or a factor of } 0.00339$$
$$I = (5 \text{ W/cm}^2)(0.00339)$$
$$I = 0.0169 \text{ W/cm}^2 \text{ or } 16.9 \text{ mW/cm}^2$$

SUMMARY

A reduction in ultrasound intensity occurs as the wave propagates through tissue. Scattering, absorption, and reflection contribute to the overall energy loss. In the absence of reflective interfaces, the intensity loss is expressed mathematically as the product of the attenuation coefficient, frequency, and distance traveled in the medium. The attenuation coefficient is determined by tissue type. Lung and bone are highly attenuating, while blood and water-like fluids are weakly attenuating. The rate of energy loss generally increases linearly with frequency. Intensity change is measured on a logarithmic scale in units of the decibel. Total decibel loss along the beam path composed of multiple tissue types is equal to the sum of the individual decibel losses for each path segment. Three essential equations of sonography (instantaneous intensity, relative intensity in decibels, and intensity loss along the propagation path) were introduced.

Single-Element Transducers: Properties

4

Chapter Objectives

To describe the important design features of an ultrasound transducer
To state the major components of the transducer and describe their function
To list the parameters that characterize pulsed-wave operation
To recognize the relationship between Q-value and bandwidth

Key terms

Backing material
Bandwidth
Center frequency
Duty factor (DF)
Fractional bandwidth
Lead zirconate titanate
   (PZT)

Matching layer
Piezoelectric effect
Pulse duration (PD)
Pulse repetition frequency
   (PRF)
Pulse repetition period
   (PRP)

Q-value
Scan range
Spatial pulse length (SPL)

TRANSDUCER DESIGN

A transducer is any device that transforms one kind of energy into another (e.g., mechanical to electrical). The ultrasound transducer must convert an electrical signal into an ultrasound wave, which is transmitted into the patient's body and then convert the returning echo into an electrical signal for processing and display. The first type of transducer, which is still in use today, employs a single-element circular disk to both transmit and receive ultrasound.

The information obtained from ultrasound scanning depends in large part on the beam characteristics, which in turn are governed by transducer design. The properties of the single-element transducer serve as a prerequisite for understanding the modifications that have been made in the modern transducers discussed in the following chapters. Numerous parameters shown in Table 4-1 characterize transducer output.

Design criteria for ultrasound transmission with an imaging transducer include proper frequency in the megahertz range, capability for pulsed-wave operation, directional control, uniform intensity, and limited spatial extent (beam width and pulse length). For positional information utilizing the echo-ranging principle, a short burst is required, and thus the sound beam must be turned on and off rapidly. A unidirectional beam (analogous to a flashlight beam versus a porch light) with limited physical dimensions is important to accurately identify the location of the reflector. Small beam width and spatial pulse length (related to frequency) restrict the region in which the returning echo can be formed. Automated scanning with a narrow beam allows sampling throughout the field of view. Uniform intensity is desirable, so that structures with similar reflectivity produce echoes of similar strength.

Table 4-1	Physical Descriptors and Symbols	
Parameter		**Symbol**
Bandwidth		Δf
Center frequency		f_c
Duty factor		DF
Maximum pulse repetition frequency		PRF_{max}
Number of cycles		n
Pulse duration		PD
Pulse repetition frequency		PRF
Pulse repetition period		PRP
Scan range		R
Spatial pulse length		SPL
Mechanical coefficient		Q-value

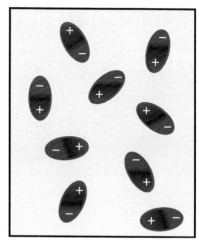

Figure 4-1 Random arrangement of dipoles (natural state).

In echo detection, reflected mechanical vibrations from an interface are recorded. The time is measured for short pulses (which may be a single vibration) to travel from the point of sound origin to the object and back to the receiver. For example, if a Chinese gong were allowed to move only once after being struck and then cushioned with a pillow to shorten the duration of the vibration, a single-cycle sound wave would be produced. The transmitted wave would move out to some distant object, undergo reflection, and then return toward the listener. In such circumstances, the echo is also a single-cycle vibration. Since the position of any object in space can be determined only to an accuracy of about half a wavelength, a resolution limit is imposed by wavelength. The ability to distinguish two objects separated by a small distance along the direction of propagation is called axial resolution. Because frequency and wavelength are inversely related, shorter wavelengths, which produce finer resolution, correspond to higher frequencies. The question then becomes what frequencies are needed to produce the resolution required in diagnostic ultrasound.

If one wavelength is a good approximation of the smallest detectable object, what frequency is required for a resolution of 1 mm in tissue? In nature, bats and certain other animals (porpoises, moles, and some grasshoppers) generate ultrasound waves having frequencies of around 100 kHz or a wavelength of 1.54 cm. Thus sources of this frequency cannot provide the desired spatial resolution. Frequencies above 1.5 MHz are necessary to generate waves with wavelengths less than 1 mm. For medical diagnostic ultrasound, it is evident that the operating frequency must be in the megahertz range.

PIEZOELECTRIC PROPERTIES

Nothing in nature can be readily adapted to transmit ultrasonic energy in the megahertz frequency range. Consequently, the transducer must be manufactured. The construction of a high-frequency transducer relies on a phenomenon first studied by Pierre and Marie Curie in the 1880s and known as the piezoelectric effect. This phenomenon is commonly found in crystalline materials that have regions of positive and negative charge on each molecule (called dipoles). In the normal crystalline lattice structure, these randomly arranged dipoles cannot migrate (Fig. 4-1). If the material is heated above a temperature called the Curie temperature, however, the molecules are free to move and rotate. When a pair of charged plates (one positive and one negative) is placed across the heated crystal, the negative region of each molecule orients toward the positive plate and the positive region toward the negative plate (opposite charges attract, like charges repel). The positive and negative regions of the molecules are slightly offset from the applied electrical field because of thermal motion. If the material is then cooled below the Curie temperature while the electrical field is still applied, the molecules will maintain their alignment. *Ultrasound transducers should not be autoclaved, because this destroys the piezoelectric properties of the material by raising its temperature above the Curie temperature and returning the dipoles to their random arrangement.*

The molecular arrangement of the dipolar molecules gives piezoelectric materials their unique properties. Conducting plates are placed on the opposite faces of the crystal. When a voltage is applied to the conducting plates, the molecules twist to align themselves with the electrical field (positive molecules toward the negative electrode, negative molecules toward the positive electrode), thereby thickening the crystal (Fig. 4-2). If the plates are reversed in polarity, the molecules will twist back in the opposite direction, creating a decrease in the crystal thickness. The actual movement is only a few microns. Alternating polarity causes expansion and contraction of the crystal, which creates mechanical vibrations. When the expanding and contracting crystal is placed in contact with the skin, sound waves are transmitted into the body. Thus a voltage applied across the piezoelectric material creates mechanical motion (sound waves). In this way the generation of the ultrasound beam can be regulated by the transducer.

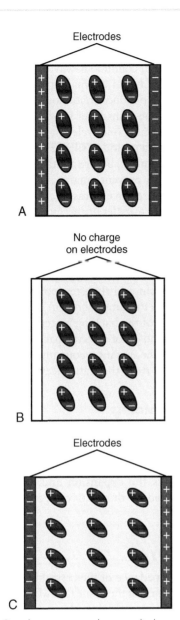

Figure 4-2 Crystal response to voltage applied across the excitation electrodes. **A,** Contraction of the crystal caused by movement of the dipoles trying to align with an applied electrical field. **B,** Normal thickness with no applied electrical field. **C,** Expansion of the crystal caused by movement of the dipoles trying to align with an applied electrical field. The polarity is reversed from that depicted in **(A)**.

The piezoelectric effect enables the same crystal to also act as a receiver of an ultrasonic echo (high-frequency pressure wave). Ultrasound waves returning from reflectors in the body strike the crystal and induce voltage variations. These signals are processed and ultimately displayed.

Natural Vibrational Frequency

If left alone, the transducer would ring in a manner similar to a tuning fork. Note that if a tuning fork is to ring at 2000 Hz, it does not have to be struck 2000 times each second to maintain the sound (although this is a possibility, particularly for continuous-wave generation). Instead,

a natural vibrational frequency occurs in which the wave is transmitted back and forth (from prong to prong) at a set frequency that depends on wave interference. If a crystal suspended in air is struck with a voltage pulse, ultrasound waves are generated. Multiple wavefronts are formed and radiate away from each face. These waves undergo constructive and destructive interference within the crystal, depending on the crystal's thickness. The crystal has a natural vibrational frequency (just as the tuning fork does) that is related to the distance between those two surfaces. To have constructive interference so that a single wave moves back and forth across the crystal, the distance from one surface to the other must be equal to half the wavelength. The natural resonant frequency increases as the crystal becomes thinner (Fig. 4-3). At high frequencies, the crystals become very thin.

Frequency does not change when the ultrasound wave enters one medium from another. The same frequency generated by the transducer is transmitted into the patient. However, a change in wavelength occurs between the crystal and the tissue; this is caused by velocity differences in the two media (1540 m/s for tissue and approximately 4000 m/s for the crystal).

Piezoelectric Materials

For diagnostic medical applications the material almost universally used in transducers is lead zirconate titanate (PZT). PZT represents a family of piezoelectric ceramics with various additives that change the properties to match a particular application. PZT is used in medical transducers because it has the desirable properties of efficient energy conversion, proper frequency range, and ability to be molded in a particular size and shape. These ceramics are brittle and can easily be damaged if dropped or bumped. Polymer material, such as polyvinylidene difluoride, is manufactured in flat membranes for use in hydrophones.

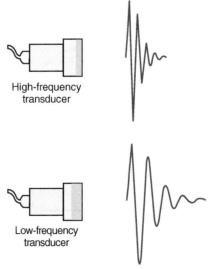

High-frequency transducer

Low-frequency transducer

Figure 4-3 Natural resonance frequency is controlled by crystal thickness *(gray region).*

TRANSDUCER CONSTRUCTION

Figure 4-4 is a cross-sectional view of a simple single-element transducer. The major component of a transducer is a crystal of piezoelectric material with electrodes placed on opposite sides to create the changing polarity. A thin film of metal is plated on the crystal surface, forming the electrodes. To improve the transfer of energy to and from the patient, the matching layer is located next to the crystal on the exit side. Crystal ringing is diminished by the introduction of the backing material, which adjoins the surface electrode opposite the exit side. The entire crystal assembly—including the electrodes, matching layer, and backing material—is housed in an electrically insulating casing (usually some type of plastic). This casing also provides structural support. To reduce the electromagnetic interference, a radiofrequency shield composed of a hollow metallic cylinder is placed around the crystal and backing material and electronically grounded to the front electrode's surface. An acoustic insulator, made of rubber or cork, coats the inner surface of the radiofrequency shield to prevent the transmission of ultrasound energy into the casing.

Backing Material

The backing material is placed behind the crystal in the transducer to dampen ringing of the crystal; its composition depends on whether the transducer is designed for continuous- or pulsed-wave operation. Continuous-wave output results if natural ringing (resonance) occurs in the crystal, in which case the backing material should have an acoustic impedance different from that of the crystal.

Maximum reflection at the backing material-crystal interface causes the crystal to ring. Air is commonly employed as the backing material for continuous-wave transducers. The crystal may be driven by an alternating voltage source of the correct frequency to induce continuous-wave output.

For imaging, the transducer sends out a short burst of ultrasound (preferably one cycle but usually two to five cycles), followed by a period of silence to listen for returning echoes (receiving mode) before another sound pulse is generated. Ideally, to prevent ringing, the backing material should effectively remove ultrasonic energy from the crystal. *For maximum transfer of energy to occur (from crystal to backing material), the backing material must have an acoustic impedance identical to that of the crystal.* Also, the backing material should readily absorb ultrasonic energy to prevent it from reentering the crystal. A combination of epoxy resin and tungsten powder is used for the backing material to damp (shorten) the ultrasonic pulse. The rear surface of the backing material is slanted so that the reflected sound is not directed back toward the crystal. Ringing lowers the instantaneous intensity of the output ultrasound wave from the transducer.

Dynamic Damping

Dynamic damping is an electronic means to suppress ringing. A voltage pulse of opposite polarity is applied to the crystal immediately following the excitation pulse. This counteracts the expansion and contraction of the crystal stimulated by the first voltage pulse, and ringing is inhibited.

Matching Layer

The acoustic impedance of the crystal is large (30 Mrayls) compared with that of the tissue (1.6 Mrayls), which results in a large reflection (81%) at the crystal-tissue interface. Only 19% of the ultrasonic energy enters the tissue (percent transmission). The acoustic impedance mismatch creates a long pulse and reduces the intensity of the beam that enters the patient. Both of these effects are undesirable for imaging. *In order to shorten the pulse and improve energy transfer across the crystal-tissue interface, a material with intermediate acoustic impedance is placed between the crystal and the patient.* This material, called the matching layer, is mounted in the transducer on the exit side of the crystal (Fig. 4-5). However, the matching layer must have low-loss properties, since high attenuation would counteract the desired effect of high transmission.

The acoustic impedance of the matching layer is made to reduce the amount of reflection at the crystal-matching layer and matching layer-tissue interfaces. This is accomplished by taking the geometric mean of the acoustic impedances for the crystal and tissue (the square root of the product of the acoustic impedances):

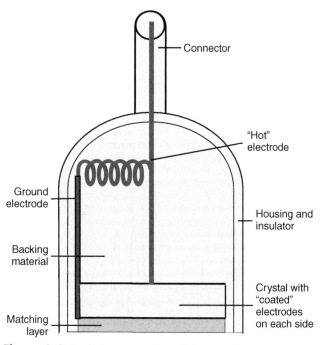

Figure 4-4 Single-element transducer. PZT crystal, electrodes, matching layer, backing material, and acoustic insulator are shown.

Connector

"Hot" electrode

Ground electrode

Housing and insulator

Backing material

Crystal with "coated" electrodes on each side

Matching layer

4-1

$$Z_{ml} = \sqrt{Z_c Z_t}$$

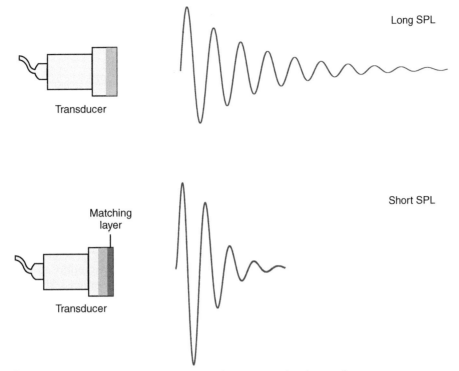

Figure 4-5 Matching layer *(dark gray region)* between crystal and tissue allows greater instantaneous intensity to enter the patient and reduces the pulse length.

The introduction of a single matching layer increases the total sound energy transferred into the tissue to 37% (the product of transmission coefficients, which is 61% through each interface). Improvement above 19% transmission without the matching layer is evident.

A specific thickness of the matching layer is also necessary. A thickness equal to integer multiples of the quarter wavelength provides maximum reinforcement of the ultrasound wave reflected from the interface. This enhances the intensity of the ultrasound wave transmitted into the body. Normally, the one-quarter layer (which causes less attenuation than a three-quarter layer or any other quarter multiple) is adjusted for the center frequency of the transducer. A transducer with a quarter-wavelength matching layer is referred to as a quarter-wavelength transducer.

Because pulsed systems produce ultrasound waves of many frequencies (frequency distribution is described by the bandwidth) and each frequency has its own associated wavelength, the optimal single matching layer for transmission or reception is difficult to design. The quarter-frequency matching layer allows maximum transmission for a single frequency of the ultrasound wave. Additional improvement in performance can be achieved by using multiple matching layers. These matching layers taper the acoustic impedance from that of the crystal to that of tissue. Indeed, the efficiency of transmission is so improved that in many cases the backing layer is no longer needed. Ringing is reduced because the energy is efficiently transferred to tissue and does not remain in the crystal for multiple reflections at the crystal interfaces.

PULSED-WAVE OUTPUT

In echo-ranging systems, the transducer must pause after sound transmission to "listen" for the returning echoes. Because the crystal cannot send and receive simultaneously, it must be pulsed for transmission after an appropriate listening time has elapsed (Fig. 4-6).

The excitation waveform for most modern instruments is a short, square wave burst consisting of one to three

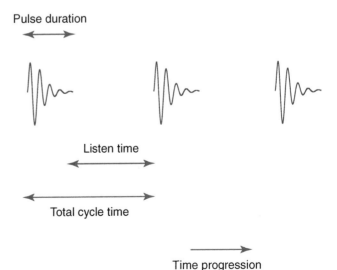

Figure 4-6 Temporal representation of pulsed-wave output. The time-dependent output from a transducer alternates between actively generating a five-cycle pulse of short duration and a longer time interval of no transmission, which allows reception of returning echoes.

cycles with a radiowave frequency equal to the desired center frequency. The driving frequency must be within the frequency operating range of the transducer (bandwidth).

PULSE REPETITION FREQUENCY

The number of times the crystal is pulsed or electrically stimulated per second is called the pulse repetition frequency (PRF). The maximum pulse repetition frequency (PRF_{max}) is limited by the maximum depth (R) to be sampled and by the velocity of ultrasound (c) in the medium, as shown by the eighth essential equation:

4-2
$$PRF_{max} = \frac{c}{2R}$$

The factor 2 accounts for the total distance traveled to the reflector and back to the transducer, which is twice the depth of sampling.

Equation 4-2 illustrates that the PRF_{max} can be increased if the velocity in the medium is increased or the scan range (the maximum depth from which an echo can be detected) is decreased. Typically, the acoustic velocity in the medium does not change (being nearly constant for all types of tissue) and cannot be adjusted by the sonographer. The sonographer can sometimes alter the scan angle to correspond with a shallower region of interest by reorienting the transducer. Patient exposure considerations and transducer heating often dictate that the operation is less than the maximum pulse repetition frequency for a given set of conditions. In designing their systems, manufacturers usually vary the pulse repetition frequency with the depth. A single independent control for PRF is normally not available to the operator.

Example 4-1

Assume that the maximum depth of interest in tissue is 10 cm. What is the maximum PRF?

$$PRF_{max} = \frac{c}{2R}$$

$$PRF_{max} = \frac{1540 \text{ m/s}}{2(0.1 \text{ m})}$$

$$PRF_{max} = 7700 \text{ 1/s}$$

PRF is often expressed in units of Hz or kHz (corresponding to 1000 pulses per second). PRFs ranging from 1 kHz to 12 kHz are used for B-mode and Doppler units.

PULSE REPETITION PERIOD

The time required to transmit a pulsed ultrasound wave plus the time devoted to listening for the returning echoes from that wave is called the pulse repetition period (PRP). It is equal to the reciprocal of the pulse repetition frequency:

4-3
$$PRP = \frac{1}{PRF}$$

Example 4-2

What is the PRP if the PRF is 1 kHz? Using Equation 4-3 and substituting a value of 1000 pulses per second for the PRF,

$$PRP = \frac{1}{PRF}$$

$$PRP = \frac{1}{1000 \text{ 1/s}}$$

$$PRP = 0.001 \text{ s}$$

SPATIAL PULSE LENGTH

Ideally, for each pulse, a short packet of ultrasound energy of the appropriate frequency (i.e., 3.5 MHz for a 3.5-MHz transducer) is directed into the body. In practice, the pulse is composed of a range of different frequencies that encompass the labeled operating frequency. The operating frequency is also called the center frequency, which represents the most dominant frequency. The physical extent of this short-duration pulse (distance along the direction of propagation at one instant in time) is called the spatial pulse length (SPL) and equals the product of the wavelength (λ) associated with the center frequency and the number of cycles (n) in the pulse:

4-4
$$SPL = n\lambda$$

For example, spatial pulse length is 1.54 mm for a transducer with a center frequency of 3 MHz that produces a pulse 3 cycles in duration.

For good axial resolution, a pulse of short duration is necessary. To shorten the pulse spatially, the number of cycles must be reduced (Fig. 4-7) or the frequency must be increased to decrease wavelength (Fig. 4-3).

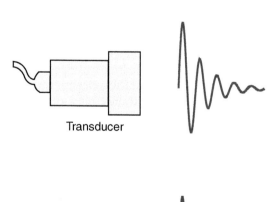

Transducer

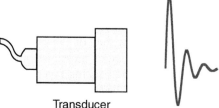

Transducer

Figure 4-7 For the same center frequency, a five-cycle pulse has longer duration than a three-cycle pulse.

Pulse Duration

The pulse duration (PD), or temporal pulse length, is the time interval for one complete transmitted pulsed wave. It describes the actual time during which the transducer is generating the ultrasonic pulse. The effectiveness of the matching layer to transfer the energy into tissue and the ability of the backing material to quickly dampen the pulse affect the pulse duration.

The pulse duration (PD) is calculated from the number of cycles in the pulse (n) and the period (τ) of the wave:

4-5
$$PD = n\tau$$

The three-cycle pulse from a 3-MHz transducer with an SPL of 1.54 mm has a pulse duration of 1 microsecond. The SPL varies directly with the pulse duration, the constant of proportionality being equal to the velocity in the medium:

4-6
$$SPL = (c)(PD)$$

Duty Factor

A typical unit with a pulse duration of 1 μs and a PRF of 1 kHz transmits ultrasound only 0.1% of the time. Most of its time by far (99.9%) is spent in a receive mode. The duty factor (DF) is the fraction of time during which the unit is active and is calculated as the ratio of the pulse duration and the pulse repetition period:

4-7
$$DF = \frac{PD}{PRP}$$

Both the PD and the PRP are expressed in units of time (either seconds or microseconds), but duty factor is dimensionless. It is merely the fraction of time during which the pulse is actively generated to the time between transmitted pulses. Recall that the pulse repetition period is equal to the reciprocal of the pulse repetition frequency; thus Equation 4-7 can be expressed in the form

4-8
$$DF = (PD)(PRF)$$

Duty factor is important in the determination of the temporal average intensity.

Example 4-3

Calculate the duty factor for a 3-MHz transducer that produces three cycles per pulse. The PRF is 1500 Hz.

$$DF = \frac{PD}{PRP} \text{ or } (PD)(PRF)$$

$$DF = \frac{1\ \mu s}{670\ \mu s} \text{ or } (1\ \mu s)(1500\ Hz)$$

$$DF = 0.0015$$

Q-VALUE

The Q-value, or mechanical coefficient, assesses an essential dependent relationship of the transmitted ultrasound beam: pulse duration and bandwidth. Bandwidth describes the range of frequencies that compose the transmitted wave. The Q-value can be thought of as having two separate definitions describing the two affected beam characteristics. These definitions are

4-9
$$Q = \frac{\text{Energy stored per cycle}}{\text{Energy lost per cycle}}$$

and

4-10
$$Q = \frac{\text{Center frequency}}{\text{Bandwidth}}$$

A high-Q transducer retains energy in the crystal and therefore loses very little each cycle. After being stimulated by the voltage pulse, vibrations continue for an extended time, producing a long-duration pulse. High-Q transducers (700 or greater) are necessary for continuous-wave ultrasound. A low-Q transducer, on the other hand, generates a short pulse after excitation because most of its energy is loss from the crystal and converted to sound during the first few vibrations. Pulsed-wave ultrasound in imaging requires low-Q transducers, the Q-value being approximately 2.

BANDWIDTH

From Equation 4-10, it can be seen that the Q-value is indirectly proportional to the bandwidth. For a transducer operating with a continuous output, only a single frequency is generated. *For a pulsed system, however, because of the complex nature of the damped pulse, a range of frequencies is generated.* Many waves of differing frequency combine to form the pulse. Fourier analysis enables a complex waveform (e.g., pulsed ultrasound wave) to be divided into its various frequency components. An algebraic summation of sine waves of varying frequency yields the original waveform; in other words, any complex waveform can be considered a series of sine waves with different frequencies and amplitudes.

The frequency spectrum can be analyzed by measuring the signal strength as a function of time for an electrical signal induced by an echo returning from a flat steel target located a fixed distance from the transducer in a nonattenuating medium. The frequency distribution in the transmitted pulse shows a centrally peaked spectrum, with the center frequency (f_c) having the greatest amplitude (Fig. 4-8).

Pulse Duration and Bandwidth

Pulse duration and bandwidth are inversely related. That is, pulse duration is inversely proportional to the bandwidth. *A low-Q transducer has a short pulse length (rapidly damped) and a broad bandwidth* (Fig. 4-9). A high-Q transducer has a long pulse length (from crystal ringing) and a narrow bandwidth. In diagnostic ultrasound imaging, trade-offs exist between good reception and good transmission, but generally low-Q transducers with broad bandwidths are desirable.

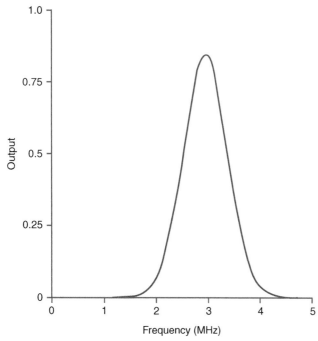

Figure 4-8 Frequency distribution of the transmitted pulse. The center frequency (f_c) is the dominant component in the transmitted output (3 MHz for this distribution).

Calculation of Bandwidth

The center frequency is the natural resonance frequency of the transducer, which depends on the crystal thickness. Equation 4-10 rewritten with symbols becomes the ninth essential equation of sonography:

4-11
$$Q = \frac{f_c}{\Delta f}$$

where Δf is the bandwidth between the half maximum points on each side of the center frequency (f_c).

From the frequency spectrum, the frequency corresponding to 50% of the maximum output is marked on each side of the center frequency. The bandwidth is calculated by subtracting the low frequency at 50% maximum output from the high frequency at 50% maximum output (Fig. 4-10). This process of determining the width of the frequency distribution at 50% maximum output is called *full width at half maximum* (FWHM).

A transducer operating at a center frequency of 7.5 MHz with a bandwidth of 3.75 MHz yields a Q-value of 2. When the second definition of Q-value for a transducer is used, it becomes evident (as stated by Equation 4-11) that a high-Q transducer has a very narrow bandwidth, whereas a low-Q transducer has a broad bandwidth.

Fractional Bandwidth

Bandwidth is often expressed as a fraction of the center frequency:

4-12   Fractional bandwidth $= \dfrac{\Delta f}{f_c} \times 100\%$

A transducer operating at a center frequency of 7.5 MHz with a Q-value of 2 yields a fraction bandwidth of 50%.

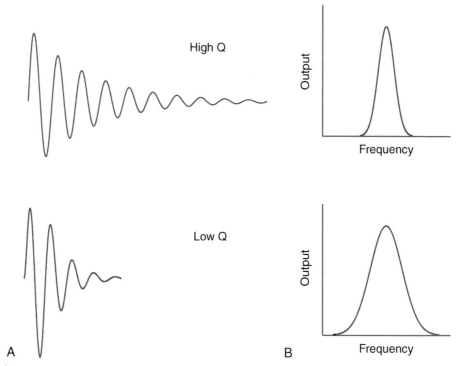

Figure 4-9 Relationship between Q-value, pulse length, and the frequency spectrum. **A,** Output versus time, illustrating pulse length for rapid damping (low-Q) versus slow damping (high-Q). **B,** Relative importance of various frequencies present in each pulse in **(A)**. This illustrates the principle that as the pulse duration is shortened, additional frequency components contribute to the transmitted pulse.

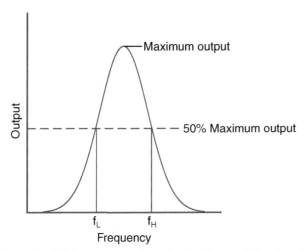

Figure 4-10 Determination of bandwidth. This is calculated as the difference between the high and low frequency limits corresponding to half the output at the center frequency (labeled as f_H and f_L). This analysis applied to Figure 4-8 yields a bandwidth of 1 MHz.

The fractional bandwidth can also be estimated using the number of cycles in the pulse (n):

4-13 $\text{Fractional bandwidth} = \dfrac{1}{n} \times 100\%$

Matching Layer Effect on Bandwidth

The presence of multiple matching layers enhances the transmission of energy into the patient and shortens the pulse duration. Thus the frequency distribution is shifted toward a broader bandwidth. The axial resolution is improved because the larger bandwidth normally produces a shorter spatial pulse length. To form a short spatial pulse, multiple frequency components are necessary.

FOCUSING

Divergence of the ultrasonic beam causes a decrease in intensity with increasing distance from the transducer. This is easily understood by considering a constant amount of energy spread over a larger and larger area. The amount of energy incident on a unit area reflector will decrease as the distance between the reflector and the transducer increases. The reflected beam will also diverge, returning to the transducer and creating a partial "miss" of the ultrasound wave at the transducer (Fig. 4-11). Thus divergence is responsible for intensity loss for both the transmitted and the reflected beam.

The transmitted waves can be directed to converge at a specific point. This manipulation, called focusing, narrows the beam width and raises the intensity over a small area at a specific distance from the transducer. Compared with a nonfocused beam, the focused beam produces a stronger echo whose spatial origin can be more accurately determined. However, this is true only for structures within the focal zone of the transducer, where beam width is narrow. Focusing techniques and the resulting ultrasonic fields are discussed in the next chapter.

COMPOSITE PIEZOELECTRIC MATERIALS

A composite transducer element is formed by dicing the piezoelectric material into an array of rectangular pillars and filling the interspace with epoxy resin (Fig. 4-12). Each pillar is small, measuring one third of a wavelength in cross-section. The pillar-to-pillar separation is twice the dimension of the pillar. Epoxy is less dense and more flexible than the replaced piezoelectric material, which causes a reduction in the acoustic impedance to 10 to 20 megarayls (Mrayls). Since acoustic impedance more closely approaches tissue, good transmission is obtained. The composite material has a very wide bandwidth, which enables the same transducer to operate over a range of center frequencies or to produce pulses of very short duration. Also, the higher sensitivity of these composite materials improves echo detection. Finally, the composite material is easily shaped for the desired configuration for geometric focusing.

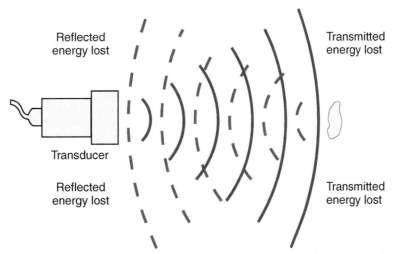

Figure 4-11 Energy loss due to divergence. Energy is lost in both transmitted *(solid lines)* and received *(dashed lines)* directions.

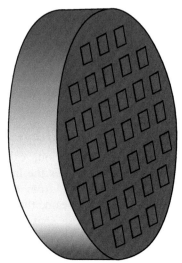

Figure 4-12 Composite piezoelectric element. Rods of PZT material (red) are configured in a periodic array and the spacing between rods is filled with epoxy.

SUMMARY

The purpose of the transducer is to produce an ultrasound wave of the proper frequency, which can be directed into the patient. The transducer also functions as a receiver for

Table 4-2	Characteristics of Imaging Transducers
Parameter	**Characteristic**
Waveform	Pulsed
Q-value	Low (~2)
Frequency	2-20 MHz
Pulse Duration	Short (1–5 cycles) (~1 μs)
Frequency Distribution	Wide bandwidth (>50%)

the returning echoes. Matching layer and backing material are incorporated into the transducer to enhance energy transmission and reduce ringing. Pulse duration and spatial pulse length describe the temporal and spatial extent of the ultrasound pulse. The rate of pulse generation is the pulse repetition frequency. The frequency distribution in the transmitted pulse is characterized by the bandwidth and Q-value. Low Q-value and wide bandwidth associated with a short duration pulse are most suitable for imaging applications. The desirable characteristics for an imaging transducer are summarized in Table 4-2. Two essential equations of sonography (maximum pulse repetition frequency and Q-value) were introduced.

Single-Element Transducers: Transmission and Echo Reception

5

Chapter Objectives

To describe the limitations of spatial sampling with a pulsed ultrasound beam
To characterize the ultrasonic field with respect to the near and far fields
To state the two focusing methods for single-element transducers
To describe the sequence of processing steps applied to echo-induced signals

Key terms

A-mode
Axial resolution
Beam width
Depth of field
Dynamic range

Far field
Focal length
Focal zone
Focusing
Lateral resolution

Near field
Noise
Signal processing
Spatial pulse length (SPL)

SPATIAL PULSE SIZE

Spatial mapping of the detected echoes depends in large part on the beam characteristics, which in turn are governed by transducer design. At an instant in time the transmitted pulse occupies a three-dimensional volume in space (the region in which the molecules are participating in the mechanical energy transfer). The spatial extent of the pulse is described along the direction of propagation (spatial pulse length) and perpendicular to the direction of propagation (beam width). The pulsed wave is the detector window, which establishes the limits of spatial sampling (the ability to perceive fine spatial detail). Reflectors that lie anywhere within the pulse generate echoes; those that lie outside the pulse do not. Spatial pulse length, beam width, and focal length characterize transducer performance. Physical descriptors and the corresponding symbols discussed in this chapter are listed in Table 5-1.

AXIAL RESOLUTION

The Q-value of a transducer in conjunction with the transducer's frequency determines the spatial pulse length (SPL), which in turn defines the axial sampling length of the transmitted pulse. The axial resolution (also called range resolution and depth resolution) specifies how close together two objects can be along the axis of the beam and still be detected as two distinct entities. Axial resolution also indicates the smallest object whose size can be accurately registered along the axis of the beam.

The smallest separation between objects that can be resolved is half the spatial pulse length. Figure 5-1 illustrates this concept. The beam leaves the transducer with an axial length of one SPL and is directed toward two interfaces spaced SPL/2 apart. The pulsed wave strikes the first interface, which causes a fraction of the ultrasonic energy to be reflected toward the transducer. The remaining energy of the pulsed wave is transmitted through the interface and advances toward the second interface, at which point some of the energy is again reflected. The echo with the pulse length of

Table 5-1	Physical Descriptors and Symbols
Parameter	**Symbol**
Beam aperture	2a
Beam width	w
Crystal diameter	D
Focal length	F
Near field depth	NFD
Spatial pulse length	SPL

the spatial pulse length and improves the axial resolution (Fig. 5-2). Note that a trade-off occurs. Although the resolution is enhanced at higher frequencies, the depth of penetration is decreased because of the frequency dependence of the attenuation coefficient. For a constant wavelength, as ringing is reduced, the axial resolution is also improved (Fig. 5-3).

Spatial pulse length is established at transmission and is not altered by attenuation along the beam path. *Axial*

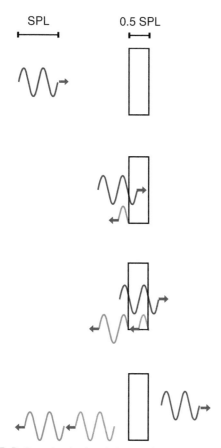

Figure 5-1 Spatial pulse length (SPL) with minimum resolution. Two objects *(vertical sides of the rectangular box)* are separated by 0.5 SPL. The respective echoes from each interface are shown by the green and orange colored lines. The objects are just resolvable.

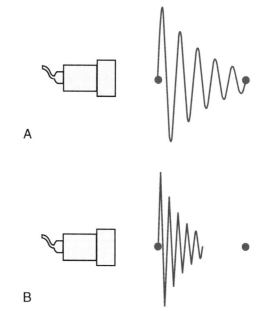

Figure 5-2 Spatial pulse length (SPL) shortened by increasing the frequency. **A,** The five-cycle pulse from a low-frequency transducer includes both objects (dots) within the SPL. **B,** The five-cycle pulse from a high-frequency transducer has a shorter SPL and can resolve objects located more closely together.

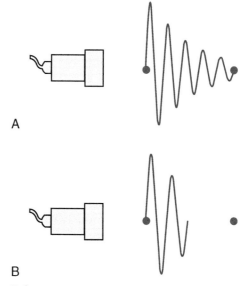

Figure 5-3 Spatial pulse length shortened by decreasing ringing. **A,** A five-cycle pulse includes both objects (dots) within the spatial pulse length. **B,** A two-cycle pulse at the same frequency has a shorter spatial pulse length and does not include both dots.

one SPL leaving the first interface has traveled a distance of SPL/2 when the pulsed wave strikes the second interface. As the reflected sound wave from the second interface moves toward the first interface, the echo from the first interface continues to proceed toward the transducer. When the echo from the second interface arrives at the first interface, the first echo has moved a distance of one SPL, and therefore the echoes from the two interfaces are separated in both distance and time when detected by the transducer.

The spatial pulse length depends on the frequency of the transducer. For a constant number of cycles, as the frequency is increased, the shortened wavelength decreases

Table 5-2	Ways to Decrease Spatial Pulse Length	
Parameter		**Change**
Frequency		Increase
Q-value		Decrease
Damping		Increase
Pulse duration		Decrease

axial resolution is essentially constant throughout the scan range (independent of depth). Factors affecting spatial pulse length and hence axial resolution are summarized in Table 5-2.

BEAM WIDTH AND LATERAL RESOLUTION

One of the fundamental objectives in transducer design is to generate a beam that is directional. If a very small crystal is used, the transmitted waves move radially outward from the source. The beam from a large-diameter crystal is unidirectional, with planar wavefronts and the lateral extent of the beam being nearly the same as the diameter of the crystal (Fig. 5-4).

Lateral resolution describes the ability to distinguish, as separate entities, two objects adjacent to each other

oriented perpendicular to the beam axis. It also refers to the ability of the ultrasound beam to depict the spatial extent of a single small object perpendicular to the direction of propagation. An object smaller than the beam width produces a signal the entire time it is within the beam; thus the object appears to be the same size as the width of the beam. Decreasing the beam width improves the lateral resolution by allowing objects close together to be resolved and by providing a more accurate spatial representation of small objects.

THE ULTRASONIC FIELD: NEAR FIELD AND FAR FIELD

A circular sound source with a diameter equal to one wavelength produces spherical wavefronts originating from the face of the crystal (Fig. 5-5). The beam diverges rapidly from the crystal face and the lateral resolution deteriorates. If the diameter of the crystal is increased to several wavelengths, each small area (one wavelength in size) becomes an individual vibrating sound source and thus produces its own spherical wavefronts. These wavefronts undergo constructive and destructive interference, resulting in a very complex wave pattern (Fig. 5-6), in accordance with Huygens' principle. The area of uniform beam width extending from the transducer forms the near field before undergoing rapid divergence in the far field. The far field is called the Fraunhofer zone, and the near field is called the Fresnel zone (Fig. 5-7).

Near-Field Depth

For a nonfocused transducer, the near-field depth (NFD), or the distance that the near field extends into the patient, is dependent on the diameter (D) and frequency (f) or wavelength (λ) of the transducer according to the following formula:

5-1
$$NFD = \frac{D^2 f}{4c} = \frac{D^2}{4\lambda}$$

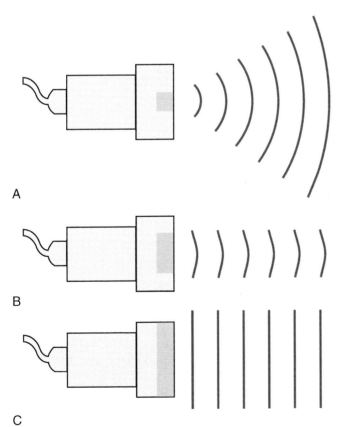

A

B

C

Figure 5-4 Effect of crystal size *(shown in gray)* on wavefronts. **A,** Spherical wavefronts produced by a small-radius source of sound. **B,** As the size of the source is increased, the wavefronts become less divergent. **C,** Large-radius transducer producing planar (directional) wavefronts.

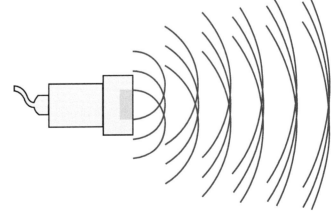

Figure 5-5 Wavefronts produced from a sound source *(gray region)* whose diameter is equal to one wavelength.

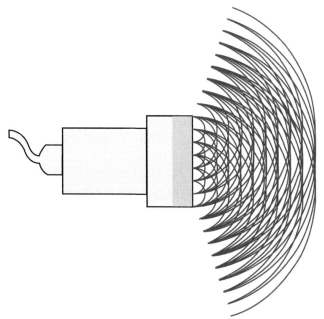

Figure 5-6 A large sound source *(gray region)* acting as multiple single-wavelength sound sources produces a complex pattern of wavefronts.

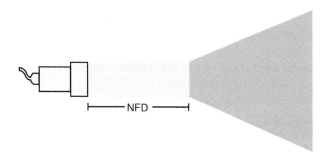

Figure 5-7 Beam pattern showing the near field *(light green)* and far field *(dark green)*. Distance NFD indicates the depth of the near field.

where c the acoustic velocity. As the frequency increases (or wavelength decreases), the near-field depth is extended from the crystal. At high frequencies, lateral resolution associated with narrow beam width in the near field is maintained at increased depth. In practice, higher frequencies are absorbed more rapidly as the beam propagates through tissue; consequently, deep structures may not be visualized because the induced signals from reflected ultrasound waves are too weak.

Example 5-1

Calculate the NFD for transducer with frequency of 5 MHz. Assume a diameter of 10 mm (0.01 m).

$$NFD = \frac{D^2 f}{4c}$$

$$NFD = \frac{(0.01 \text{ m})^2 (5 \times 10^6 \text{ 1/s})}{4(1540 \text{ m/s})}$$

$$NFD = 0.081 \text{ m} = 8.1 \text{ cm}$$

Similarly, for a constant-diameter of 10 mm, the near-field depth is 4 cm at a frequency of 2.5 MHz, but is elongated to 12 cm if the frequency is increased to 7.5 MHz. This demonstrates that the near-field depth is extended as the frequency is increased. Near-field depth is also lengthened if the crystal is made larger. The lateral resolution at shallow depths, however, is sacrificed as crystal diameter (which affects beam width) is increased.

Example 5-2

Calculate the near-field depth for transducer with a diameter of 15 mm. Assume a frequency of 5 MHz.

$$NFD = \frac{D^2 f}{4c}$$

$$NFD = \frac{(0.015 \text{ m})^2 (5 \times 10^6 \text{ 1/s})}{4(1540 \text{ m/s})}$$

$$NFD = 0.182 \text{ m} = 18.2 \text{ cm}$$

For a constant frequency of 5 MHz, the near-field depth is 8 cm. For a diameter of 10 mm, but is shortened to 2 cm if the diameter is decreased to 5 mm.

Far-Field Divergence

Beyond the near field is the region called the far field (Fraunhofer zone), where the ultrasound beam begins to diverge. The angle φ, a measure of the beam's divergence for a nonfocused transducer, is given as

$$5\text{-}2 \qquad \sin \varphi = \frac{1.22\lambda}{D} = \frac{1.22c}{Df}$$

Therefore,

$$5\text{-}3 \qquad \varphi = \arcsin\left(\frac{1.22\lambda}{D}\right) = \arcsin\left(\frac{1.22c}{Df}\right)$$

These formulas predict that as the frequency is increased (or wavelength is decreased), the angle of divergence becomes smaller. Also, as the diameter is increased, the beam diverges less rapidly.

Example 5-3

Calculate the angle of divergence (φ) for a transducer with a frequency of 4 MHz. Assume a diameter of 10 mm.

$$\varphi = \arcsin\left(\frac{1.22c}{Df}\right)$$

$$\varphi = \arcsin\left(\frac{(1.22)(1540 \text{ m/s})}{(0.01 \text{ m})(4 \times 10^6 \text{ 1/s})}\right)$$

$$\varphi = 2.7 \text{ degrees}$$

The lateral resolution deteriorates in the far-field region because of divergence of the beam. Therefore scanning areas of interest should be confined to the near field if possible. An exception to this practice may occur in scanning large patients.

Self-Focusing Effect

Before we leave this topic, the assumption that, in the near field, the beam width is equal to the diameter of the transducer crystal should be clarified. The nonfocused single-crystal transducer has a self-focusing effect, so that the beam width actually decreases to a minimal value at the transition point between the near field and the far field and then begins to diverge. In fact, the beam width at the transition point is equal to half the diameter of the crystal. The acoustic pressure actually increases at the transition point because the power is distributed over a smaller area. At a distance equal to twice the near-field depth, the beam's diameter diverges to a size equal to the crystal's diameter.

Thus the lateral resolution, based on beam width, is better than would normally be expected for nonfocused transducers. Typically, however, the beam's shape is altered by the presence of an attenuating medium; therefore, the beam's width is assumed to be equal to the crystal's diameter in the near field.

SIDE LOBES

Side lobes are secondary projections of ultrasonic energy that radiate away from the main ultrasound beam (Fig. 5-8). Output mode (continuous wave [CW] versus pulse wave [PW]), pulse shape, transducer design, and radial mode vibration all contribute to the formation of side lobes. *Radial mode vibration* (nonthickness mode) refers to the expansion and contraction of the circular disk along the radial direction. Side lobes are more prominent during CW operation, whereas PW output tends to suppress side lobes. The intensity of side lobes is normally 60 to 100 dB below that of the main ultrasound beam, which usually does not pose significant problems in imaging. If they are present at high intensity levels, however, side lobes create artifacts (presentation of off-axis structures) and degrade lateral resolution.

FOCUSING

Lateral resolution can be improved by focusing the transmitted beam. Focusing reduces the beam width compared with that dictated by crystal diameter alone. At the focal point, the beam width is most narrow. The focal length is the distance from the transducer face to the focal point. The intensity of an ultrasound beam at the focal point is expected to be greater than that for a nonfocused transducer of the same diameter because the cross-sectional area of the beam is less for the focused than for the nonfocused beam. The focal zone or axial extent of this narrow beam width is defined as the region where intensity has a value within 3 dB of the maximum. Alternatively, the focal zone is described as the region in which the beam width is less than twice the beam width at the focal point. The focal zone is closer to the face of the transducer than the nonfocused near-field depth provided the transducers are of equal diameter and frequency.

Focusing Methods

To improve the lateral resolution, a single-element transducer can be focused in two ways. Sound follows many of the same principles as light. It can be focused by an acoustic lens that works in a manner similar to a light lens. Acoustic lenses are formed from polystyrene, nylon, or aluminum and placed in front of the piezoelectric crystal (Fig. 5-9). The velocity of sound in the lens is greater than that in tissue; thus sound waves are bent toward a point in tissue (principle of refraction). The most common form of focusing for transducers uses a curved crystal (Fig. 5-10), which is an internal focusing method.

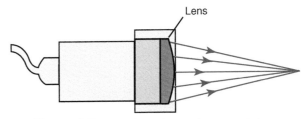

Figure 5-9 Focused transducer with an acoustic lens.

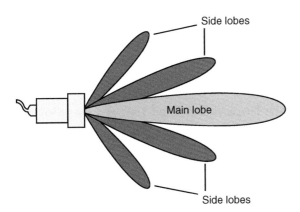

Figure 5-8 Side lobes. Sound energy radiates in multiple directions. The intensity of the side lobes is less than that of the main lobe.

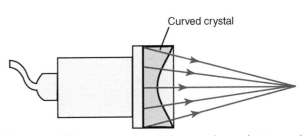

Figure 5-10 Focused transducer with a curved piezoelectric crystal.

Degree of Focusing

The degree of focusing can be changed to vary the focal length by increasing the radius of curvature of the crystal or by increasing the curvature of the acoustic lens. This allows transducers operating at the same frequency to be made with focal zones at different depths, depending on the degree of focusing (Fig. 5-11). As the degree of focusing becomes stronger, the beam width is made narrower, but the focal zone is drawn closer to the face of the transducer. The degree of focusing is expressed quantitatively as the ratio of unfocused near field depth to focal length.

A weak-focused (also called long-focused) transducer composed of a single element has a focal length of 7 to 19 cm; a medium-focused transducer has a focal length of 4 to 10 cm; and a strong-focused (short-focused) transducer has a focal length of 1 to 4 cm.

Beam Width

One of the major advantages of focusing is to reduce the beam width in the focal zone (Fig. 5-12). The beam width in the focal zone (w) is estimated by the aperture (2a), focal length (F), and wavelength (λ):

5-4
$$w = \frac{1.4\lambda F}{2a} = \frac{1.4 Fc}{2af}$$

For single-element transducers the aperture and crystal diameter are the same. However, this is not the case for other types of transducers, and aperture must be described independently of crystal dimensions, which is why notation as

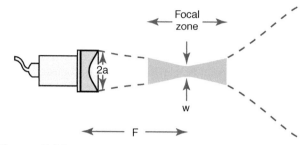

Figure 5-12 Parameters describing the ultrasonic field for a focused transducer. Aperture (2a), depth of field (focal zone), focal length (F), and beam width (w).

introduced here is distinct. As frequency and aperture size (the diameter of the crystal) are increased, beam width at a designated focal length is reduced.

Example 5-4

Calculate the beam width in the focal zone for a 1-cm diameter transducer operating at 3 MHz. The focal length is 4 cm.

$$w = \frac{1.4\lambda F}{2a}$$

$$w = \frac{1.4\,(0.51\ mm)(40\ mm)}{10\ mm}$$

$$w = 2.8\ mm$$

Depth of Field

The focal zone is the region within the ultrasonic field that provides the best lateral resolution. The length of the focal zone (or depth of field) is given by

5-5
$$\text{Depth of field} = \frac{7.1\lambda F^2}{4a^2}$$

Example 5-5

What is the depth of field for a transducer 1 cm in diameter operating at 3 MHz with a focal length of 4 cm?

$$\text{Depth of field} = \frac{7.1\lambda F^2}{4a^2}$$

$$\text{Depth of field} = \frac{7.1(0.051\ cm)(4\ cm)^2}{4(0.5\ cm)^2}$$

$$\text{Depth of field} = 5.8\ cm$$

Depth Dependence of Lateral Resolution

Lateral resolution is not constant throughout the scan range. Since the beam width changes with depth, accurate spatial representation of small objects varies with depth (Fig. 5-13). The ability to resolve adjacent structures will also depend on their location in the ultrasonic field. Factors affecting beam width and hence lateral resolution are summarized in Table 5-3.

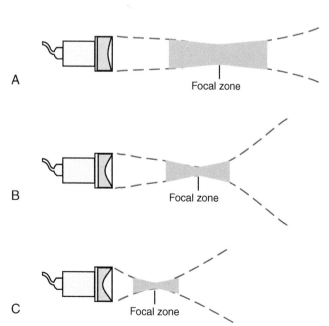

A

B

C

Focal zone

Figure 5-11 As the focusing is made stronger, the beam width decreases, the focal zone moves closer to the face of the transducer, and the intensity increases in the focal zone. **A,** Weak or long focusing. **B,** Medium focusing. **C,** Strong or short focusing.

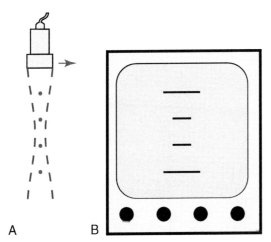

Figure 5-13 Depth dependence of beam width. **A,** Beam width changes with depth for a focused transducer. The small reflectors at different depths are not displayed with equal lateral extent **(B)**.

Table 5-3	Effects on Beam Width	
Parameter	**Change**	**Effect on Beam Width**
Frequency	Increase	Decrease
Aperture	Increase with focal length constant	Decrease
Aperture	Increase with ratio focal length to aperture constant	No change
Focusing	Increase degree of focusing	Decrease
Focal length	Decrease	Decrease

ECHO RECEPTION

Any discussion of basic ultrasonic instrumentation must include the A-mode scanner, which forms the foundation for other scanning modes. A-mode scanning is an echo-ranging technique in which an ultrasound beam is directed along a single path into the body. A transducer generates a pulsed ultrasound wave via the converse piezoelectric effect and directs that beam into the body. As the ultrasound wave strikes various interfaces in the body, some of the energy is transmitted and some is reflected, in accordance with the reflection formula. The echo returns to the transducer, and the pressure wave incident on the crystal is converted into an electrical signal and processed for display.

Detected echoes from interfaces along this path are displayed as a series of deflections from the baseline trace (Fig. 5-14). The position of the deflection along the horizontal axis denotes the depth of the interface; the height of the deflection denotes the strength of the echo. The A-mode scanner is used here as a model to demonstrate the fundamentals of echo reception and signal processing.

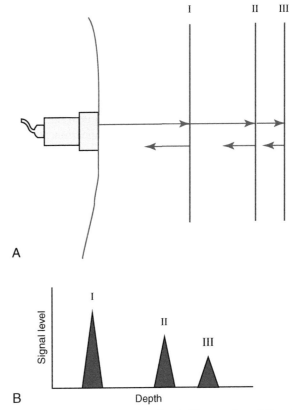

Figure 5-14 A-mode scan and display. **A,** Three interfaces (I, II, and III). **B,** Corresponding display of the interfaces.

Transmit Power

Most ultrasound units include an output or transmit power control that adjusts the excitation voltage to the crystal to regulate the intensity of the transmitted acoustic pulse (Fig. 5-15). Higher intensity results in a proportionally stronger echo from the reflector. The typical excitation voltage pulse is about 150 volts. Frequently, the control is adjustable in decibel increments or percentage of maximum power. Increased transmitted intensity enhances the detectability of weak reflectors. However, higher intensity levels increase patient exposure.

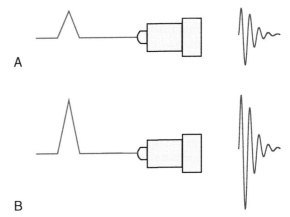

Figure 5-15 Excitation voltage regulates the transmitted beam intensity. **A,** Low voltage. **B,** High voltage.

Amplification

The echo, in the form of mechanical pressure waves, strikes the crystal and induces a radiofrequency signal via the piezo-electric effect. The waveform of the radiofrequency signal mimics the ultrasound waveform, since the voltage variations are in response to pressure-induced thickness changes in the crystal. A preamplifier located very near the piezoelectric crystal provides initial signal amplification, which enables signal transfer to the amplifier without significant degradation from spurious electronic noise. In the amplifier, the radiofrequency signal is further increased in voltage for processing. The amount of amplification is designated by the term *gain*, which equals the ratio of the output signal to the input signal. Combinations of linear, exponential, logarithmic, and variable amplifications can be used.

The most common type of receiver gain is logarithmic. The amount of gain is adjustable by the operator. Weak signals undergo greater amplification than do strong signals. The disparity in signal level between weak and strong reflectors is diminished. Logarithmic amplification reduces the dynamic range (ratio of highest signal to lowest signal) of the induced signals. Decreasing the dynamic range is called compression. Receiver gain adjusts only the amplification of the received signals and has no effect on the intensity of the transmitted ultrasound beam.

Time Gain Compensation

One problem that must be considered is the attenuation of an ultrasonic beam with depth. Equally reflective interfaces produce different signal levels, depending on their relative distances from the transducer. It is advantageous to display reflectors of similar size, shape, and reflection coefficients with equal signal strengths.

Time-dependent exponential amplification (called time gain compensation [TGC], depth gain compensation [DGC], swept gain control, depth-varied gain, distance-attenuation compensation, and sensitivity-time control) is applied to correct the signals for attenuation. This can easily be demonstrated: Assume that a phantom is composed of alternating layers of water and gelatin (Fig. 5-16, *A*) that are very similar in acoustic impedance. Each layer is the same thickness. A small fraction of the incident beam is reflected at each interface, and the percent of reflected intensity is constant for every interface in the phantom. Recall that the reflection formula does not distinguish which medium contains the incident beam.

Because of attenuation along the propagation path, however, the display shows exponentially decreasing signal strengths (Fig. 5-16, *B*) rather than signals of equal amplitude. To compensate for this attenuation, a TGC control is used to increase the amplitude of processed signals with time or depth (Fig. 5-16, *C*). The amplification is a reverse exponential function because the signals decrease exponentially (Fig. 5-17). The application of depth-varying gain also contributes to signal compression.

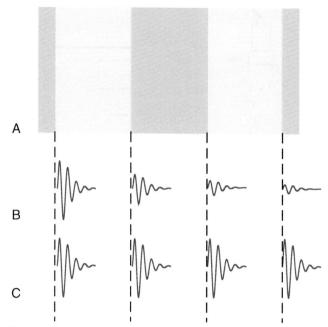

Figure 5-16 Effect of time gain compensation (TGC). **A,** Phantom composed of alternating layers of water *(blue)* and gelatin *(orange).* All interfaces have the same composition. **B,** Signal amplitude versus depth without TGC. **C,** Signal amplitude versus depth with TGC.

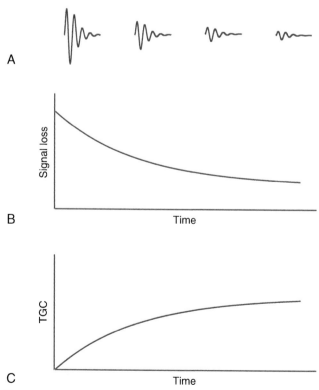

Figure 5-17 Time gain compensation (TGC). **A,** Signal amplitude versus depth without TGC. **B,** Exponential loss in signal caused by attenuation. **C,** Reverse exponential TGC variable gain to apply to the signals in **(A)**.

Time Gain Compensation Controls

Different tissues have varying rates of attenuation. The frequency response of the attenuation rate depends on the tissue type. This, along with the capability to enhance a particular area of interest, makes a variable TGC desirable. Some diagnostic ultrasound units have a combination of TGC controls. The near gain adjusts the level at which the initial signals are amplified. The delay regulates the depth at which the TGC begins. Often it is convenient not to amplify signals originating close to the transducer because they have high amplitude levels. The slope of the TGC indicates the amount of compensation that is applied with depth. The far gain represents the maximum amount that signals can be amplified. In this zone the signals are amplified by a constant amount, but they exhibit an exponential decrease because of attenuation.

Variable TGC controls are commonly configured in a slider knob arrangement in which each knob corresponds to a particular depth and movement of the knob left to right increases the applied gain at that depth. The association of each knob with depth depends on the scan range. Often, the variation of gain with depth is displayed on the monitor to provide feedback to the operator. This allows adjustment for smooth transition from one knob-controlled region to the next.

The variable TGC controls permit adjustable compensation for transducers of different frequencies, allowing greater amplification when high frequencies are used. Remember that attenuation in soft tissue is frequency-dependent. As the frequency is increased, more amplification is required to counteract the accelerated loss of beam intensity.

SIGNAL PROCESSING

The radiofrequency signal induced in the transducer by the incident echoes could be amplified and then displayed, but it would then appear similar to the transmitted acoustic pulse. If numerous interfaces are present, the interpretation of the received signals becomes confusing. For viewing ease, the goal is to process the signal before displaying it. The signal processing lowers the information content (smaller dynamic range) while it also facilitates the association of final output with physical structures.

The normal processing procedure involves rectification (converting the negative portion of the radiofrequency signal to positive) after the signal has been amplified and has undergone TGC (Fig. 5-18). Alternatively, the negative components can be eliminated rather than flipped to positive. The peaks of the radiofrequency waveform are "electronically" surrounded or enveloped, which is generally accomplished by passing the signal through a circuit with a slow time response. The overall outline of the waveform is retained, but the internal fast oscillations are lost (Fig. 5-19).

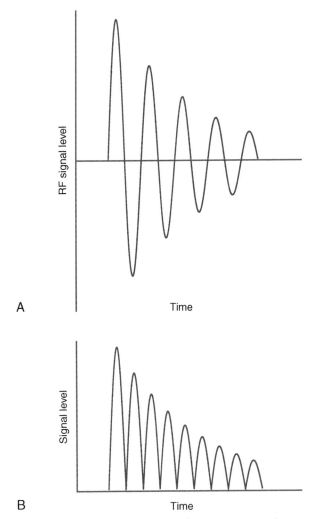

Figure 5-18 Rectification. **A,** The crystal response to an incident sound wave induces a radiofrequency signal in the receiver circuit. **B,** In the rectified signal, negative components are reversed to become positive.

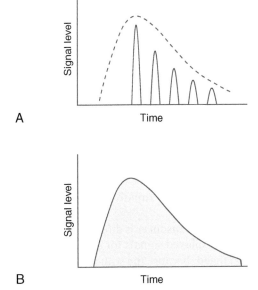

Figure 5-19 Enveloping. **A,** The induced radiofrequency signal that has been enveloped (i.e., an electronic surrounding of the peaks). **B,** The resultant enveloped signal.

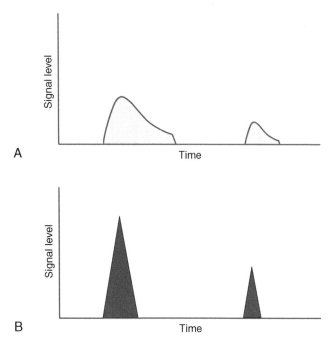

A

B

Figure 5-20 Integration. **A,** Two enveloped signals. **B,** The area under each enveloped signal, represented by the height above the baseline.

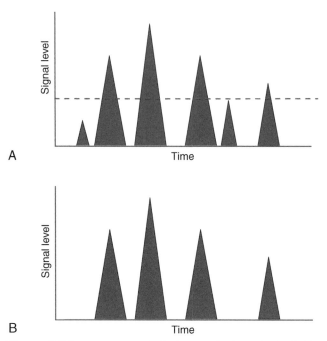

A

B

Figure 5-21 Rejection control. The four signals above the threshold in **(A)** *(dotted line)*, are processed and ultimately displayed in **(B)**. The others, below the threshold, are not.

The area under the enveloped signal is electronically measured. Determination of the area is called integration. This area is then represented by the height of the deflection from the baseline in A-mode scanning. An increase in the signal strength results in a larger area under the curve and therefore an increased height in displayed echo signal (Fig. 5-20).

A rejection control (also called threshold or suppression) eliminates low-level signals and noise below a certain level, as selected by the operator (Fig. 5-21). Rejection of signals decreases the dynamic range.

DISPLAY

For A-mode scanning, the relative signals for echoes received from different depths are displayed on a monitor in a two-dimensional format. A trace is swept horizontally across the screen at a constant rate that correlates with the speed of ultrasound in tissue. The trace, which must advance the equivalent of 1 cm on the distance scale for every 13 μs, is synchronized with the transmitted pulse. The signal detected for each interface deflects the trace in the vertical direction with the horizontal position determined by the elapsed time. Because the duration of the echo is short, the vertical deflection rapidly returns to the baseline (Fig. 5-22).

As long as the transducer is directed along the same line of sight, the displayed signals for stationary reflectors remain unchanged, because the scan is repeated many times each second. The sampling rate is equal to the pulse repetition frequency (200 to 2000 Hz). If the transducer is positioned toward a new line of sight, the displayed signals change in accordance with the interfaces encountered

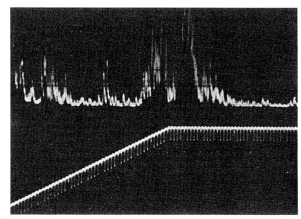

Figure 5-22 A-mode display of the liver *(top curve)* with the accompanying time gain compensation *(lower curve)*.

along this sampling direction. Once again, the scan is displayed at the rate of the pulse repetition frequency.

NOISE

If a reflector is probed repeatedly with a series of pulsed ultrasound waves, each wave creates an echo characteristic of the object. The returning echoes are detected by the transducer. Under these conditions, induced signals of equal strength are expected. In practice, however, the signal amplitude is not constant but fluctuates from one measurement to the next. This variation is known as noise.

Noise is inherent in the measurement process and cannot be eliminated. System electronics, environmental radiofrequency interference, and power line voltage fluctuations

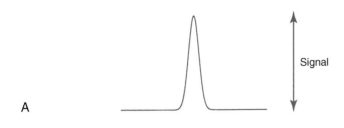

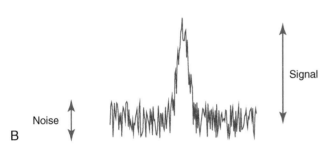

Figure 5-23 Effect of noise on the signal. **A,** Ideal signal (no noise). **B,** Noise masking the true signal.

High signal-to-noise ratios indicate strong signals, which are easily detected. A minimal signal-to-noise ratio of 3 to 5 is necessary to distinguish weak echoes from the noise. Since noise is random, signal processing cannot isolate the signal from the noise; that is, mathematical corrections applied to the detected signal to eliminate the noise are not possible. When multiple samplings of an interface are averaged together, however, the signal-to-noise ratio is increased.

SUMMARY

A piezoelectric material is electronically stimulated to produce an ultrasonic pressure wave via the converse piezoelectric effect. The transmitted pulsed wave enters the patient's body, and a portion of the incident intensity is reflected at the various interfaces encountered along the propagation path. Returning echoes strike the transducer and, because of the piezoelectric effect, induce an oscillating voltage (radiofrequency signal). The echo-induced signals undergo both amplification and TGC. The latter compensates for attenuation of the echo according to the depth of origin. The A-Mode display format of the electronically amplified and processed signals consists of signal strength in the vertical direction versus depth in the horizontal direction. A time-synchronized excitation voltage pulse to the transducer activates the timed adjustment of TGC and the time base sweep for display. A-mode sampling is repeated at 200 to 2000 Hz, and thus the pattern of deflections appears stationary to the human eye.

contribute to noise. Signals must be processed and displayed in the presence of noise (Fig. 5-23). As weaker and weaker signals approach the noise level, they become more difficult to identify. The relative amplitude of the signal compared with the noise variation is delineated by the signal-to-noise ratio.

Static Imaging Principles and Instrumentation

6

Chapter Objectives

To identify the components of a static B-mode scanner
To understand image formation in static B-mode

Key terms

Line of sight
Position generator

Registration arm
Static B-mode

OVERVIEW

Modifications are required to convert the A-mode unit into an imaging device. The two-dimensional spatial mapping of echo-induced signals was first accomplished with a static B-mode scanner. A-mode instrumentation is discussed briefly, because the basic unit was described in Chapter 5. A-mode scanning and static B-mode imaging have a very limited role in current clinical practice and have been almost totally replaced by real-time (B-mode), Doppler, and M-mode devices. Nevertheless, the principles of static imaging are essential for understanding sonography instrumentation. Multiple examples using static instrumentation illustrate basic imaging concepts and are relevant to advanced applications.

A-MODE SCANNING

The main system components are illustrated in Figure 6-1. All these subsystems are synchronized with respect to time. The block diagram shows a transducer connected to the transmitter-receiver section of the scanner. A pulsed ultrasound wave is directed into the patient's body, and the echoes generated at various interfaces along the beam path are detected. Only structures that lie along the direction of propagation within the ultrasound beam are interrogated. This sampling according to the beam path is called the line of sight or scan line. The sampling is restricted laterally by the width of the beam. The transducer, acting as a receiver rather than a transmitter, converts the ultrasound wave (returning echo) to an electronic signal that is processed and displayed. The displayed signal is related to interactions that have taken place in the body.

Coincidentally with the excitation of the crystal, the clock measures the elapsed time from transmission of the ultrasound pulse to reception of the echo. This time determines the depth of the interface based on the constant velocity of ultrasound in tissue (1540 m/s). The initialization of the display baseline sweep is also synchronized with beam transmission. The sweep rate corresponds to 1 cm every 13 microseconds.

Any special amplification based on elapsed time, such as time gain compensation (TGC), also requires knowledge of the exact time of travel for the pulse. The height of the deflection indicates the strength of the received echo; the horizontal position

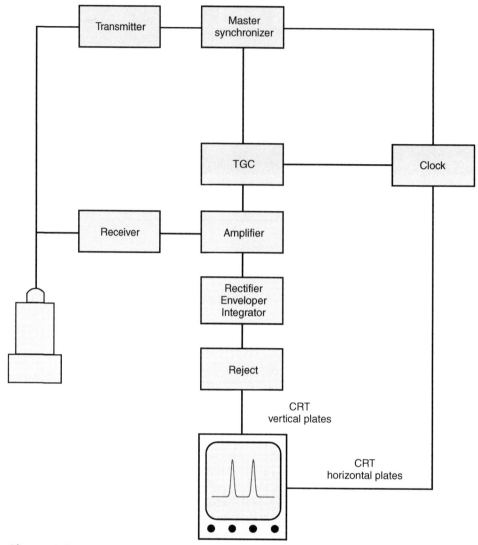

Figure 6-1 Block diagram of the A-mode scanner. The signal processing steps of time gain compensation (TGC), amplification, integration, and rejection occur before display. The output trace is controlled by elapsed time in the horizontal direction and signal level in the vertical direction.

along the trace denotes the depth of the interface. Multiple interfaces encountered along the sampling direction are detected by a series of echoes.

Variation in signal level is caused by reflectivity of the interface and the attenuation of the beam as the ultrasound wave travels to and from the various interfaces. TGC attempts to correct for attenuation loss. Without TGC, strong reflectors far from the transducer may produce signals of lower amplitude than weak reflectors near the transducer. The A-mode scan also contains spatial information; that is, it registers the distance between interfaces.

A narrow beam samples the structures along the line of sight. *Only one line can be observed at any given instant on the display.* As long as the transducer and detected interfaces are stationary, the trace appears unchanged, because the monitor is refreshed at the rate of the pulse repetition frequency (PRF). For a different line of sight to be observed, the transducer must be moved to a different position.

ILLUSTRATIVE A-MODE SCANS

A-mode scans illustrate the concepts of TGC, receiver gain, rejection, axial resolution, focusing, and lateral resolution.

Without TGC, identical reflectors at different depths have exponentially decreasing signal levels as the beam path is increased. TGC provides variable amplification based on elapsed time to correct for the effect of attenuation loss on the echo signal; thus the displayed signal level for each reflector is the same regardless of the depth of the reflector (Fig. 6-2).

Receiver gain is applied equally to all echo-induced signals so that each signal is increased in magnitude by the same factor (Fig. 6-3). This generally enhances the presentation of weak signals. The rejection control eliminates weak signals with amplitudes less than the threshold value.

When the interfaces are located close together along the direction of propagation, the displayed signals overlap

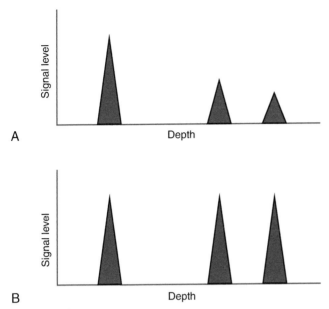

Figure 6-2 Signals from identical reflectors located at different depths. **A,** No time gain compensation (TGC). **B,** TGC applied during signal processing.

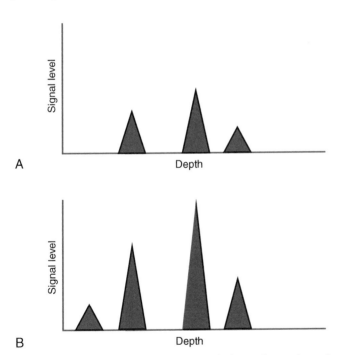

Figure 6-3 Receiver gain. **A,** Signal levels from reflectors located at different depths. **B,** Application of a factor of 2 in receiver gain. Additional weak signal is displayed.

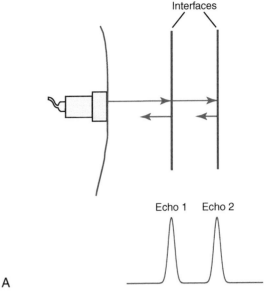

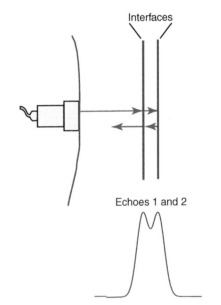

Figure 6-4 Axial resolution in A-mode scanning. **A,** Interfaces separated by a distance greater than half the spatial pulse length are depicted as two distinct deflections. **B,** When interfaces are located close together, the returning echoes strike the transducer at nearly the same time. The signals overlap and are combined into a single deflection.

(Fig. 6-4). The two echoes appear as a single vertical deflection, which is consequently interpreted as a single interface. Echoes are more likely to be resolved if the spatial pulse length is kept short (high frequency and few cycles).

An echo is generated for each object within the ultrasonic field. If multiple reflectors are present at a certain depth, multiple echoes are formed. However, echo ranging places the echo-induced signals at the same point on the time axis, and the signals are superimposed on the time axis (Fig. 6-5). By focusing the beam to reduce its width at a certain depth, only one small object in the focal zone is interrogated (Fig. 6-6).

STATIC B-MODE SCANNING

In static B-mode imaging the amplitude of the signal (detected echo strength) is represented by the brightness of a dot. The position of the dot represents the depth (time) of the reflector from the transducer (Fig. 6-7). The information contained in the two-dimensional A-mode display (signal level and depth) has been condensed to one dimension

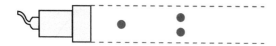

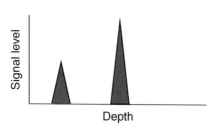

Figure 6-5 Effect of beam width. The presence of two reflectors at the same depth does not yield two separate signals but rather an increase in signal level corresponding to that depth.

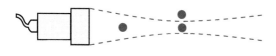

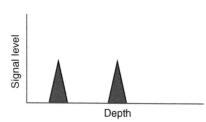

Figure 6-6 Focusing the beam allows the reflector within the focal zone to be the primary contributor to the observed signal.

B-mode signal levels

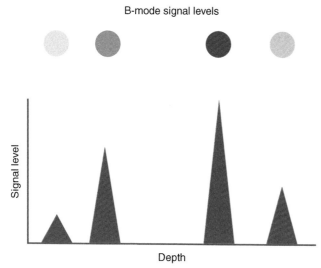

Figure 6-7 Comparison of B-mode and A-mode displays. The A-mode display shows four interfaces encountered along the line of sight, which, represented by different shades of blue, are converted to dots of varying brightness in the B-mode display.

in the B-mode display, but the relative signal level and spatial relationship of the interfaces have been maintained.

Static B-scanning, whereby multiple scan lines are combined to delineate the echo pattern from internal structures within the body, forms a two-dimensional image of the area of interest. The transducer is moved across the patient so that the patient is scanned from many different directions. A single line of sight through the patient is acquired at each position of the transducer when the pulser is activated (Fig. 6-8). The scan line is composed of a series of bright dots representing the interfaces encountered along that line of sight. The superimposition of multiple scan lines creates a composite two-dimensional image, which has the advantage of portraying the general contour of the patient and the internal organs (Fig. 6-9). Compound static B-mode scanning produces a single image that can be envisioned as a stop-action photograph of the echo-generating structures.

Scanning Requirements

Two technical requirements with B-mode scanning not present with A-mode are registration (i.e., the two-dimensional placement of an echo's origin) and storage of the scan-line information. Knowledge of transducer position is essential to the proper registration of echo-induced signals from different scan lines at the correct locations within the image. To form the final image,

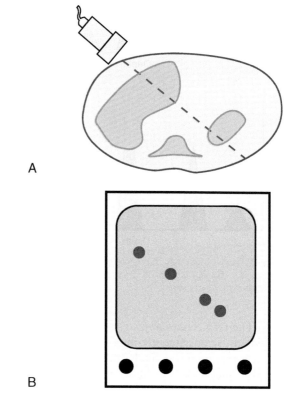

Figure 6-8 Single scan line in B-mode. **A,** The transducer position and orientation define the line of sight sampled. **B,** In B-mode, the interfaces are represented as red dots along the line of sight. On the actual gray-level monitor for image display, the brightness of each dot is varied to represent the strength of the echo originating at that location.

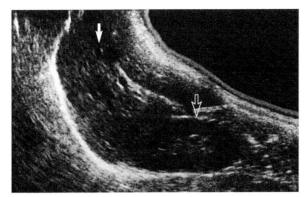

Figure 6-9 Gray-scale image of a kidney *(open arrow)* and the liver *(solid arrow)*.

information from previous scan lines must be retained in some manner.

For the accurate localization of an interface (i.e., the origin of its echo), the horizontal and vertical position of the transducer as well as its angulation must be known. Thus the transducer is mounted on a special scanning or registration arm that indicates its precise location so the time-of-flight (depth) measurements along the beam axis can be accurately recorded. Because the transducer changes its orientation frequently during scanning, this arm must be flexible; however, at the same time, it must be stable to accurately correlate collected information within the image.

Sensors mounted in the registration arm define the position of the transducer with respect to a reference point established at the time of scanning. This information is communicated to the position generator, which calculates the appropriate spatial coordinates as a function of elapsed time.

The registration arm is responsible for ensuring that the echo information from a particular interface is displayed at the same location, regardless of transducer orientation; that is, the interface should be in exactly the same location on the display when the subject is viewed from many different directions. False placement of interface position can cause the image to become blurred and distorted.

The second requirement with static B-mode scanning involves storing the signal levels at the appropriate locations for display. By moving the transducer in A-mode scanning to sample a different line of sight, the trace on the monitor is changed. The information obtained from the previous transducer position is not retained on the screen. To maintain the trace, the transducer must be kept in the same position—pointed along a single line of sight. The display is continually updated with the same information (i.e., the scan is repeated over and over at the rate of the PRF). If a scan were acquired all the way around a patient, as is the case for static B-mode scanning, the initial traces would disappear from the screen before the total scan was completed. (Five to 10 seconds are required to perform a B-mode scan.) Indeed, as soon as the ultrasound beam is directed along a new line of sight, the prior trace is lost. In addition to the scanning arm modifications already discussed, a modification for signal storage is necessary.

Analog Scan Converter

A-mode scan information is limited to depth and signal level only. Static B-mode, however, has three variables: two-dimensional spatial location within the scan plane and the signal level.

Initially, storage cathode ray tubes (CRTs) were used to display static B-mode images. These CRTs exhibit only an "on" or "off" mode. If the detected signal is strong enough, it is displayed as a light-emitting area on the phosphorescent screen. Otherwise, weak signals are read as no signals, and no light is emitted from the corresponding areas on the screen. This produces the so-called bistable image (Fig. 6-10). Most of the internal detail of organs is absent, however. Because the nonspecular reflections lost in a bistable image (i.e., when the amplitude is too low to be recorded) are desirable for sonography, new storage/display technology was developed in the 1970s to show the finer detail of internal structures. Called analog scan converters, these devices enabled different echo amplitudes (i.e., detected signal strengths) to be displayed in varying shades of gray so that the fine internal structure of various organs could be visualized. These converters represented a major innovation in the evolution of ultrasound.

Rapid alternation between the read (display) mode and the write (collect) mode enables the image to be viewed as it is being formed; that is, the scan converter switches back and forth from line-by-line acquisition during collection to raster-by-raster scanning during display. This characteristic is responsible for the name of the device—the scan converter. Once the data are collected, the image can be viewed by operating the device in a continuous read mode.

Digital Scan Converter

As already noted, digital scan converters were developed during the 1970s. These devices are essentially solid-state computer memories that are inexpensive, reliable, and versatile. Because they do not use evacuated tubes, the instability and drift associated with the analog systems is

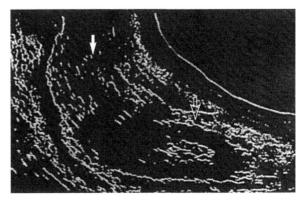

Figure 6-10 Bistable image of a kidney *(open arrow)* and the liver *(solid arrow)*. Note the loss of contrast in this image compared with the image shown in Figure 6-9.

eliminated. Prolonged viewing of acquired image data is now possible, and day-to-day variations are reduced. The spatial detail and contrast resolution obtained with a digital scan converter are superior to the fuzzy images provided by analog systems. Spatial resolution is now determined primarily by the spatial pulse length and ultrasound beam width.

The area scanned is divided into small rectangular or square picture elements called pixels, which make up a two-dimensional matrix. Each pixel contains a digital number representing the amplitude of the received echo. The placement of echo amplitudes within the matrix is designated by the position generator. The out-of-plane width of the sound beam means that each pixel actually signifies a three-dimensional volume of tissue, called a voxel. The output of the computer memory (digital scan converter) is read in a raster fashion and converted back into an analog signal, which provides the input to the display monitor.

Signal Processing

Another feature of the digital scan converter is the overwrite-protect circuit. Each interface is scanned from multiple directions during an acquisition. A variety of signal levels are detected for each pixel depending on the transducer orientation. When a signal is received, the appropriate location in the scan converter is identified via sensors in the registration arm and the position generator. The scan converter would replace the value that already exists in memory with the new signal amplitude if the overwrite-protect system were not present. Overwrite-protect processing permits the maximum-strength signal to be displayed for a particular location while rejecting other low-amplitude signals that may be received for that same location.

The overwrite-protect circuit works in the following manner: When the interface is scanned initially, the associated signal level is stored in the scan converter. As the scan continues, the approach to the interface may be closer to normal incidence for subsequent scan lines, resulting in a stronger detected signal. This signal level replaces the first value in the scan converter for that pixel. At another scan line the interface may yield a lower signal level, which is discarded, because a higher value has previously been recorded for that location. Thus an image is generated in which the maximum signal level is recorded for each pixel throughout the image.

SUMMARY

Static imaging techniques, particularly the use of B-mode gray-scale scanners, were the mainstay of ultrasound departments through the mid-1970s. The development of scan converters greatly hastened the acceptance of diagnostic ultrasound in the medical community. B-mode scanners have provided the foundation for extensive applications of ultrasound as a noninvasive diagnostic tool. The most important clinical features of static B-mode imaging are summarized in Box 6-1. Although real-time imaging with superior temporal resolution has a limited field of view and lower signal-to-noise ratio, this modality has now replaced static B-mode scanners. However, many of the same principles of operation still apply.

Box 6-1	**Important Clinical Features of Static B-mode Imaging**
Large field of view Multiangle sampling (high signal-to-noise ratio) Long acquisition time Motion artifacts Restricted transducer movement Single-depth focusing	

Image Formation in Real-Time Imaging

Chapter Objectives

To understand image formation in real-time B-mode scanning
To recognize the advantages and limitations of B-mode imaging

Key terms

Analog-to-digital
  conversion
Field of view
Frame rate

Line-of-sight sampling
Matrix size
Scan converter
Scan-line sampling

Scan line density
Scan range

FEATURES OF IMAGE FORMATION

In real-time B-mode scanning, the displayed image is continuously and rapidly updated with new echo data as a narrow, pulsed beam is repeatedly directed throughout the field of view. Field of view is the physical region interrogated by ultrasound scanning from which the detected echoes are recorded in the two-dimensional image. The depth of the field of view is the scan range and is in the direction of propagation. The width of the field of view is the lateral extent over which the beam is directed and is generally perpendicular to the central line of sight. Various brightness levels or shades of gray depict the relative reflectivities of structures. The display rate of updated information is commonly 15 or more images each second. The transducer can be moved to any scan plane without any restriction in movement. Instant feedback with respect to anatomic structures included within the field of view facilitates sonographic procedures. The major disadvantage of B-mode imaging is that the limited field of view makes anatomic identification more difficult and/or excludes nearby structures from the image.

PRINCIPLES OF REAL-TIME IMAGING

Real-time B-mode imaging depicts the reflectivity of structures within the field of view and continually updates this information for display by repeating the data acquisition process. A succession of two-dimensional images is formed rapidly to give the perception of motion if structures are moving within the sampled region. It can be compared with other dynamic modalities (motion-picture films) in which a series of stop-action shots are taken and then viewed rapidly one after another to depict motion. Or, if the transducer is being moved, the succession of two-dimensional images shows the anatomy portrayed by the changing scan plane.

   Data collection for each frame is a combination of echo ranging and directional beam scanning. The time delay between the transmitted pulse and the received echo determines the distance of the reflector from the transducer. This distance is measured along the beam axis (direction of propagation). A series of echoes following the

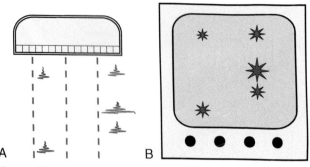

Figure 7-1 Image formation in real-time ultrasound. **A,** Echo-ranging data measured with three scan lines acquired sequentially allows spatial mapping of detected echoes. The origin and amplitude of each echo along the respective beam paths (dashed lines) are shown. **B,** Image display on monitor. The brightness of the dot represents the strength of the detected echo.

transmitted pulse allows placement of multiple interfaces encountered by the beam along that path. Only structures that lie along the direction of propagation within the beam are interrogated. This linear sampling according to the beam path is called line-of-sight or scan-line sampling. An image is composed of multiple scan lines by acquiring echo-ranging data along different straight-line paths by scanning the beam (Fig. 7-1). Displayed brightness for a reflector is controlled by the intensity of the detected echo.

A pulsed-wave narrow beam is first directed along a straight-line path; after the echoes are received, the ultrasound beam is then moved to a new sampling direction. Beam orientation is controlled by mechanical or electronic means in a repetitive, automated fashion without intervention by the sonographer. A single image is formed by sweeping pulsed sound beams along multiple sampling directions throughout the field of view. Every scan line requires one pulse of ultrasound waves to probe interfaces along its path. This process is repeated to produce successive images of the region.

As motion becomes more rapid within the field of view, a faster frame rate is necessary to display the structures without jerkiness (abrupt transitions from one location to another, or blurring). The time for the pulse to travel to the depth of interest and back to the transducer—along with the need for good spatial resolution provided by a large number of lines of sight in each image—imposes a restriction on the frame rate. Commonly 120 to 150 scan lines compose noncardiac images at rates of 15 to 30 frame per second.

SCAN CONVERTER

Multiple lines of sight are the building blocks of each image. As discussed further on, each line of sight represents a particular position of the crystal or activation of a group of crystals in the transducer array, which is established by the scanning mechanism. The ultrasound beam is directed into the patient in a well-defined pattern. Hence, no external reference is necessary to determine the position of the

line of sight. A digital scan converter assembles the echo-induced signals from each scan line and then deciphers this information during readout into the two-dimensional image format for display. The digital representation of signal levels allows image processing to aid interpretation.

ANALOG-TO-DIGITAL CONVERSION

The information content of the echo wavetrain must be changed to a digital format for the write/read functions of the scan converter. Some accuracy is sacrificed when a signal is digitized, as occurs in the translation of information from the detection system (signal amplitude and spatial location of the reflector) to a form that is understood by the computer. The translation process is called analog-to-digital conversion and is limited by the number of bits available in the digitization process. The analog signal is a continuously variable entity, whereas the digital signal is expressed in discrete steps.

Height Conversion

Imagine that there are two ways (via a staircase or ramp) of ascending to the second floor from the first floor in a building. By using the stairs, a description of your position (height above the first floor) consists of the number of the step you are standing on multiplied by the height of a single step. You are constrained to standing on one of the steps; a position between steps is not possible. If you stand on step number 2 and each step is 2 feet high, your location is designated as 4 feet above the first floor. At step number 3, you move to a height 6 feet above the first floor. The description is limited to discrete intervals of distance established by the size of the step (in this case increments of 2 feet). However, by taking the ramp, you would reach any height above the first floor.

If we replace each step in the staircase with two smaller steps, we can now describe the height as increments of 1 foot. In Figure 7-2, a height 5.75 feet above the first floor can be represented precisely by the ramp, but it would be approximated by step number 2 in staircase A (at a height of 4 feet) or by step number 5 in staircase B (at a height of 5 feet). An error is introduced in the quantitative description of the variable (in this case position), because discrete values are used. If we divide the discrete values into smaller and smaller steps, however, the accuracy of the conversion process is improved. In general, staircase B provides a more accurate assessment of position than does staircase A, because many more steps are used in the conversion process. The same effect is achieved by employing more bits in the digitization of analog signals.

In medical imaging, the analog signal is a voltage waveform generated by the detector. Increased signal strength is represented by an increased value of the voltage. The transformation of this analog signal to a digital format is limited to discrete steps, the size of each step being dictated by the bit depth of the analog-to-digital converter

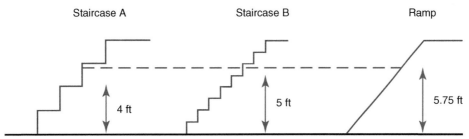

Figure 7-2 Comparison of analog and digital representations. The 5.75-foot height above the floor *(dotted line)* can be represented exactly by the ramp but is only approximated by the staircases. Staircase A (with large steps) is less accurate in its representation than staircase B. The fifth step in staircase B is closer to the actual height than the second step of staircase A.

Ultimately, the bit depth in the imaging chain affects both contrast and dynamic range.

Serial Sampling

In the previous examples, one digital value was assigned to the analog signal. Other applications may require that the time dependence of the analog signal be preserved. The analog signal is repeatedly sampled during the time interval, and the instantaneous value at each sampled point is digitized. Figure 7-3 illustrates the digitization of a voltage waveform varying in time. Once more, the analog-to-digital conversion process yields discrete steps (in this case with respect both to voltage and to time).

SPATIAL REPRESENTATION

The information obtained from a scanned area is divided into small square picture elements called pixels, which are combined to form the image. Each pixel corresponds to a particular region, designated by spatial coordinates, and is associated with the signal strength from that region. The amplitude of the received signal is converted to a digital number (ones and zeros) by the analog-to-digital converter before placement in scan converter. The number of pixels available depends on the matrix size, which denotes the number of rows and columns in the pictorial representation. For example, a 512 × 512 matrix has 512 rows and 512 columns. The image is composed of a total of 262,144 individual pixels (the number of rows multiplied by the number of columns).

For the digitized representation of the echo signal to be placed at the correct location in the image matrix, the spatial coordinates (row and column) must be specified. This is accomplished by a position generator, which uses the time of travel for the ultrasound pulse and element position (mechanical scanners) or element selection/phasing (multiple-element arrays) for beam direction. The signal amplitude and position coordinates for multiple lines of sight are temporarily placed in the buffer before they are written to the scan converter. The format is changed from signal levels along successive lines of sight to the matrix notation, which represents a composite of all scan data. Figure 7-4 shows two successive line-of-sight samplings of a scanned region. Three reflecting structures of varying amplitude are detected. The contents of the buffer corresponding to the two lines of sight are listed in Table 7-1, where the signal level is recorded as a function of the Cartesian spatial coordinates. Alternatively, the beam angle and elapsed time could be placed in the buffer to indicate position (with the spatial coordinates calculated from these two parameters).

The signal amplitudes are assigned to the appropriate pixels in an 8 × 8 matrix (Fig. 7-5). The spatial coordinates dictate the location within the matrix and the signal level dictates the numerical value of the pixel. In this

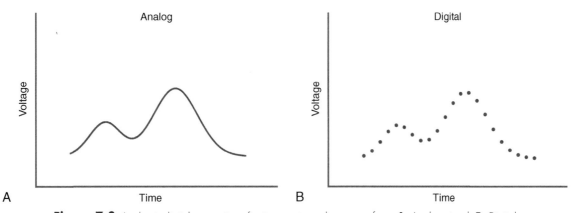

Figure 7-3 Analog-to-digital conversion of a time-varying voltage waveform. **A,** Analog signal. **B,** Digital signal.

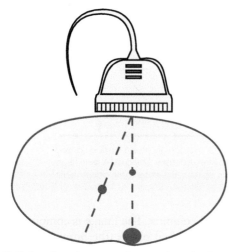

Figure 7-4 Sampling of a patient along two lines of sight. Note that the two interfaces are detected along the central line of sight. The size of the red dot is directly proportional to the intensity of the reflected echo.

Table 7-1	Contents of the Buffer for Successive Scan Lines	
Signal Amplitude	**X Position**	**Y Position**
000	5	1
000	5	2
000	5	3
000	5	4
001	5	5
000	5	6
000	5	7
111	5	8
000	5	1
000	5	2
000	4	2
000	4	3
000	3	4
010	3	5
000	2	6
000	2	7
000	1	8

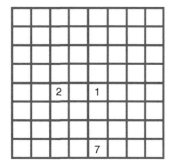

Figure 7-5 An 8 × 8 matrix depicting the three structures observed in Figure 7-4. Note that the pixels corresponding to the various interfaces are assigned different values based on the intensity of the reflected echoes.

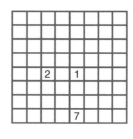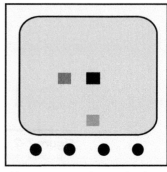

Figure 7-6 Image matrix in digital format is converted to gray levels pixel by pixel for display.

example the pixel locations corresponding to the various interfaces are assigned different values based on the intensity of the reflected echoes.

On display, each pixel is depicted as a uniform shade of gray based on the pixel value and a lookup table that translates pixel value to brightness (gray-scale map). The distribution of different shades of gray for all pixels composes the image (Fig. 7-6). Each pixel has a single shade because only one value is stored in the scan converter for that pixel. The same value is assumed to exist throughout the spatial extent represented by the pixel. This assumption is most appropriate for pixels with small physical dimensions. Once more, some accuracy is sacrificed by the digital representation of spatial location. As the matrix size increases, the system has the potential of presenting more spatial detail, which is demonstrated by the digitized picture of Abraham Lincoln in varying matrix sizes (Fig. 7-7). Currently, matrix size for B-mode imaging is 350 × 750, 480 × 640, 600 × 800, or 720 × 960, depending on manufacturer and model. At a viewing distance of 18 inches, the individual pixel elements are not distinguished and the image appears spatially continuous.

IMAGE DISPLAY

Solid-state flat panels such as liquid crystal displays have become the preferred display monitors for most applications. The screen is divided into pixels, similar to the scan converter matrix that holds image information. The light level or color for each screen pixel is individually controlled. Computer monitors do not comply with the information rate transfer restrictions imposed by television broadcast standards. This enables an increased number of pixels in both dimensions and higher frame rates than are available when a commercial TV video signal is used.

The video interface converts the digital image to an analog format for video transmission. Each pixel in a row of the image matrix is read sequentially left to right to form one raster line. After the readout for one row is completed, the pixels in the next row are read sequentially to form another raster line. This row-by-row readout sequence continues, such that a raster line is formed for each row in the image matrix. Data obtained for a raster line in the image

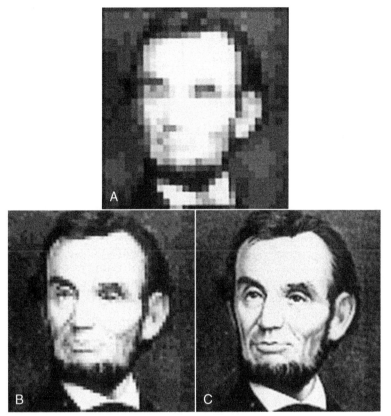

Figure 7-7 Matrix representation of a portrait of Abraham Lincoln. **A,** 32 × 32 matrix; **B,** 64 × 64; **C,** 128 × 128.

matrix are shown as one raster line across the screen. The brightness of light on the screen is dictated by the level of the input signal (stored pixel value) and the position is governed by the raster scanning sequence. Because raster scanning of the image matrix and raster scanning of the screen are synchronized, the signal level in the image matrix—and therefore the echo measurements—is converted into a visual image. The refresh rate for computer monitors is 60 to 120 times per second.

TIME CONSIDERATIONS

For each line of sight, one pulse of ultrasound waves is transmitted to detect interfaces located along the beam path. A finite amount of time is necessary for the ultrasound wave to move away from the transducer, probe the region of interest, and return as an echo to the transducer (13 microseconds for every centimeter of tissue). Every scan line requires a similar sequence of events. Extension of the scan range requires increased measurement time to acquire the echo-ranging data for each scan line (Fig. 7-8).

The following analogy illustrates the concept of image formation in real-time ultrasound. A company wants to determine the effectiveness of advertising in attracting customers to its stores. Imagine that three stores are each located one block away from a central starting point in the directions of north, east, and west. A sonography student,

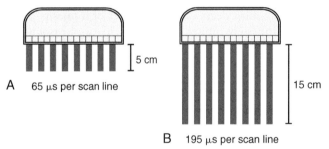

Figure 7-8 Time to acquire a scan line depends on scan range. **A,** a 5-cm scan range. **B,** a 15-cm scan range.

who is also an employee of the company, is assigned to monitor the number of customers in each store and then report these findings. The student walks east to the first store, counts the customers, and returns to the starting point, where the information is recorded. Other stores are evaluated sequentially in the same manner. However, customer number is accurate only for the time at which the observation occurred. Customers will enter and leave a store. To obtain the current status, the student would have to return to each store repeatedly.

In this analogy the number of customers indicates the reflectivity of the interface, and the directions east, north, and west represent different beam paths (a total of three scan lines). Obviously customer data are not obtained instantaneously; travel time to and from each store limits the rate at which the information can be collected.

By constraining the sonography student to walk at a constant velocity along the straight-line paths, the time required to obtain customer data from all stores is well defined. Similarly, the acoustic velocity of ultrasound in soft tissue is constant and imposes a restriction on the frequency of sampling. The scan range is set at one block. However, if the stores were located farther away, the sonography student would have to travel a longer distance and the information updates would be less frequent. As scan range is increased, more time must be allotted to accumulate data for a scan line. Compare the total time to collect an image consisting of eight scan lines for the different scan ranges shown in Figure 7-8. The total times for scan ranges of 5 and 15 cm are 520 and 1560 microseconds respectively.

Frame-Rate Limitations

Since a finite amount of time is necessary to form one image, the number of images that can be acquired and displayed each second (frame rate) is limited. The maximum frame rate (FR_{max}) is given by the 10th essential equation of sonography:

7-1 $$FR_{max} = \frac{c}{2Rn}$$

where c is the velocity of ultrasound in the medium, R the scan range, and n the number of lines of sight per frame (lpf). Equation 7-1 indicates that, if the scanning depth and/or number of lines of sight is increased, the maximum frame rate must decrease. The number of frames per second is ultimately limited by the velocity of ultrasound in tissue (1540 m/s).

For instance, assume that the field of view extends to a depth of 10 cm. The data collection time for each line of sight is 130 µs. If 100 lines of sight compose each image, the maximum frame rate becomes 77 fps. Extension of the depth of interest results in a reduced maximum frame rate. If 100 lines of sight are to be maintained for a change in scan range from 10 to 20 cm, the maximum frame rate is decreased to 38 fps.

Example 7-1

What is the maximum frame rate (FR_{max}) if the scan range is 15 cm and 150 lines compose each frame?

$$FR_{max} = \frac{c}{2\,Rn}$$

$$FR_{max} = \frac{1540\ m/s}{2(0.15\ m)(150\ lpf)}$$

$$FR_{max} = 34\ fps$$

To achieve a faster maximum frame rate, the scan range and/or number of lines of sight must be reduced. Table 7-2 demonstrates the relation between number of lines of sight, depth of scanning, and maximum frame rate. The time required for data collection for each frame equals the reciprocal of the maximum frame rate.

| Table 7-2 | Maximum Frame Rate versus Depth and the Number of Lines of Sight |

Depth (cm)	Maximum Frame Rate			
	25 LS	**50 LS**	**100 LS**	**200 LS**
5	616	308	154	77
10	308	154	77	38
15	205	103	51	26
20	154	77	38	19
25	123	61	30	15
30	103	51	25	12

LS, lines of sight.

The number of scan lines per frame and PRF determine the actual frame rate (FR), which is often less than the maximum frame rate.

7-2 $$FR = \frac{PRF}{n}$$

B-mode scanners usually operate at PRFs between 2000 and 5000 Hz, but this figure can be as high as 12,000 Hz to preserve lateral resolution while maintaining a high frame rate. Some sacrifice in scanning depth may be required at higher PRFs. The manufacturer sets the frame rate, scan range, scan width, and number of lines of sight based on the clinical application. These default values are likely to produce reasonable image quality for the average patient. Several approaches are possible to compensate for an increase in scanning depth. The real-time unit may automatically decrease the frame rate but maintain the same number of lines. On the other hand, both frame rate and number of lines may be adjusted downward. The number of lines may be reduced without a loss in resolution by narrowing the field of view. Often, several transducers with different center frequencies are available for use with a single ultrasound unit. Each frequency is optimized with respect to the number of lines of sight and frame rate as a function of sampling depth according to the clinical application.

BEAM WIDTH

The design criteria for an imaging transducer include directional beam transmission with a narrow beam width. These characteristics are desirable because small objects can be probed individually and distinguished as separate entities.

A single object smaller than the beam width produces an echo when it is intercepted by the transmitted pulsed wave. An echo is created regardless of the lateral position of the object in the ultrasonic field (Fig. 7-9). The lateral dimension of the object in the image is defined as the same size as the beam width. Multiple small objects displaced laterally but equidistant from the transducer are not resolved when encompassed by the beam (Fig. 7-10). Remember, axial displacement of objects can be detected

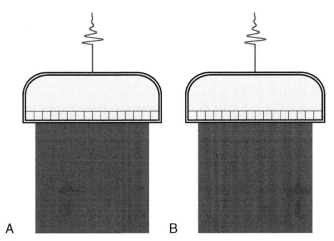

Figure 7-9 Generation of an echo by small object within the ultrasonic field using a broad beam *(red region)*. **A, B,** At constant depth, the induced signal is the same regardless of lateral location.

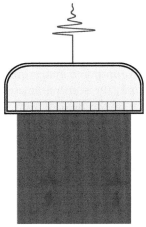

Figure 7-10 Generation of echoes by two small objects within the ultrasonic field using a broad beam *(red region)*. Since the depth is the same and the echoes arrive at the transducer simultaneously, the induced signal does not indicate the presence of two structures. The signal strength is twice that in Figure 7-9.

by altered echo times. Multiple samplings with successive narrow beams enable the objects to be observed as separate entities (Fig. 7-11).

Sampling is restricted laterally by the width of the beam. Objects located outside the beam do not contribute signals for that scan line. Scanning with a narrow beam width throughout the field of view enables an accurate depiction of interrogated structures in the lateral direction.

LATERAL RESOLUTION

Lateral resolution describes the ability to resolve two objects adjacent to each other that are perpendicular to the beam's axis. Decreasing the beam width improves the lateral resolution by allowing objects close together to be resolved and by providing a more accurate representation of small objects. *Line density also affects lateral resolution.*

Returning to the analogy involving the student sonographer, suppose, instead of three stores in the survey,

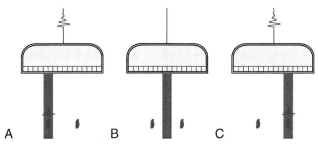

Figure 7-11 By narrowing the beam and collecting echo-range data along multiple scan lines *(three separate red regions)* separated in time, signals that indicate the lateral positions of the objects are generated. **A-C,** Time sequence for signals received along different beam paths. The time interval for each scan line equals scan range multiplied by 13 μs/cm.

numerous stores were distributed throughout the city. If travel were restricted to the directions of north, east, and west, respectively, then only stores located along these three paths would be encountered—other stores would be missed. To include all stores in the survey, the student sonographer would have to walk in many different directions. For real-time image formation, increasing the number of scan lines improves the spatial sampling in the direction perpendicular to beam propagation. The effect of line density on image quality is illustrated in Figures 7-12, 7-13, and 7-14.

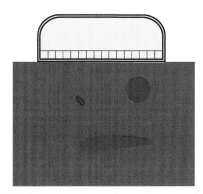

Figure 7-12 Phantom containing three objects. Each object has a unique size and shape.

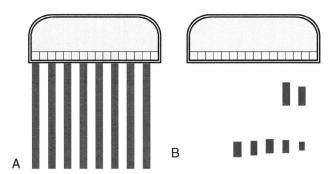

Figure 7-13 Effect of line density on lateral resolution. **A,** Scan lines *(total of eight denoted by red regions)*. **B,** Image formed by probing the phantom in Figure 7-12 along the scan lines in **(A)**. Note that the smallest object is not observed because low scan line density creates sampling voids within the field of view.

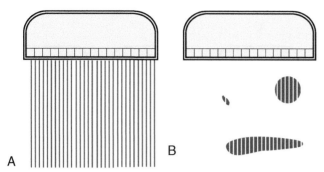

Figure 7-14 Lateral resolution is improved by increasing line density. **A,** Scan lines *(total of 31 denoted by red regions)*. **B,** Image formed by probing the phantom in Figure 7-12 along the scan lines in **(A)**.

In practice, lateral resolution is affected when the separation between two scan lines is greater than the beam width. Reducing the number of scan lines to achieve a high frame rate sometimes creates this situation. Furthermore, if the scan range and PRF are unchanged, expansion of the width of the field of view decreases the density of the scan lines. Scan line density is the number of scan lines per distance or angular arc in the width direction. Extending the scan range while maintaining the frame rate and the width of the field of view often has a similar effect of reducing scan-line density. However, adjustments in PRF (up to the maximum for that scan range) may be applied to maintain frame rate and number of scan lines.

TEMPORAL RESOLUTION

As motion becomes more rapid within the field of view, a faster frame rate is necessary to display the structures without jerkiness (abrupt transitions from one location to another). The finite transit time for the ultrasound pulse to travel to the depth of interest and back to the transducer, as well as the need for good spatial resolution provided by a large number of lines of sight in each image, imposes a restriction on the frame rate. Often, spatial resolution is sacrificed to improve the temporal resolution of fast-moving structures.

SUMMARY

Image formation is based on echo ranging and beam scanning. A major advantage of real-time ultrasound is the rapid updating of echo data within the field of view without intervention by the operator. Also, excellent temporal resolution of moving structures can be achieved. Maximum frame rate depends on scan range and number of scan lines. Beam width and scan-line density affect the lateral resolution. To optimize image quality for different clinical applications, the scan parameters of frame rate, scan range, width of the field of view, and line density are adjusted. The tenth essential equation in sonography (maximum B-mode frame rate) was introduced.

Real-Time Ultrasound Transducers

8

Chapter Objectives

To describe the various types of real-time transducers
To understand the principle of electronic focusing with multiple element arrays
To recognize the limitations in spatial sampling with the focused pulsed beam

Key terms

Annular phased array
Apodization
Channel
Compound linear arrays
Curvilinear arrays
Dynamic receive focusing

Electronic focusing
Endosonography
Footprint
Grating lobes
Linear arrays
Phased arrays

Receive-beam formation
Sector scanner
Side lobes
Slice thickness
Subdicing
Vector arrays

CLASSIFICATION OF SCANNERS

Real-time ultrasound imaging, now commonly called B-mode, has replaced static B-mode imaging. Classification of real-time transducers is based on the method by which the ultrasound beam is focused and directed through the field of view. Mechanical sector scanners, the first major class, are normally the simplest and least expensive. Mechanical motion of single or multiple crystals sweeps the beam back and forth over the region of interest to collect different lines of sight for images in rapid succession. Focusing is achieved by fixed mechanical means. The second major class, multiple-element transducers, directs and focuses the beam electronically. A seldom used transducer, the annular phased array, mechanically steers the electronically focused beam through the field of view.

MECHANICAL SCANNERS

The mechanical sector scanner has one or more piezoelectric crystals attached to a stepping motor that moves the crystal(s) to various locations throughout an arc. The changing positions of a crystal allow scan data to be collected from multiple lines of sight. In addition to the previously mentioned limitations of pulse repetition frequency on frame rate, the mechanical motion of a crystal restricts the acquisition rate to about 30 frames per second. Mechanical real-time units typically employ one or more fixed focused crystals.

Often the crystal is mounted within a liquid medium to eliminate any air interfaces between the moving crystal and the protective front surface of the transducer. The ultrasound path across the liquid medium is narrow (< 3 mm). Gel is also placed between the transducer face and the patient to remove air-tissue interfaces.

One of the first real-time mechanical scanners employed a disk-shaped focused crystal attached to a motor (Fig. 8-1). It oscillated or wobbled back and forth during data collection and with a frame rate of 15 frames per second subtended an arc of 15

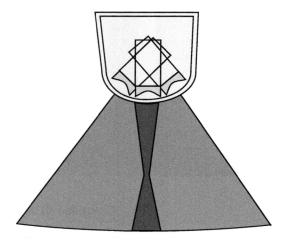

Figure 8-1 In a mechanical sector transducer a single crystal with a fixed focal length is swept back and forth across the field of view by a motorized arm.

to 60 degrees. Some of the early systems vibrated so much, in fact, that they were uncomfortable for both the patient and the sonographer.

When the crystal is at the extreme left position, data collection begins. The crystal is excited, and the transmitted beam moves outward along that line of sight, a fraction of its energy being reflected at various interfaces along its path. After an interval equal to the time needed for the wave to travel to the maximum depth of interest and return to the transducer (13 µs per centimeter), the crystal is moved to the next line of sight by the stepping motor and again excited. This sequence repeats itself until the last line of sight is collected for one image (i.e., the crystal is at the extreme right position). The time required to collect one image depicting information from a depth of 15 cm with 200 lines of sight is 39 milliseconds, and the process is repeated for the next image, which in the present example achieves a frame rate of 26 images per second. The time to collect scan data for each frame establishes the upper limit of the frame rate.

Focusing to a specific depth along each line of sight is done mechanically. The focal zone for a particular transducer is fixed and cannot be changed. Because beam width is not constant along the scan line, lateral resolution and slice thickness are not uniform throughout the field of view. The focal length of the transducer must be matched to the depth of the structures of interest. In the clinical setting, this requires multiple interchangeable transducers, each with a different focal length. Lateral resolution is also affected by scan-line density. Line density is varied by adjusting the speed of rotation of the crystal. Mechanical sector transducers offer the advantage of high line density.

In another version of the mechanical scanner, multiple crystals are mounted on a rotating wheel. The technique for acquiring echo data is very similar to that used with the oscillating sector scanner. A crystal is positioned at the extreme left and is excited, and the ultrasound beam probes interfaces along that line of sight. The wheel then

moves, and the crystal is excited for the next line of sight. When the crystal moves to the extreme right, the last line of sight is collected for one frame. The neighboring crystal on the rotating wheel is then in position at the extreme left to begin the acquisition for the next frame. This technique enables faster frame rates.

Oscillating or rotating-wheel contact scanners produce an image with a sector or pie-shaped format. The field of view is narrow near the transducer and expands with depth. Because these sector scanners are physically small, scanning in tight areas between ribs, behind ribs, and elsewhere is possible. The limited number of crystals and mechanical steering enable manufacture of these transducers at relatively low cost.

Problems with mechanical sector transducers do exist, however: Their small size limits the field of view and may make anatomic identification difficult. Their fixed focal length restricts the best lateral resolution to a limited range of depths. The scan line density is reduced with distance from the transducer face. There are more lines of sight crossing a given area near the top of the sector than in an equal area near the bottom. Streams of water radiating from a showerhead demonstrate a similar effect. Near the source, they are close together, and they become less concentrated as distance from the showerhead increases.

In practice, lateral resolution is affected when the distance between two lines is greater than the beam width. Reducing the number of lines to achieve a high frame rate sometimes creates this situation. Furthermore, increasing the sector angle to encompass a larger field of view decreases scan line density (provided that the scan range and frame rate are unchanged) and degrades lateral resolution.

LINEAR ARRAYS

An important advance in medical diagnostic ultrasound instrumentation occurred in the late 1970s with the development of electronic multiple-element transducers. These devices produce high-quality images with high frame rates and the possibility of high line density without the limited lifetime caused by mechanical wear. More importantly, the transducer is manipulated electronically to focus as well as to direct the ultrasound beam throughout the field of view.

Linear arrays contain multiple rectangular crystals arranged in a straight row. Each crystal is independently controlled to produce an ultrasound beam and then to receive the returning echoes for data collection. The crystals are activated in a sequential fashion to form the individual lines of sight (Fig. 8-2). The number of crystals in the array determines the maximum number of scan lines for each image. If the array contains 130 individual crystals that are fired (excited) one at a time in sequence, 130 lines of sight can be acquired.

The first crystal in the array is excited, and then a time delay for collection of the returning echoes is imposed

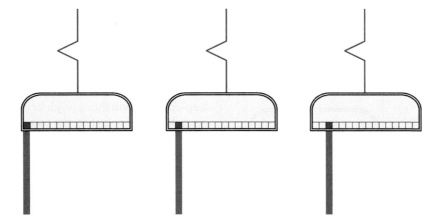

Figure 8-2 Beam scanning with a linear array. The direction of the beam is determined by element selection during transmission. The first three scan lines are shown. For a scan range of 15 cm, each crystal is fired 195 μs after the preceding crystal.

before the next crystal is fired. The duration of the delay is set by the scan range (13 μs is required for every centimeter of depth). For example, assume that a maximum viewing depth of 15 cm is desired. The first crystal is electronically stimulated to produce an ultrasound beam; 195 μs later, the second crystal is excited. After another 195 μs, the third crystal is fired. This sequence continues until all 130 crystals are fired and corresponding echoes detected to form one image. The timed activation sequence for the 130 crystals is repeated for the next image. The time required to collect scan data for one image is set by the scan range and the number of scan lines, which establishes the maximum frame rate. The 15-cm depth limits the pulse repetition frequency to 5000 pulses per second. With 130 lines per frame, the maximum frame rate is 19 frames per second.

Recall that the physical dimensions of the crystal dictate the width of the ultrasound beam in the near field. Linear arrays consist of many small crystals along a row. The major problem with a linear array is that the small crystal size produces a short, narrow near field and a rapidly diverging far field. As demonstrated with single-element transducers, large crystal diameter extends the near field depth and produces a less rapidly diverging far field. Multiple small crystals activated together in the linear array behave in a similar manner to a single crystal of equivalent size (Fig. 8-3).

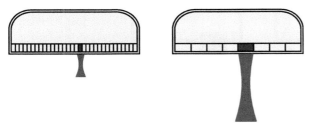

Figure 8-3 Crystal size in the transducer array affects the beam pattern. Small crystals create a short near field and a rapidly diverging far field. Large crystals produce a wider but deeper near field and a less diverging far field.

When a group of crystals in the linear array is stimulated, the respective ultrasonic fields from all crystals in the group act in concert to provide a more favorable beam pattern by maintaining beam width over an extended range. This scheme, however, while superior to a small, single crystal acting alone, creates fewer lines of sight for the same scan plane width, which causes the spatial registration to deteriorate. For example, assume that 16 individual crystals are fired in groups of four. The first four crystals are excited simultaneously and then 195 μs elapse before the next four crystals in a group (numbers 5 through 8) are fired. By using adjacent blocks of four crystals, four lines of sight that are spaced widely apart can be created (Fig. 8-4). This is less than ideal, although the beam width for sampling each line of sight at increased depth is improved.

To achieve good lateral resolution throughout the field of view, a combination of narrow beam width associated with the near field and high line density is required. This is accomplished by varying the crystals that compose the group. Figure 8-5 shows the excitation sequence for the first three lines of sight for a 16-crystal linear array. The number of lines of sight is increased by firing crystals 1 through 4, waiting 195 μs, and then firing crystals 2 through 5. After another 195 μs, crystals 3 through 6 are excited. In other words, a set of four crystals is fired as a group to produce the desired beam pattern, and, by overlapping groups, the number of lines of sight can be increased. This approach produces 13 lines of sight for the 16 crystals shown, rather than 4 lines of sight obtained by fixed groups of four.

The linear array with 200 to 500 piezoelectric elements produces good temporal resolution (high frame rate) and good spatial resolution (beam width and number of scan lines). The field of view is presented in a rectangular format, with the in-plane width equal to the physical length of the array. The linear array has a flat face, which causes difficulty in maintaining transducer-patient contact when a wide field of view is desired. Nevertheless, this step-down technique improved the image quality of real-time

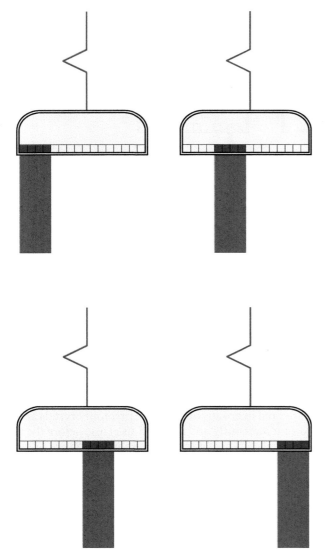

Figure 8-4 Lines of sight for a linear array. Four elements compose a group, and the group is shifted by four elements for each successive transmission. For a 15-cm scan depth, each group of four crystals is fired 195 μs after the preceding group. For a 16-element array, four lines of sight are produced.

scanners dramatically, although additional adjustments in focusing are necessary to narrow the beam width further so the spatial resolution will be optimal.

ELECTRONIC FOCUSING TECHNIQUES

Regardless of whether a single crystal is excited or a group of crystals is fired together; the rectangularly shaped radiating surface creates a near field with the in-plane beam width equal to the aperture (Fig. 8-6). However, the ultrasonic field for a linear array is not symmetrical; therefore, the beam dimension along the row of crystals (in-plane) and perpendicular to the row of crystals (elevation) must be specified separately. As previously stated for single-element transducers, ultrasound beams are focused to improve the lateral resolution and sensitivity. Because a linear array has a rectangular format, focusing must be applied in two directions to narrow the beam width perpendicular to the direction of propagation (Fig. 8-7). Focusing along the in-plane direction affects the lateral resolution. Focusing along the elevation direction (out of plane) determines the thickness of tissue represented by the cross-sectional image.

Mechanical focusing is used to reduce the width of the ultrasound beam in the elevation direction. Mechanical focusing is achieved either by curving the crystal or, more commonly, by placing an acoustic lens in front of the crystal. The beam is most narrow at a specified depth, which is fixed by the lens or curvature of the crystal. Focusing in the elevation direction is applied uniformly to each crystal in the array. The slice thickness varies along the scan line but is typically 3 to 10 millimeters within the focal zone. For the in-plane direction, electronic focusing narrows the beam width to 1 millimeter or less, and the depth of focus can be varied.

Focusing Dynamics

The sequence of firing one group of crystals and then firing the next group prohibits mechanical focusing of the ultrasound beam in the in-plane direction. The relative position

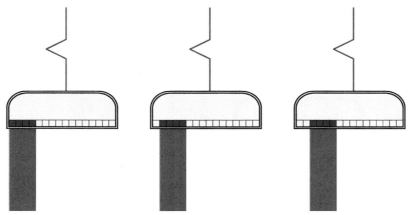

Figure 8-5 Lines of sight for a linear array. Four elements compose a group, and the group is shifted by one element for each successive transmission. The total number of lines of sight for the 16-element array is increased to 13 by overlapping segments.

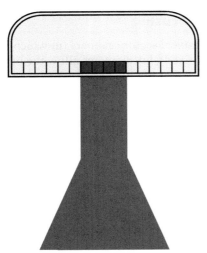

Figure 8-6 The ultrasonic field from a segment of crystals in an array is similar to that from a single crystal circular transducer.

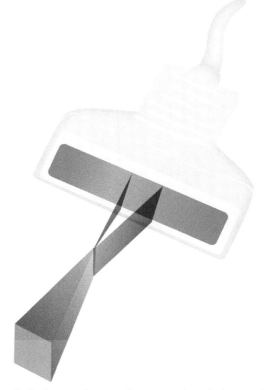

Figure 8-8 Electronic focusing of an array reduces the beam width in the in-plane direction.

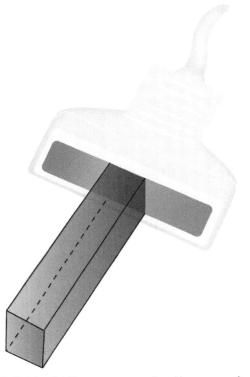

Figure 8-7 Near-field beam pattern produced by a group of crystals in the linear array in the absence of focusing.

of a crystal in the group dictates the focusing requirements for that crystal. *Because most crystals in the array belong to multiple firing groups, the focusing requirements change and cannot be achieved by static mechanical means.* For example, crystal 3 is the center of a five-crystal firing sequence involving crystals 1 through 5; when crystals 2 through 6 are fired, crystal 3 occupies the second position; and when 3 through 7 are fired, crystal 3 moves to the first position. This changing position dictates different

focusing requirements for that crystal and thus prohibits fixed mechanical focusing in the in-plane direction.

Fortunately, linear arrays can be electronically focused in the in-plane direction (Fig. 8-8), which (when combined with mechanical focusing in the elevation direction) creates a narrow beam in the matched focal zones (Fig. 8-9). Focusing in the in-plane direction is variable, which allows narrow beam width in this direction at any specified depth along the scan line, whereas the beam width in the elevation direction is not changeable. The spatial sampling volume has three components (Fig. 8-10).

Principles of Focusing

Electronic focusing involves the superimposition (algebraic summation) of ultrasound waves. Each crystal produces a particular wave pattern, and the overall pattern derived from a group of crystals is the summation of all the wave patterns from the individual crystals (Huygens' principle). For a group of crystals, the main beam axis is centered at the middle crystal. Electronic focusing is accomplished by offsetting the firing sequence of various crystals in a group by well-defined time delays. These delays are small compared with the time required for the sound beam to travel to the depth of interest. The firing sequence is accomplished by delay lines, which are electronic devices that hold the signal from the pulser for a specified period. The exact time delay depends on the

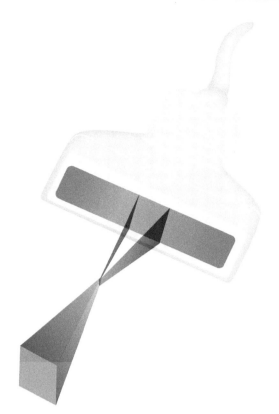

Figure 8-9 Resultant beam pattern from both mechanical focusing and electronic focusing. Slice thickness is most narrow at a depth within the focal zone of the mechanically focused crystals.

Transmit Focusing

Unlike mechanical sector scanners (in which depth of the focal zone is fixed), linear arrays allow the operator to select one of several possible focal lengths (transmit focal zones) within the scan plane. *The depth of the focal zone is altered by varying the delay times between crystal excitations.* The field of view is scanned with a depth of focus specified by the operator. After review of the real-time image, a new focal zone may be selected (by modifying the delay line timing) to rescan the same area with different focal length in the scan plane. This technique is called transmit focusing. Electronic control of the elements allows variable focusing along the scan line, which, in turn, narrows beam width in the in-plane direction at the focal zone (Fig. 8-12).

High line-density images with multiple focal zones throughout the image are also possible using these adjustable delay lines (Fig. 8-13). Multizone transmit focusing typically slows the frame rate, because data must be collected for all the scan lines across the array with a set focal zone depth before the scan lines are repeated with a different focal zone depth. For example, assume that the unit can be focused to three different depths for the same "image." In reality, three separate images, each focused to a particular depth, must be collected before they are combined into one "final image" for viewing. Since the field of view is scanned multiple times to compose each real-time image, frame rate is reduced significantly.

Aperture Focusing

Electronic focusing during transmission is also accomplished by varying the number of crystals activated in the segment (Fig. 8-14). Focusing must occur within the near field of the excited crystal group. As with single-element transducers, the depth of the near field is a function of the dimensions of the active elements and the frequency. The aperture is increased to maintain near-field beam width for longer focal lengths.

For example, two crystals are fired as a group to produce a very short, narrow near field and a rapidly diverging far field (designed to enhance the focal zone near the transducer). If more crystals are added in the group, then the depth of the near field is extended and the beam width near the transducer is broadened. Importantly, at increased depth, the beam is made narrower by increasing the aperture. *Large aperture extends the depth of focus.* Manufacturers employ combinations of time-delayed firing and changing beam aperture to optimize focusing at different depths.

The extent of the focal zone (depth of field) for a multiple-element array depends on aperture size, focal length, and frequency (Fig. 8-15). To maintain the depth of field as focal length is increased, the aperture must also increase. This is accomplished by using a small group of crystals at short focal lengths and more elements at longer

crystal position and the focal zone depth desired. The wavefronts generated by all crystals in the group are made to arrive at a specific point simultaneously, and the result is a focused beam at that point.

Figure 8-11 demonstrates electronic focusing with five crystals of an array. The positions of the crystals are arranged so the distance from either crystal 1 (r_1) or crystal 5 (r_5) to the point of interest is the same but greater than the distance from either crystal 2 (r_2) or crystal 4 (r_4). Distances r_2 and r_4 are equal but greater than r_3 (the distance from crystal 3 to the point of interest). The wavefronts from each of the five crystals must arrive at the focal point at exactly the same time. This is accomplished by firing crystals 1 and 5 first, delaying a short time before firing crystals 2 and 4, and finally waiting another short time before firing crystal 3. The ultrasound beam thus is focused in the in-plane direction, producing a narrow width over a limited depth near the focal point. The next segment of crystals (2 through 6) is fired in the same manner (2 and 6, 3 and 5, then 4) to produce another similarly focused beam, but directed along a different line of sight. The remaining segments across the array are also focused by this delayed firing technique. A narrow beam is swept throughout the field of view to collect an image using a set focal length. Improved spatial detail (lateral resolution) is thus obtained within the focal zone corresponding to a particular depth in the image.

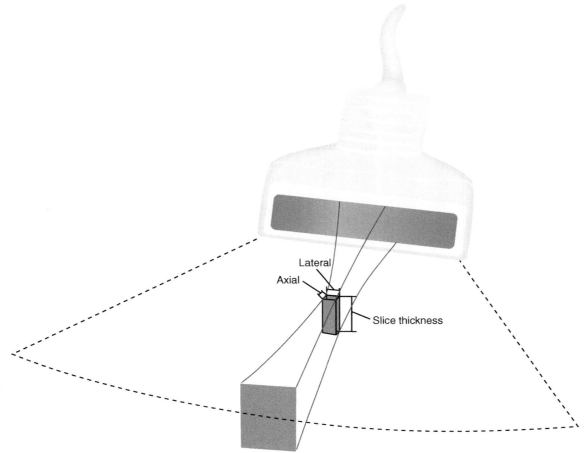

Figure 8-10 Spatial sampling. In-plane focusing affects lateral resolution. Mechanical focusing in the elevation direction determines the slice thickness. Axial resolution is determined by the spatial pulse length.

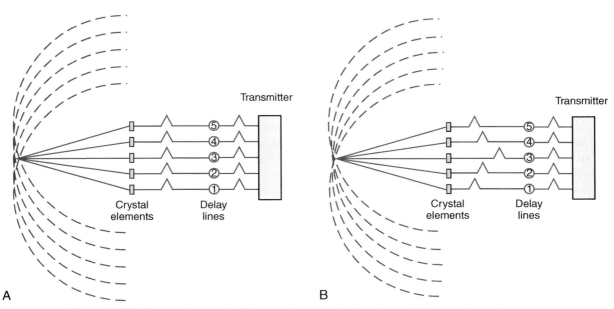

Figure 8-11 Electronic focusing. **A,** If five crystals are stimulated simultaneously, the wavefronts do not arrive simultaneously at the target, because the distances of travel for each wavefront is not the same. **B,** Transmit delay lines are used to excite the crystals at slightly different times (nanosecond delays between firings). The wavefronts arrive exactly simultaneously at the target point, and the result is a focused beam. Crystals 1 and 5 are stimulated first, then 2 and 4, and then 3. When the time delays are changed, other points are allowed to become the center of focus.

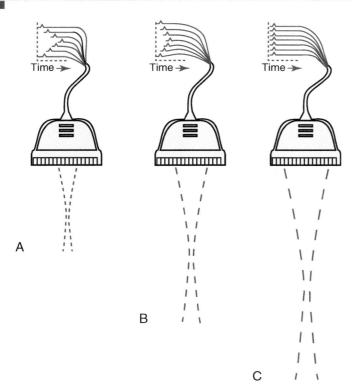

Figure 8-12 Variable delay lines allow focusing at different depths. The delay lines stagger the timed-excitation pulses to the crystals, depending on the degree of focusing desired. **A,** Short focus. **B,** Medium focus. **C,** Long focus.

focal lengths. Since the depth of field is inversely proportional to the square of the aperture, at a specific focal length increasing aperture size creates a strongly focused beam and improves lateral resolution.

Dynamic Receive Focusing

Another means to reduce the effective sampling volume is dynamic focusing in the receive mode. The principle of receive focus is difficult to conceptualize. The following analogy may help: Three runners of equal ability begin a race at the same starting point but follow different routes to the finish line. At the finish line, an observer is assigned to each runner and must shout the point of origin when the runner crosses the finish line. Because the distance traveled by each runner is not identical, three separate shouts are heard as the race is completed. If an obstacle, such as a wall, is placed in the path of each runner, the sequence of finish can be regulated. The height of the wall is adjusted depending on the distance between the starting point and finish line. To increase the delay before crossing the finish line, the obstacle is made greater. In this case, the shortest route would incorporate the tallest wall. For a certain combination of obstacles, the runners finish the race simultaneously, and one loud shout is heard from all the observers identifying the point of origin. The race can be made more complex by varying the starting point. The heights of

the obstacles can be adjusted according to the change in distance. Now the observers are given a chart that denotes the starting point based on the elapsed time of the race. This is possible because the participants run at the same speed. The shouts of the observers at the finish line are still synchronized; only the words to identify the starting points vary. Dynamic receive focusing works in a similar manner.

By means of time-delay circuitry in the receiver, the returning sound beam-induced signals are refocused when multiple crystals receive the echo. Dynamic focusing is not limited to one fixed depth per transmitted pulse, as transmit focusing is, but is applied for all depths. In Figure 8-16, five crystals are activated to receive the ultrasound beam reflected toward the transducer from the object. The ultrasound beam diverges during its return to the transducer. The wavefront intercepts crystal 3 first, then crystals 2 and 4, and finally crystals 1 and 5. Through the use of receive-time delays, the echo-induced signal at crystal 3 is delayed until the wavefront reaches crystals 1 and 5. Similarly, the echo-induced signals from crystals 2 and 4 are delayed until the wavefront reaches crystals 1 and 5, although the delay time is shorter than for crystal 3. The actual time delay is determined for each crystal by simple geometry and an assumed constant velocity of ultrasound in soft tissue. The wavefront from the object appears to be in phase for all five crystals, resulting in a "focused" beam from that depth of interest. This delay and sum strategy is called receive-beam formation.

The same principle applies to an object located farther from the transducer, as in Figure 8-17, but because of the greater depth, the wavefront strikes the crystals with less variability. A shorter series of receive delay times focuses the detected signals from the object. The elapsed time from transmission to reception determines the delay times for each crystal. The depth for receive focus is always known; thus receive delay times are constantly changed to yield a continually focused beam at all depths. That is, during the acquisition of scan data, the receive time delays are varied dynamically to sweep the focal zone to each point along the scan line. Hence the name of this technique is dynamic receive focusing.

The received beam width is uniformly narrow along the line of sight. In essence, therefore, lateral resolution is improved by restricting the tissue volume that contributes to each scan line in the image. A dynamic aperture adjusts the number of receiving crystals along the array to optimize focusing as a function of depth. Additional elements are included in the aperture as the depth of the focal zone is increased (Fig. 8-18). *Dynamic receive focusing is achieved without a loss in frame rate or line density.*

Each independent element with the associated electronics for transmission and reception constitutes a channel. Focusing is improved as the number of channels is increased. Compare the spatial resolution at a depth of 8 cm for the sonograms obtained with 64 versus 128 receive channels (Fig. 8-19).

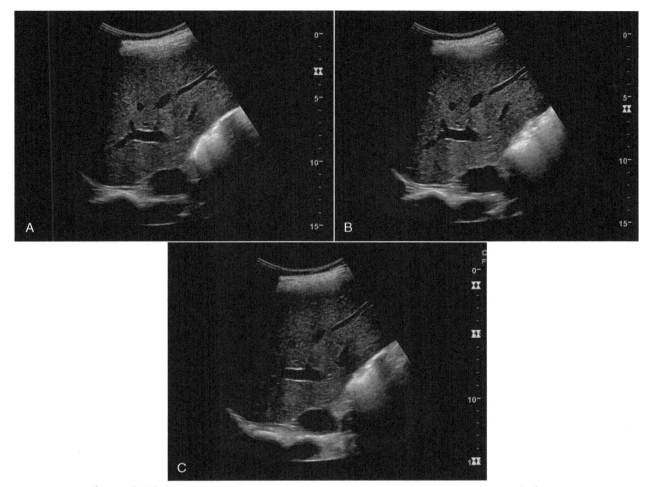

Figure 8-13 Improvement of image quality with transmit focusing. **A,** Single focal zone at a depth of 3 cm. **B,** Single focal zone at a depth of 6 cm. **C,** Multiple transmit focal zones throughout the scan range (1 cm, 5 cm, 15 cm).

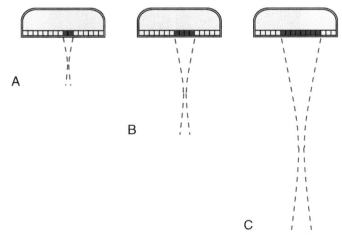

Figure 8-14 Aperture focusing. Two crystals are fired for short focus (**A**), four crystals for medium focus (**B**), and eight crystals for long focus (**C**).

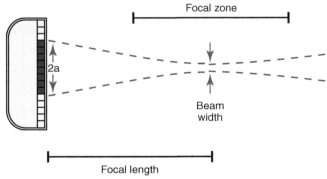

Figure 8-15 Depth of field (focal zone). Beam width is most narrow with the focal zone, which is affected by aperture size (2a), focal length, and wavelength.

Effective Beam Width

Linear arrays use both transmit focusing and dynamic receive focusing. The effective beam width is the product of the transmit focal zone beam width and the received beam width. As the number of fixed transmit focal zones increases, the composite effective beam width becomes narrower. Each segment along the line of sight is optimized for a certain focal length. Since the ultrasound beam diverges rapidly beyond the focal zone, multiple transmit focal zones are necessary to maintain a narrow beam width along the entire scan line.

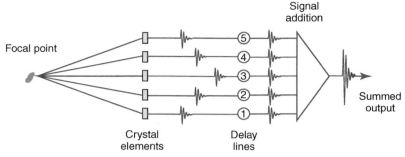

Figure 8-16 Dynamic receive focusing. The echo wavefront from the object arrives at crystal 3 first, then at 2 and 4, and finally at 1 and 5. By delaying the individual echo signal at each crystal until the wavefront has arrived at all five crystals, focusing is applied to the received signals to produce a summed output.

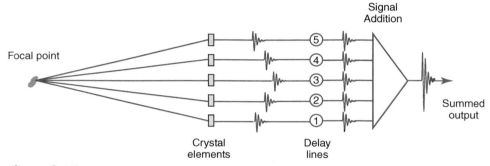

Figure 8-17 Dynamic receive focusing. The delay times change with respect to depth. Compare the signal spacing in time with that shown in Figure 8-16.

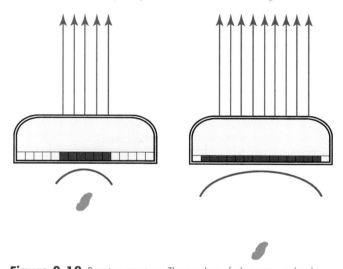

Figure 8-18 Receive aperture. The number of elements used in beam formation increases with depth.

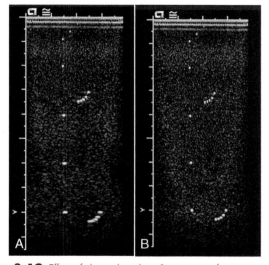

Figure 8-19 Effect of channel number. Sonograms of a tissue-mimicking phantom with 64 receive channels **(A)** and 128 receive channels **(B)**. (Courtesy of Rob Steins.)

CURVILINEAR ARRAYS

In the past few years curvilinear arrays (also called convex or curved linear arrays) that portray a large trapezoid-shaped field of view have been developed. The array contains 128 to 256 crystal elements arranged along an arc in a linear fashion. The radius of curvature is usually 25 to 100 mm. A large radius of curvature extends the width of the field of view. Unlike the case with linear arrays, the width of the field of view is not restricted to the physical size of the array. As is the case with other multielement arrays,

the physical dimensions of the crystal elements and the number of elements excited influence the beam pattern.

As linear arrays do, curvilinear arrays direct the beam by select activation of multiple crystals in a group, stepping down after the appropriate delay and then firing the next group. The curved crystal arrangement provides lines of sight that are perpendicular to the array surface (Fig. 8-20). No loss of focus occurs at the edges of the field of view; however, beam divergence may limit the useful

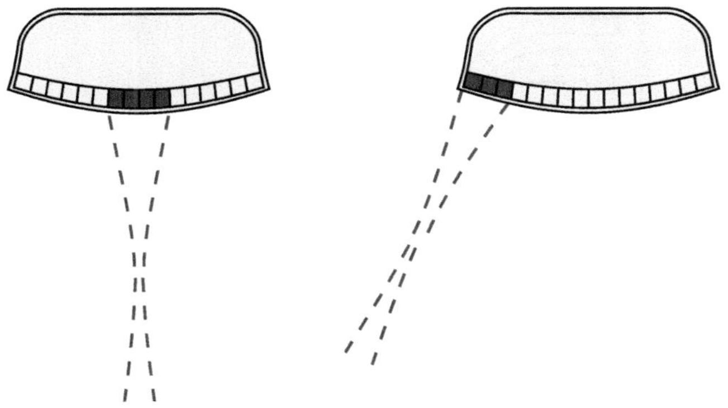

Figure 8-20 Curvilinear array. Ultrasonic beams are directed perpendicular to the array surface.

depth. Analogous to sector scanning, line density is decreased at depth with curvilinear arrays, and a loss of lateral resolution can occur.

PHASED ARRAYS

Another electronic real-time system, the phased array, was developed to overcome certain limitations inherent in the linear array. Image formation with a linear array produces a rectangular format in which the width of the field of view is determined by the physical length of the row of elements in the array, and the maximum number of scan lines corresponds to the number of elements in the array. The relatively low number of scan lines per frame allows high frame rates, but lateral resolution is sacrificed. The large footprint (size of the radiating surface of the transducer) may be several centimeters in length, which prevents access to structures where a narrow acoustic window is available (e.g., between the ribs for cardiac imaging).

Phased arrays also contain multiple rectangular crystals arranged in a straight row. The phased array can have a small footprint with few crystals, but typically it is composed of 128 elements. To generate and direct the ultrasonic beam, all (or most) of the crystals in the array are excited nearly simultaneously. This contrasts with linear arrays, in which the crystals are stimulated in groups. The design produces a sector format with a sector angle as large as 90 degrees. Scan lines diverge with depth; therefore, scan line density is not constant throughout the field of view. A small sector angle (e.g., 30 degrees) enables a higher frame rate or increased scan line density. For example, an image composed of 150 scan lines can be updated 30 times per second if the scan range is 15 cm. Phased arrays are commonly employed in echocardiology because their small size (10 to 30 mm in length) enables better access to the heart.

Electronic steering of the beam throughout the field of view allows data collection along different lines of sight. Additional small time adjustments are applied for transmit focusing purposes as the beam is steered. The phased array can also be dynamically focused in the receive mode. Outside the central field of view, lateral resolution

deteriorates, because electronic focusing becomes more difficult when large-angle beam steering is performed. As with linear arrays, phased arrays are mechanically focused in the elevation (slice thickness) direction.

Transmit Steering

The entire phased array produces only one line of sight each time the crystal elements are excited. Electronic steering relies on the interference of waves for reinforcement to produce planar wavefronts, thus the name phased array. By altering the timing sequence of the excitation pulses, the direction of propagation of the transmitted beam can be varied to any desired scan angle (Fig. 8-21). The scan angle is denoted as the angle between the direction of propagation and the normal to the central element in the array.

Figure 8-22 illustrates the principle of transmit steering using a five-element phased array. Elements are stimulated in sequence according to the prescribed time delay between excitations. Each crystal produces a circular wavefront, which moves into tissue. Since the origins of the individual wavefronts are shifted with respect to location and time, they will add together to create a resultant planar wavefront. The planar wavefront propagates through tissue at a constant scan angle.

Transmit Focusing

The concept of beam formation can be extended to include focusing of the transmitted beam at a specific depth along the direction of propagation. In Figure 8-23 the distance between each array element and the point of interest (focal point) is different. The time for sound to travel from element 5 to the focal point is shorter than that for element 4, and the time for sound to travel from element 4 to the focal point is shorter than that for element 3, and so forth. If the delay time between elements is set equal to the time difference for travel, then the wavefronts arrive simultaneously at the focal point.

Note that the respective time delays between elements are not linear but rather spherical. The range of the time delays is decreased for longer focal lengths.

As with linear arrays, transmit focusing is limited to one focal point for each transmitted beam. Once data have been collected along this scan line, the focal point can be changed (by modifying the delay-line timing) to rescan this line of sight with a new focal point. In this manner the transmit focal zone can be positioned at different depths. This improves the lateral resolution. However, multiple-zone transmit focusing slows the frame rate because multiple-transmit pulses are necessary to compose each scan line.

Dynamic Focusing

Dynamic focusing during reception, as described for linear arrays, is also possible. Analogous to transmit focusing with respect to the timing sequence, the time for the echo

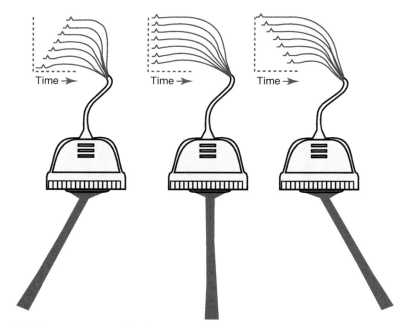

Figure 8-21 Beam steering with a phased array. Each crystal is connected to an adjustable delay line. The excitation sequence is changed to steer the beam in different directions.

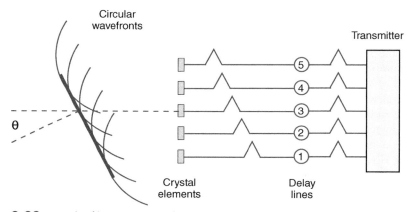

Figure 8-22 Principle of beam steering. After stimulation, each crystal produces a circular wavefront. The wavefronts from all crystals combine to create a planar wavefront that propagates through tissue at scan angle θ.

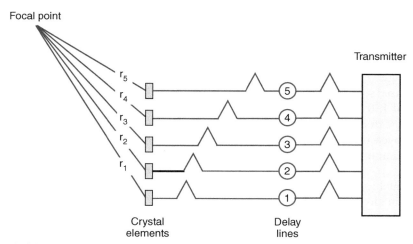

Figure 8-23 Transmit-beam focusing. The distance between the focal point and the element (r_i) determines the delay time before excitation for that element ($i = 1, 2, 3, 4,$ or 5).

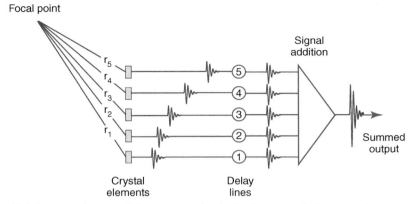

Figure 8-24 Receive focusing. Echoes generated at the focal point reach elements in the array at slightly difference times. Each induced signal is delayed by an amount corresponding to the difference in travel distance. The signal from element 5 is detected first and must undergo the longest delay before signal addition.

created in the focal zone to reach an array element depends on the distance to the element in the array. By delaying the output from each element by the time difference from the longest path, the signals induced by echoes originating from within the focal zone are synchronized in time. The outputs from all received elements are then summed to produce a large-amplitude signal (receive beam formation). Figure 8-24 illustrates that the array is initially focused to a single spatial location during reception. After all echoes associated with this focal region have been received, the time delay for each channel is changed to create a new focal zone distal to the previous focal zone.

COMPOUND LINEAR ARRAYS

Vector arrays (also called compound linear arrays and virtual convex) incorporate characteristics from both the linear array and the phased array. In fact, this transducer is classified as a phased array by some manufacturers. Multiple crystals are fired at one time to direct the beam along different paths. Scan lines for the central field of view are obtained by selective excitation of elements so that the beam path is perpendicular to the array. At the extremes of the field of view, the ultrasound beam is steered at wide angles by the phased method. The timed excitation of a large number of crystals is controlled by delay lines. An enlarged effective field of view that extends beyond the physical length of the array is created. Areas of overlapping data are manipulated by the scan converter to form a composite image. The footprint is smaller than that for the curvilinear array, and the field of view is trapezoidal in shape.

ANNULAR PHASED ARRAYS

An annular phased array, when viewed end-on (Fig. 8-25), has a central, circular disk surrounded by concentric rings of additional crystals. For each transmitted pulse, each crystal is excited in such a fashion as to permit electronic focusing to a very small region (1 to 3 mm) at a specified depth along the scan line. When the timing sequence is

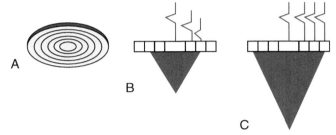

Figure 8-25 Annular array. **A,** End view of an annular array showing six crystal elements. Note that all except the innermost crystal are doughnut-shaped. **B,** Side view to show focusing at shallow depth. **C,** Side view to show focusing at increased depth.

changed, the focal zone is placed at various depths along the beam axis. Dynamic receive focusing is also possible, although an annular phased array must be mechanically steered to collect different scan lines.

The ultrasound beam converges symmetrically to the focal point. The beam width is the same in both the slice-thickness direction and the in-plane direction (similar to a single-element, circular disk). This symmetrical beam should be contrasted with ultrasound beams generated by linear arrays, which have varying dimensions depending on the focusing technique, pulsing sequence, and crystal size.

SECONDARY LOBES

Secondary lobes originate at the transducer and radiate outward at various angles to the main beam. There are two types of secondary lobes: side lobes and grating lobes. Side lobes, which are present with all transducers (single or multiple crystals), result from nonthickness mode vibrations (radial mode vibrations for circular and annular transducers), immediate reverberations at crystal-tissue interfaces, and interference phenomena. They are typically lower in intensity compared with the main beam. A technique called apodization reduces the intensity of side lobes in electronic arrays. Apodization employs a variable-strength voltage pulse to the crystals across the aperture during transmit focusing. The excitation voltage

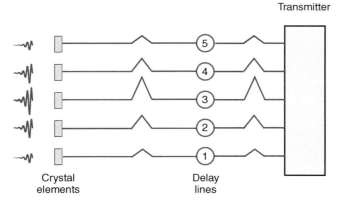

Figure 8-26 Apodization demonstrated by varying the strength of the voltage pulse to each crystal (represented by different peak heights in a five-crystal segment). The highest voltage is applied to the center crystal.

to the individual crystals of each segment is maximized at the center and reduced toward the periphery (Fig. 8-26). During reception, the contribution to the overall signal from crystals is modulated according to the position in the segment. High frequency and a large number of similar elements in the active area of an array (effectively creating a larger radiating surface) reduces the intensity of side lobes.

Another secondary lobe problem unique to crystal arrays is *grating lobes*, which are caused by the regular periodic spacing of elements within the array. Grating lobes are oriented at an angle to the main beam. When this element-to-element distance is decreased to less than one wavelength, the angle of the grating lobes becomes greater than 90 degrees with respect to the main beam, and thus the grating lobes are eliminated.

Unfortunately, the elements of the array are often spaced greater than one wavelength from center to center; however, design engineers have found that the grating lobes can be suppress by a technique called subdicing. In this technique, the normal element of an array is divided into many smaller subelements, with the subelements electronically connected to form the original-size element. The subdiced elements act in concert as a single crystal, but the element divisions effectively reduce the center-to-center distance between transmission points.

Phased arrays have a more severe problem with grating lobes, because the steering of an ultrasound beam at large angles increases the number and intensity of grating lobes as compared with the beam from a linear array. The grating lobes are a result of the summation of side lobes from the individual crystals. When multiple crystals are pulsed for steering, low-intensity side lobes are added together and create significant secondary lobes of energy.

CRYSTAL ELEMENT ISOLATION

Another consideration with multiple-element arrays is interelement isolation, in which the stimulation of one element in an array may affect adjacent elements. When a

voltage pulse excites one element, the other elements should not respond. The same holds true when a crystal receives an echo. No communication (cross-talk) should take place between each crystal element and the neighboring crystals. Electrical and mechanical coupling exists between the array elements and cannot be completely eliminated. The array elements are isolated electrically by separate ground wires and separate signal electrodes for each element (including subdiced elements). Nevertheless, the elements are not completely isolated electronically, because they act as tiny capacitors. Mechanical isolation is a much more difficult problem to overcome, because the elements are mechanically coupled by the matching layers, focusing lenses, and backing material. Even the housing itself, which is used for electrical and acoustic insulation, serves to couple the elements together. Return echoes pass through the matching layers and focusing lens before striking the crystal element to induce a radiofrequency signal. The return echoes are dispersed and also strike the adjacent crystals; thus low-amplitude signals are induced in these elements.

Furthermore, crystals must be mechanically isolated to prevent ultrasound transfer between crystals. Air, as a spacing material, partially eliminates this coupling. Any sound produced by a crystal from length-mode vibrations is reflected back into the crystal rather than transmitted to the adjacent crystals. An alternative method of isolating crystals is to design the width and length dimensions to be dramatically different from the thickness. An aspect ratio (thickness/length or thickness/width) of 2:1 provides significant cross-talk reduction.

DIGITAL BEAM FORMER

The function of focusing during transmission and reception is executed by a digital beam former. The complex combination of time delays, aperture, and apodization are most effectively applied with digital electronics during both transmission and reception. Compared with analog devices, digital beam formers allow greater flexibility in beam manipulation with regard to ultrasonic field shape, beam width, direction, and intensity.

SMALL-FOOTPRINT TRANSDUCERS

Phased arrays with small physical dimensions are desirable for neonatal applications and small-parts scanning. However, by necessity, these transducers have a limited area for assembling the piezoelectric elements. Electronic focusing becomes suboptimal as scan range is extended beyond a depth equal to twice the active length of the array. Small-footprint transducers, because of their limited range, operate at high frequency (5 to 20 MHz) and have excellent axial resolution (Fig. 8-27). Additional advantages of small-footprint transducers are their reduced weight and relatively wide field of view (90-degree sector format).

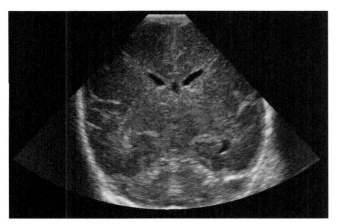

Figure 8-27 Sonogram of a neonate head acquired with a vector transducer.

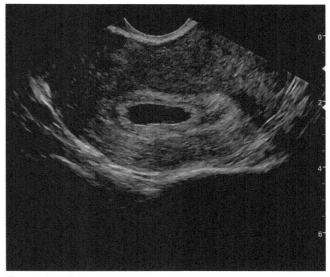

Figure 8-28 Sonogram of gestational sac acquired with a transvaginal transducer.

ENDOSONOGRAPHY

Endosonography transducers—such as endovaginal (transvaginal), endorectal, and transesophageal transducers—are specially designed real-time mechanical, linear array, or phased array transducers mounted on probes that can be inserted into various body cavities.

Endovaginal transducers are available in which a single focused crystal is mounted at the end of the probe. This crystal is mechanically swept up and down to produce a 45- to 110-degree sagittal sector. By rotating and tilting the probe, different planes can be imaged.

Linear array and phased array endosonography transducers work in the same manner as the corresponding contact real-time transducers; they are just much smaller. Multiple lines of sight for each image are collected, either by mechanical or electronic means. Because the crystals are close to the tissues of interest and there is thus minimal sampling depth, many lines of sight can be collected to improve the spatial mapping (Fig. 8-28). The obvious necessity of keeping the transducer crystal(s) small creates problems in maintaining a narrow beam, but restricted sampling depth overcomes this difficulty. Both electronic focusing and dynamic receive focusing are possible. High-frequency transducers are used to optimize axial and lateral resolution. By pulsing at very high frequencies, rapid framing rates can be obtained, which is particularly valuable for transesophageal imaging of the heart. Scan data from multiple planes are acquired throughout the area of interest by rotating or moving the probe within the body cavity.

The transesophageal transducer is a small phased array inserted down the esophagus to acquire two-dimensional images of the heart (Fig. 8-29). Because the transducer is close to the heart, high frequency, high line density, and high frame rates are achievable. Acoustic coupling devices (e.g., water-filled condoms) are not necessary because the esophagus tends to collapse around the probe.

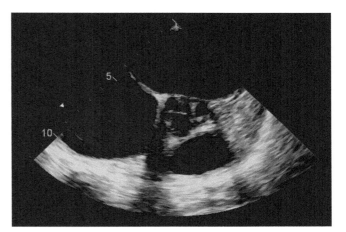

Figure 8-29 Sonogram of aortic valve obtained with a transesophageal transducer.

TRANSLUMINAL TRANSDUCERS

Extremely small crystal arrays are mounted on the end of a catheter to inspect the interior of vessels visually for vascular plaques. These transducers, which operate at 10 to 20 MHz, produce very highly detailed images that aid in the placement of balloons for plaque reduction or laser obliteration. Such probes have proven to be valuable in echocardiology for assessing valves and cardiac vessels, particularly in postinfarction procedures. Placement of catheters through the umbilical cord to the fetal heart may have applications in fetal cardiology. Transluminal probes are also inserted into the fallopian tubes to evaluate the status of a fertilized oocyte.

1.5D ARRAY TRANSDUCERS

A major weakness of linear arrays is the inability to apply dynamic focusing to control the slice thickness of the transmitted beam. Focusing in the elevation plane is commonly accomplished by acoustic lenses with fixed focal lengths. Within the focal zone, the slice thickness is 3 to 5 mm; but outside the focal zone, slice thickness can increase significantly. Compare this with an in-plane beam width of about 1 mm, which is achievable by electronic focusing. This relatively large elevation beam width creates partial volume artifacts when small structures are being imaged. Contours may be blurred, and the detected signal level is a combination of the small reflector and the surrounding tissue. The 1.5D array transducer provides electronic focusing in the elevation plane.

The single row of elements in the conventional linear array is replaced by three to seven rows of smaller elements in the 1.5D array (Fig. 8-30). The interelement spacing is half of the wavelength and the interrow spacing is 10 times the wavelength. Beam direction is determined by element selection. The additional crystal elements with time-delay channels enable electronic focusing in the elevation plane.

HANAFY LENS

An alternative method to control beam width in the elevation plane is to use a variable-thickness crystal called a Hanafy lens. The central portion of the crystal in the elevation direction is thin, resonates at high frequency, and forms a superficially focused beam. The crystal becomes

thicker, resonates at lower frequency, and contributes to focusing at progressively deeper depths as the outer boundary of the crystal is approached. This technique produces an extremely broad bandwidth pulse with narrow slice thickness along the scan line.

2D ARRAY TRANSDUCERS

Electronic steering in three directions to sample a volume without moving the transducer is the motivation for the development of matrix phased (2D) array transducers. Available modes of operation include 3D and 4D but also B-mode, in which the operator can orient the scan plane in any direction within the scanned volume. The matrix phased array is formed by crystal elements configured in multiple rows forming a rectangular plane. Total elements number between 2000 and 9000. Each element must have a separate electrical connection for independent control. Transmit focusing with multiple crystal rows (similar to 1.5D) narrows the in-plane and elevation beam widths as the beam is steered (Fig. 8-31). Several factors, but primarily cost and transducer heating, have limited the clinical introduction of 2D arrays. In the newest designs, scanning electronics are incorporated into the scan head to reduce the size and weight of the transducer.

Capacitive micromachined ultrasonic transducers (CMUTs) have been developed as a potential replacement for traditional transducers with piezoelectric crystal elements. In the most common design, an electrode is embedded in a dielectric membrane, which is mounted over a thin vacuum cavity enclosed by a second electrode. The membrane is made to vibrate rapidly when an alternating voltage is applied to the electrodes. Each membrane element is very small, with a diameter of 30 microns. The element packing is denser than can be achieved with piezoelectric materials (minimal size is 100 microns). Integrated circuit technology allows fabrication of a thin two-dimensional array of thousands of elements. The advantages of CMUTs include high frequency (6 to 40 MHz), wide bandwidth, low cost, and excellent acoustic coupling with tissue. Lower sensitivity and high cross-talk are current limitations of this technology.

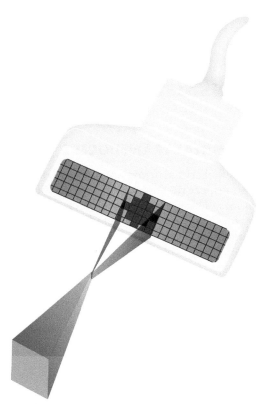

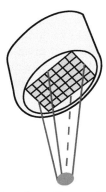

Figure 8-30 1.5D transducer. By subdividing each crystal in a linear array to form multiple rows of crystals, it becomes possible to focus in the elevation direction at different depths.

Figure 8-31 Matrix transducer. The two-dimensional array of crystal elements enables focusing and steering of the beam throughout the sampled volume.

TRANSDUCER CARE

A transducer is susceptible to damage if it is dropped or sustains an impact. A cracked transducer surface is potentially dangerous to both the operator and patient and must be removed from service (Fig. 8-32). The repeated twisting and bending of the cable can lead to transducer malfunction. During transport of the unit, care must be taken to prevent damage to the cables.

Many external transducers are not watertight; thus immersion in a liquid can damage the transducer. The preferred cleaning method is a damp cloth moistened with soap and water. If decontamination of bodily fluids is required, then disinfecting and sterilizing solutions—usually containing glutaraldehyde—are used. Intracavitary probes are soaked *for a prescribed time* in the disinfecting liquid. Extended immersion in the liquid can damage the intracavitary probe. The sonographer should always check the manufacturer's recommendations for cleaning.

Gas sterilization, ultraviolet sterilization, dry heat sterilization, autoclaving, and soaking in chlorine bleach can damage the transducer and must be avoided. If sterility is required, then the transducer is placed in a sterile sleeve filled with sterile coupling gel.

Chemical agents containing acetone, mineral oil, iodine, or oil-based perfume can also damage the transducer. Coupling gels with these chemical agents should not be used. The manufacturer usually provides a list of approved products.

SUMMARY

Many different types of transducers have been developed for real-time imaging, including mechanical sector and five types of arrays: linear, phased, curvilinear, vector, and annular phased. All these transducers with the exception of the mechanical sector contain multiple crystal elements, which are individually controlled for beam formation during transmission of the ultrasound beam and reception of tissue-generated echoes. Characteristics of each transducer type are summarized in Table 8-1.

Electronic sequencing/steering and focusing for a multiple-element array are applied only within the scan plane. Geometric focusing with a lens or curved crystal elements determines slice thickness. The curvature of the elements determines the depth of focus in the elevation direction, which is unchangeable.

Transmit focusing is limited to one focal zone for each transmitted pulse directed along a specific scan line. Dynamic receive focusing is applied to echo-induced signals from multiple elements to focus the resultant signal to a particular point along the scan line. Beam formation during reception is a dynamic process in which focusing is swept along all depths of the scan line as a function of elapsed time. After data collection for one scan line is completed, the transmitted pulse is directed along a new scan line and the beam formation processing is repeated.

Multizone transmit focusing improves the lateral resolution of B-mode image by narrowing the in-plane beam width throughout the scan line. This is accomplished by using multiple focal zones, each with a different depth of focus along a single scan line.

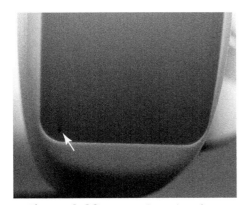

Figure 8-32 Damaged transducer face.

Table 8-1	Transducer Characteristics					
Type	**Scanning Mechanism**	**In-plane Focusing**	**Slice Thickness**	**Image Format**	**Footprint**
Mechanical sector	Mechanical	Mechanical	Mechanical	Sector	Pointed
Linear array	Electronic sequencing	Electronic	Mechanical	Rectangular	Flat
Curvilinear array	Electronic sequencing	Electronic	Mechanical	Trapezoidal	Curved
Phased array	Electronic steering	Electronic	Mechanical	Sector	Flat
Vector array	Electronic sequencing and steering	Electronic	Mechanical	Trapezoidal	Flat
Annular phased array	Mechanical	Electronic	Electronic	Sector	Pointed

Real-Time Ultrasound Instrumentation

9

Chapter Objectives

To understand various operational modes in real-time imaging
To describe the principle of receive-beam formation
To state the function of operator controls: power, gain, time gain compensation, scan range, freeze frame, and cine loop

Key terms

3D ultrasound
4D ultrasound
Cine loop
Coded excitation
Elastography

Extended field of view
Frequency averaging
Freeze frame
Nonlinear propagation
Phase aberration
Receive beam former

Spatial compounding
Tissue harmonic imaging (THI)
Transmit beam former
Voxel Zone sonography

OPERATIONAL MODES

Advances in real-time instrumentation (broadband frequency response, miniaturization of electronics, high-speed digital components, and increased sensitivity) have improved real-time image quality and led to the development of new scanning techniques, such as tissue harmonic imaging, coded excitation, extended field of view, elastography, zone sonography, spatial compounding, and volume scanning.

IMAGE ACQUISITION

B-mode image formation is a multiple step process, executed in real-time but dependent on operator input. Figure 9-1 is a block diagram of a B-mode scanner with a multiple-element transducer. For example, a scanner with 128 channels requires 128 pulsers, 128 transmit/receive switches, and 128 crystals in the array. High channel number improves beam steering/sequencing, focusing, and the spatial registration of the detected echo signals. Multiple operator controls allow optimization of the image to compensate for tissue variations among patients.

The transmit/receive switch is designed to isolate the sensitive receiver amplification stage from the high voltages associated with crystal excitation. On command by the transmitter and as directed by the transmit beam former, the pulsers generate short voltage oscillations, which are directed to the appropriate crystals within the array for beam formation. Beam formation in the transmit mode consists of both beam steering/sequencing and focusing, including aperture selection, generation of time delays, and apodization. The stimulated crystals generate an ultrasound pulse of short duration and send it into the body. During reception, the crystal elements convert the returning echoes from reflectors along the scan line to electronic signals that can subsequently be

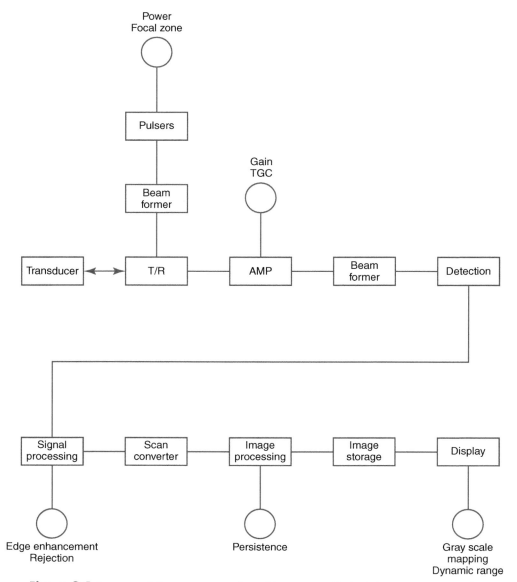

Figure 9-1 Image-acquisition components of a real-time scanner. Circles indicate operator controls.

processed and displayed. The processing sequence for the received signal is time gain compensation (TGC), gain, beam formation (receive mode), signal processing, scan conversion, image processing, image storage, and display.

TGC is variable gain applied as a function of elapsed time to compensate for attenuation caused by sound propagation through tissue. The amplifier increases the relatively weak induced signals for analog-to-digital conversion, which usually takes place in the receive beam former. It executes dynamic receive focusing of the detected echo across several crystal elements. The beam-sum signal is then modified by applying logarithmic compression and edge enhancement before envelope detection.

Scan data acquired line by line must be compiled in a 2D image format for viewing. This takes places in the scan converter, which is essentially an image matrix in computer memory. Finally, the digital signals in the scan converter

are communicated to the monitor for real-time display as a series of 2D images. Additional processing such as gray-scale mapping and persistence are applied to enhance the displayed image according to operator preference. Storage of a single image (freeze frame) or multiple images (cine loop) in a buffer allows prolonged viewing following acquisition.

Signal and image processing are discussed in more detail in the next chapter. Digital beam former, scan converter, operator controls, and system design are examined in the following sections.

RECEIVE BEAM FORMER

In the receive beam former, time gain-compensated radiofrequency signals from the crystals undergo analog-to-digital conversion before interpolation, time delay, apodization, and summing (Fig. 9-2). Interpolation increases

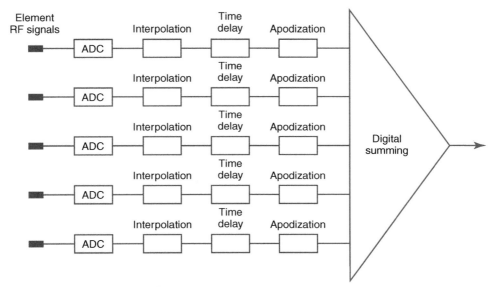

Figure 9-2 Digital receive beam former.

the effective sampling rate to allow nanosecond time delays for dynamic receive focusing. Channel-specific time delays are applied as a function of elapsed time and crystal position so that echoes from the receding transmitted pulse stay continuously in focus. Weighting of the channel signals (dynamic apodization) minimizes side-lobe intensity levels and enhances focusing.

In a hybrid design, analog processing of multiple channels with appropriate analog time delays occurs before digital conversion and beam summing. The reduced number of analog-to-digital converters lowers cost. In general, analog delay lines degrade beam former performance, resulting in limited accuracy and variations with time and temperature. Digital beam formers are more stable and offer greater flexibility.

IMAGE MATRIX

For the digitized representation of the echo signal to be placed at the correct location in the image matrix, the spatial coordinates (row and column) must be specified. This is accomplished by a position generator, which uses the time of travel for the ultrasound pulse and position sensors (single-element transducers) or element selection/phasing (multiple element arrays) for beam direction. The beam sweeps through the region of interest either electronically or mechanically in a repetitive fashion. The signal amplitude and position coordinates for multiple lines of sight are placed temporarily in the buffer before transfer to the scan converter. The format is changed from signal levels along successive lines of sight to the matrix notation, which forms a composite of all scan lines. The buffer also serves to hold the scan data acquired at a very rapid rate until the computer can store the information in memory.

OPERATOR CONTROLS

Several operator-adjustable controls are available to optimize the two-dimensional image. The most important instrument settings are scan range, transmit power, transmit focal zone, receiver gain, TGC, dynamic range (compression), edge enhancement, rejection, persistence, and gray scale map. Additional manipulation of the scan data may also be applied (as discussed in Chapter 10).

Transmission

The depth control sets the scan range for the field of view. Scan range also influences the frame rate and line density, which may not be under direct operator control.

The power control adjusts the intensity of the ultrasound beam transmitted into the patient. Power levels are commonly expressed in decibels or percentage (e.g., 0 dB or 100% indicates full power and −3 dB or 50% indicates half maximum power). Increased transmitted intensity improves the signal-to-noise ratio and enhances sensitivity (weak reflectors can be observed as shown in Fig. 9-3). On many scanners a change in the power setting is accompanied by an automatic commensurate adjustment of gain so that the overall image brightness remains constant.

The number and position of transmit focal zones can be selected by the operator to minimize the beam width at the depth of interest. Multiple transmit focal zones improve the lateral resolution throughout the field of view; however, the frame rate is generally reduced (Fig. 9-4).

Receiver Gain

Receiver gain modifies the amplification of signals during signal processing and often is expressed in decibels or in percentage. Noise and signal are amplified by the same

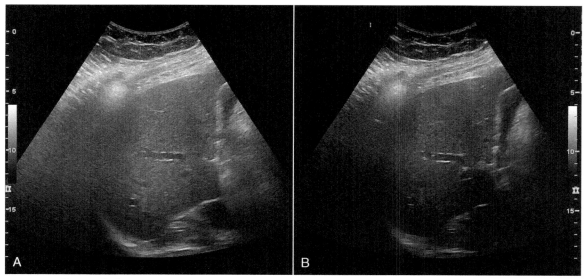

Figure 9-3 Effect of power setting in the acquisition of a sonogram of the liver. **A,** High power. **B,** Low power. Note the loss of weak tissue scatterers at a depth of 15 cm.

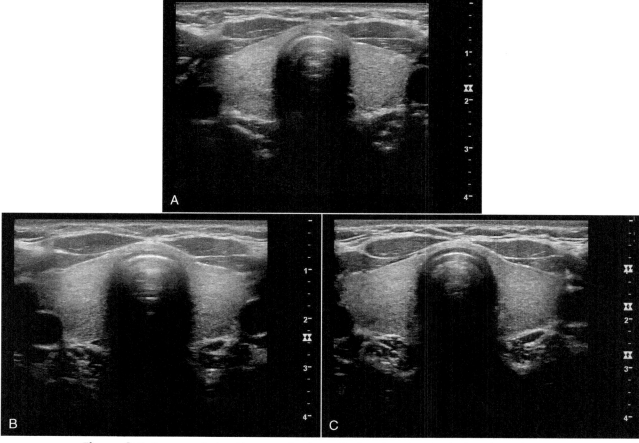

Figure 9-4 Illustration of selectable transmit focal zone. The hourglass along the depth markers indicate the transmit focal zones. **A,** Short focus. **B,** Medium focus. **C,** Multiple-zone focus.

amount and thus, the signal-to-noise ratio is unchanged by gain. Consequently gain is used to establish the proper brightness level for image display, but it generally does not improve the detection of weak reflectors.

Time Gain Compensation

Time gain compensation is also a type of receiver gain that is varied according to time delay to correct for attenuation along the beam path. Manual slide controls allow fine-tuning of depth amplification, but they must be readjusted when the depth of scanning or scan plane is changed.

Signal Processing

Because the scan converter and display device are unable to process the extremely wide dynamic range of echo-induced signal levels, compression is necessary. In general, the digitized signal levels are placed in an eight-bit scan converter. The range of values of the received signals after beam formation, however, may extend over four or more orders of magnitude. A logarithmic transformation of the signal levels is employed to compress the signal levels to a narrower range.

Ultrasound imaging is ideally suited to the detection of boundaries between structures. Edge enhancement is a filtering technique that can be applied to the line-of-sight data to further emphasize a change in signal level generated at tissue boundaries.

Rejection control, by accepting signals greater than a prescribed amplitude, reduces low-amplitude noise. Weak signals from scatterers along the scan line are also eliminated. In some circumstances acoustic noise exceeds the threshold value and contributes to the image.

Persistence

Persistence is a noise-reduction technique that applies temporal averaging to individual pixels. The operator selects the number of frames during which averaging is applied. Variations in noise at each pixel location tend to offset each other with time, whereas echo-induced signals tend to be reinforced. Fast-moving objects become blurred in the image when persistence is increased.

Freeze Frame

Real-time imaging depicts motion of moving interfaces, which is lost during freeze-frame display of one real-time image. The freeze-frame control allows the operator to select an image of interest for prolonged viewing. Scan data acquisition is discontinued while the freeze-frame option is activated.

Cine Loop

The cine loop function allows the operator to review a sequence of acquired images. Many frames (200 to 2000 or more, corresponding to an acquisition time of several seconds) can be stored in computer memory for immediate playback using the cine loop function. The rate of playback can be adjusted to coincide with or deviate from the real-time acquisition rate. The slow-motion (frame-by-frame) review capability allows the sonographer to select an appropriate image for study as well as hard-copy recording if desired.

SYNTHETIC APERTURE

Lateral resolution is improved as the number of processing channels is increased. A linear array can easily contain several hundred elements. However, it is expensive to maintain a dedicated processing channel for each element. The number of channels in the receive beam former can be reduced to half the number of elements if a two-pulse sequence is used for transmission-reception (synthetic aperture). Half the elements participate in receive-beam formation following the first transmit pulse and form a series of echo-induced signals along the scan line. These scan data are stored and delayed until the echo-induced signals from the second transmit pulse are similarly acquired and processed by the beam former. The two sets of echo data are then combined (Fig. 9-5). The high crystal number is maintained with the synthetic aperture for excellent lateral resolution, but the time for image composition is increased.

MULTIPLE BEAM FORMERS

All the previous discussions regarding beam formation and transmit focusing have emphasized that the maximum sampling rate is one scan line per transmitted pulse. Multiple beam formers now provide the ability to acquire multiple scan lines per transmitted pulse (up to four). The width of the transmission beam is expanded to include an area that would be sampled by multiple scan lines. Dynamic receive focusing of the returning echoes by each of the different beam formers permits the transmitted beam width to be subdivided into smaller effective beam widths. Each beam former then contributes one scan line to the image. An example of parallel beam formation is illustrated in Figure 9-6.

Multiple scan-line generation per transmitted pulse reduces the acquisition time per frame and can increase frame rate. Alternatively, lateral resolution can be improved by increasing scan line density. Parallel processing with multiple beam formers in transmit mode using multiple focal zones can also improve lateral resolution without a loss in frame rate.

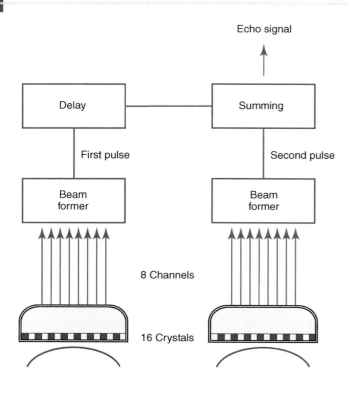

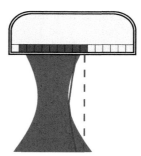

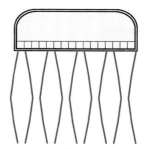

Figure 9-7 The receive scan line *(dotted line)* with multiple beam formers is offset from the transmitted beam. The effective sampling path *(solid line)* is a curved combination of the transmitted beam width and receive aperture.

Figure 9-5 Synthetic aperture. The number of channels is half of the number of crystals. Radiofrequency signals from two transmitted pulses are summed to compose the received focused echo signal along one line of sight.

Figure 9-8 Scan-line geometry for multiple beam formers. Nonparallel scan lines compose the image.

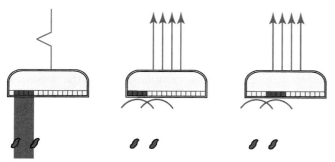

Figure 9-6 Multiple beam formers permit multiple receive scan lines for each transmitted pulse. The transmitted beam extends over several crystals. Echoes from reflectors at the same depth strike the array at different center points. Two receive apertures of four crystals each acquire data along different lines of sight. An independent time delay for each aperture focuses the signal along the respective scan line.

COHERENT IMAGE FORMATION

Multiple receive-beam formation from a single excitation creates a subtle geometric distortion. The narrow receive focusing and the more broad transmission beam do not share a common axis but rather are offset from one another. The net effect is that sampling along the scan line is curved (Fig. 9-7). Mapping of the echoes in the image

matrix assumes parallel scan lines. Image composition with curved scan lines degrades spatial detail (Fig. 9-8).

Coherent image formation corrects scan-line curvature by manipulating the sampling data from multiple receive-beam formers to compile synthetic straight scan lines. The time-varying summed signal from each beam former is retained and assembled in two dimensions. Coherent image processing includes both axial data along individual scan lines and lateral data from adjacent scan lines. Since time-varying information is used, this technique is often described with the term *phase*.

The echo amplitudes for a pair of oppositely curved interrogation lines are averaged, depth-by-depth, to produce the fabricated radiofrequency signal along the synthetic line (Fig. 9-9). This processing occurs before rectification and enveloping and is a good approximation for the signal that would have been obtained for a straight scan line located midway between the acquired curved scan lines.

Any phase change between the pair of interrogation lines caused by beam steering or aperture must be corrected before averaging. The same method of delay and summing of radiofrequency signals used in beam formation also applies. Since processing includes spatial phase information, accurate echo signal data in the lateral dimension are possible.

PHASE ABERRATION

Beam forming applies time delays based on geometric considerations (path-length differences from point of focus to the respective elements) and an assumed constant acoustic

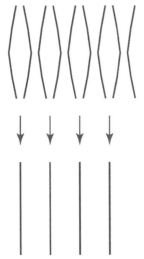

Figure 9-9 Curved scan lines are acquired across the field of view. Lines with opposite curvature are paired and combined to form a synthetic scan line. The synthetic scan lines are used to compose the image.

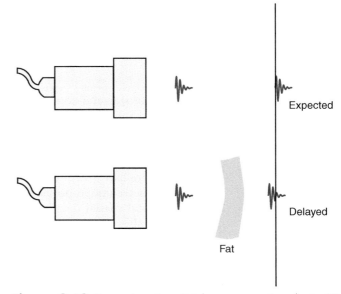

Figure 9-10 Phase aberration. Fat has an acoustic velocity 8% slower than that of soft tissue. Fat along the beam path causes a delay compared with the anticipated arrival time based on a uniform path of soft tissue only.

velocity. However, acoustic velocity in tissue can differ from 1460 m/s in fat to 1665 m/s in collagen. If the tissue velocity is not uniform along the path, as when fat is present near the skin layer, the ultrasound pulse arrives at a later time than expected (Fig. 9-10). This delay causes a loss of signal coherence during beam formation, which is called phase aberration (Fig. 9-11). Phase aberration reduces the signal-to-noise ratio and degrades sensitivity. Correction for phase aberration is performed by adjusting the time delay applied independently to each crystal in the active aperture of a multiple element transducer.

BROADBAND TECHNIQUES

Real-time units with limited bandwidth have relatively poor axial resolution and cannot perform signal and image processing based on frequency information. Broadband transducers provide flexibility in operation such that image acquisition parameters can be changed during scanning. As the frequency bandwidth becomes wider, the possibility of matching optimal image acquisition parameters with the desired clinical information is

improved. Broadband techniques include multifrequency imaging, confocal imaging, dynamic frequency filtering, and frequency compounding.

MULTIFREQUENCY IMAGING

In multifrequency imaging the available broad bandwidth is subdivided into two or more frequency ranges for transmission and reception of sound waves. The operator selects the center frequency appropriate for the examination. The high-frequency portion provides the best spatial detail. The low-frequency portion affords maximum tissue penetration. An intermediate-frequency bandwidth between these two extremes is also possible.

The outcome of multifrequency imaging with different center frequencies is the same as if three independent transducers were supplied within the same housing. The distinct advantage is one of convenience in that one variable-frequency transducer views the patient's anatomy

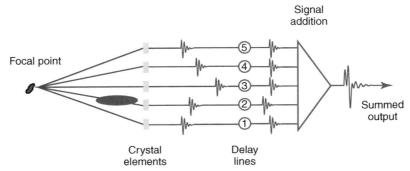

Figure 9-11 Loss of signal coherence in beam formation when phase aberration is present.

while the center frequency is adjusted. The optimal frequency range can be selected without losing the clinical point of interest in the scan plane.

CONFOCAL IMAGING

Confocal imaging is an extension of transmit-zone focusing, except that each transmit focal zone is formed with a different center frequency. In this imaging scheme the available broad transmit bandwidth is split into multiple frequency ranges. Multiple small transmit bandwidths with different center frequencies are used to collect echo data along each line of sight. This technique provides a very narrow beam width with good spatial detail at all depths. Since multiple transmit pulses are necessary for each line of sight, the frame rate generally decreases.

DYNAMIC FREQUENCY FILTERING

Dynamic frequency filtering uses the total transducer bandwidth for the transmitted pulse and then adjusts the receiver center frequency and bandwidth to lower frequencies as deeper depths are sampled. Since tissue attenuation is frequency dependent (higher frequencies are absorbed more rapidly), a frequency shift occurs as the ultrasound wave propagates through tissue. The center frequency and bandwidth of the echo decrease as the depth increases. By continuously and automatically matching the receiver with the frequency characteristics of the detected echo based on elapsed time, this technique provides additional focusing at various depths and improved noise reduction.

High-definition imaging can alter the transmitted bandwidth depending on the scanning range in conjunction with dynamic frequency filtering. High-frequency components may be eliminated in the transmitted pulse to extend the depth of penetration. Lateral resolution at shallow depths is improved by removal of the low-frequency components.

FREQUENCY COMPOUNDING

If the bandwidth of the receiver is matched with that of the transmitter, then during reception the short echo pressure variations can be faithfully converted into radiofrequency signals with broad bandwidth. In frequency compounding (or frequency averaging) the echo frequency spectrum is subdivided into frequency bands by filters, processed separately, and then recombined to form a composite image. The summing of frequency images can be adjusted to emphasize penetration, resolution, or tissue texture. A common application is acoustic noise reduction to improve contrast resolution.

SPATIAL COMPOUNDING

The amplitude of the echo-induced signal depends on the angle of incidence and the geometry of the boundary. Normal incidence maximizes the intensity of the reflected echo. During the examination the sonographer reorients the transducer, changing the relative beam direction with respect to an interface to maximize the reflectivity from a particular interface. In so doing, however, the less favorable beam orientation for other reflectors throughout the field of view causes their respective signals to be decreased. Spatial compounding, by acquiring multiple beam angles and averaging the data, reduces acoustic noise while improving border definition of specular reflectors. Manufacturer's descriptors of this technique include *sonoCT* and *cross beam*.

An array with a high number of elements and channels is required. A group of elements is stimulated to steer the beam at a specific angle. The active aperture is moved along the length of the array until all scan lines with that beam angle are obtained. The procedure is repeated three to seven times for different beam angles. One frame of the field of view is acquired at each beam angle. The steering angles may range ±20 degrees. Figures 9-12 and 9-13 illustrate the sampling for three beam angles.

Spatial averaging of the frames is accomplished in real time with no loss of frame rate. Figure 9-14 shows a sequence of sampled frames using three distinct beam angles. The displayed image is an average of the three most recently acquired frames. In this manner the displayed image is always composed of pixels insonated from multiple directions. Since the displayed image is refreshed when a new frame is obtained, no reduction in frame rate occurs.

A wideband transducer is necessary to lower the center frequency for large angle steering in order to reduce grating lobes. The fully compounded region does not occupy the entire field of view; the scan lines for all beam angles

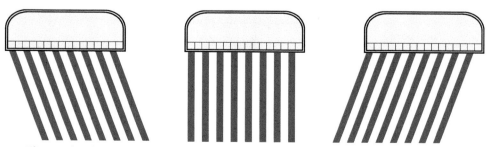

Figure 9-12 Spatial compounding with the transmitted beams oriented at three different angles.

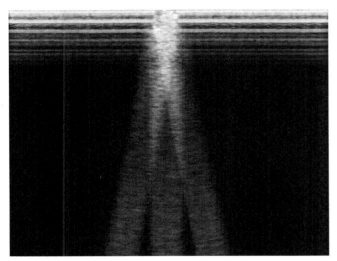

Figure 9-13 B-mode visualization of the transmitted beams oriented at three different angles.

do not overlap at the periphery, which becomes more pronounced with depth. In this case the displayed image is formed on scan data from a reduced number of beam angles. The extent of the fully compounded region depends on system design considerations including the number of elements, transmitted frequency, distance between elements, width of the spacing between elements, and element angular response.

A weighted average of the scan lines is necessary to compensate for differences in amplitude caused by sensitivity variation in the angular response of the elements, differences in aperture, and changes in center frequency. Maximum amplitude detection from all scan lines at each pixel may be used as an alternative to averaging, but noise reduction is diminished.

Spatial compounding improves the depiction of tissue boundaries and reduces noise variations (Fig. 9-15). Shadowing from strong reflectors and enhancement from

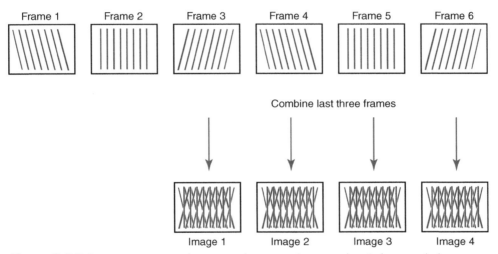

Figure 9-14 Frame composition and averaging during spatial compounding. In this example the previous two frames are combined with the current frame to compose the displayed image.

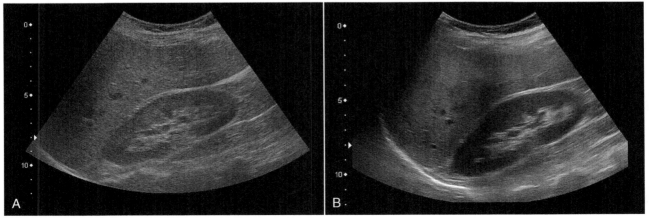

Figure 9-15 Sonogram of the kidney. **A,** No spatial compounding. **B,** Spatial compounding.

weak reflectors are less pronounced. Increasing the number of angles of insonification amplifies the compounding effect. However, since the sampling occurs over more frames, the potential for motion blur also increases.

EXTENDED FIELD OF VIEW

The advantages of real-time ultrasound include excellent temporal resolution (high frame rate), focusing using multiple element arrays, and freedom to position the transducer. However, static B-mode enabled a large anatomic region to be displayed in a single image. Real-time field of view is limited by transducer width (linear array) or sector scanning angle (mechanical sector, annular phased array, phased array, curvilinear array). To establish spatial relationships throughout a large region, the sonographer must often acquire several small field-of-view frames and then compose a mental picture of the anatomy.

Real-time ultrasound with extended field of view attempts to overcome this limitation by combining successive frames to form a panoramic image as the transducer is moved across the patient. The field of view of the panoramic image is larger than the field of view of a single real-time frame and can be generated in real time. An alternative method acquires real-time images in a cine clip and then processes the successive frames to form the panoramic image. Sonograms of a placenta and a neck acquired with extended field of view are shown in Figures 9-16 and 9-17.

In static B-mode, lines of sight are mapped in the image based upon the location and orientation of the transducer. The positional information is obtained by sensors in the articulating arm after a reference point has been defined. The presence of position-sensing devices inhibits flexibility. Extended field-of-view real-time imaging employs computer analysis of image features to determine transducer location without sensors or an articulating arm.

Image Registration

As the transducer is moved slowly across the patient, individual frames are obtained at a rapid rate (15 to 20 frames per second). Sequential frames have many common image

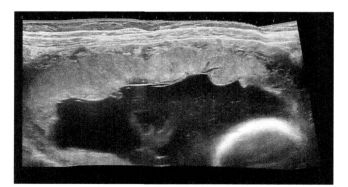

Figure 9-16 Sonogram of a placenta obtained with extended field of view.

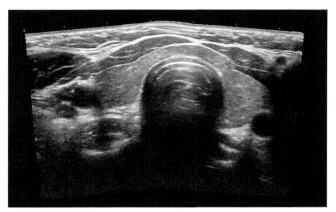

Figure 9-17 Sonogram of a human neck obtained with extended field of view.

features, because much of the anatomy examined by each frame is the same. The overlapping region for two frames acquired sequentially as the linear array is translated to the right is shown in Figure 9-18. Each frame is depicted individually in Figure 9-19; then the frames are superimposed on one another, as shown in Figure 9-20. Examination of the superimposed image identifies the club and triangle as common image features, which have moved linearly right to left from the first to the second frame (direction opposite to the motion of the transducer). The speed of the transducer movement determines the magnitude of the displacement of common image features.

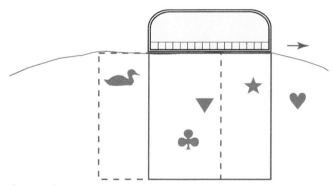

Figure 9-18 Multiple frames are obtained as a linear array moves across the patient. The first frame is denoted by the dashed-line border. The second frame is denoted by the solid-line border.

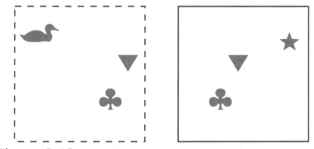

Figure 9-19 Image features present in each frame acquired in Figure 9-18.

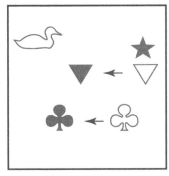

Figure 9-20 Individual frames in Figure 9-19 superimposed on one another. Structures in the first frame are denoted by the solid-line outline of the geometric shape. Arrows indicate the change in position of common image features.

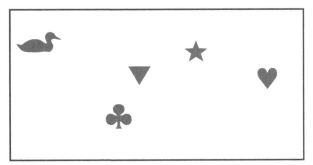

Figure 9-21 Extended field of view of scan data acquired in Figure 9-18.

By measuring the geometric shift and rotation of common image features, the motion of the probe can be established. Once the probe motion is known, each successive frame can then be registered with respect to all previous frames that form the panoramic image. Figure 9-21 depicts the extended field of view as the probe is moved across the region shown in Figure 9-18.

Computer matching of image features in successive frames is accomplished by dividing the most recently acquired frame into blocks and then searching the prior frame for a region with similar properties corresponding to an individual block. The search initiates at the location of the block and proceeds radially outward. The change in position of the common image features is small if the sampling rate is rapid and tissue motion is minimal. The matching region is expected to be near the block location and thus is the logical point at which to begin the search. Parallel processing allows multiple blocks to be analyzed simultaneously, which reduces the time to register the frame.

Each block is assigned a motion vector based on matching with the reference image. A map of local motion (velocity) vectors is created. If the probe moves linearly, as illustrated in Figure 9-18, image feature displacements are in the same direction and at the same distance throughout the superimposed frames. However, a curved body surface would cause the probe to rotate as it is moved across the patient. If the probe translates and rotates,

the image feature displacements change with depth. Image feature displacements are not the same for all blocks throughout the velocity map. The difference in local motion vectors near the top versus near the bottom of the velocity map allows determination of the overall probe motion. The current frame is translated and rotated to properly position the image data within the panoramic image.

The extended field of view composed in real time has both real-time and static components. The real-time component advances with the probe motion and shows the anatomy currently being imaged. The static component displays the anatomy that has been scanned. Using Figure 9-18 as an example, the extended field-of-view image combines frames left to right as the probe advances, but the right side portion displays the current real-time image. All frames used to compose the extended field-of-view image are placed in cine buffer so that the individual frames may be viewed.

The fidelity of registration process is corrupted by actions that reduce image feature similarity. The primary factors that can cause artifacts are large-scale tissue motion and off-plane rotation. Tissue motion contributes to the displacement of common image features and results in improper registration of the current frame. Off-plane rotation shifts the imaging plane at an angle into or out of the plane of the reference image. The sampled anatomic region is changed, which eliminates common image features. Small-scale off-plane rotation inherent in freehand scanning is usually tolerated in extended field-of-view imaging.

CODED EXCITATION

Coded excitation employs long waveforms during transmission to improve the signal-to-noise ratio, penetration, or both. Two common methods to encode the transmitted waveform are frequency modulation and binary encoding. Since the total transmission time is 20 μs or longer, axial resolution would be poor unless the received signal induced by the echo wavetrain were manipulated mathematically to identify the reflectors along the beam path. The processing determines reflector location and reflectivity of the interface. These decoding techniques are described as matched filtration or deconvolution.

Binary Encoding

The applied voltage for a single transmitted pulse is represented by a square wave in the voltage waveform. These binary-coded pulses now comprise the burst during transmission (Fig. 9-22). Coded burst transmission for B-mode imaging is composed of 8 to 22 separate pulses, each with a specified intensity. The binary code in Figure 9-22 is described as 200301.

The transmission burst has a known binary-coded sequence. Each reflector along the scan line produces a

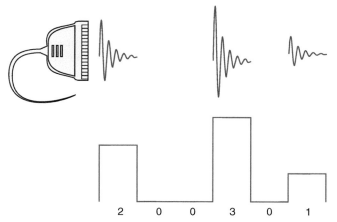

Figure 9-22 Transmit pulse burst formation in coded excitation. A 200301 coded sequence is depicted.

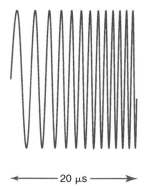

$\longleftarrow$ 20 µs $\longrightarrow$

Figure 9-23 Frequency-modulated transmitted pulse in coded excitation. The frequency increases during transmission time. Pulse duration is 20 µs.

similarly coded sequence in the echo wavetrain. Long-duration echoes from nearby reflectors overlap one another. The time-varying, echo-induced signal is analyzed (in a process called deconvolution) for the coded pattern to yield a short, well-defined echo of a few cycles for each reflector. This would correspond to the echo-induced signal if a conventional short-duration transmission pulse of less than 1 microsecond were used.

Sometimes the reverse process is easier to understand. Suppose there are two reflectors separated by a few centimeters along the beam path. During echo ranging with a short-duration pulse, each reflector generates a short-duration echo, which is separated in time in the echo wavetrain. If a binary-encoded burst were to replace the short-duration transmitted pulse, each echo would be similarly elongated by the same coded sequence and the echoes could easily overlap. Mathematically, if each reflector location were replaced by the coded sequence, the echo wavetrain during reception would be obtained. Fortunately mathematical techniques and knowledge of the transmitted coded sequence allow the processing of the echo wavetrain to identify the individual reflector components without prior knowledge of the reflectors along the beam path.

Frequency Modulation

Frequency modulation of the transmitted pulse is achieved by varying the emitted frequency with time (Fig. 9-23). Imagine that the initial transmitted frequency is at the lower limit of the bandwidth and is subsequently increased linearly with time. This creates a long-duration pulse, but all frequency components within the bandwidth are contained in the pulse. If transmission of each frequency is matched in time (e.g., time offset is equal to zero), the traditional short duration pulse is obtained. In this method frequency is used to encode the pulse. Upon reception, the frequency encoding is removed to time-compress the waveform. This is accomplished by the

convolution of the received signal with the time-reversed transmitted pulse. Axial resolution does not depend on the duration of the chirp pulse but rather on the fractional bandwidth. Since the transmitted pulse is composed of all frequencies throughout the bandwidth, axial resolution is maintained.

Compared with traditional echo ranging, more energy per unit time without higher peak intensity is present in the coded waveform. This is the source of the improvement in signal-to-noise ratio. Since the spatial pulse length is 3 cm for a 20-microsecond pulse duration, image formation at shallow depths less than 1.5 cm is compromised. Traditional echo ranging is more appropriate for superficial structures. Artifacts in the form of repeating echoes from strong reflectors are sometimes encountered. Side lobes are a major consideration and can be reduced by proper weighting of each frequency and the window function (range of frequencies) in pulse formation.

ZONE SONOGRAPHY

The serial format of the line-by-line acquisition for conventional B-mode imaging imposes a time constraint for image formation and thereby limits the frame rate. Transit time for a scan line is fixed by the path length and acoustic velocity, and each scan line with a single receive beam former requires at least one pulse/receive cycle. In zone sonography the acquisition time for a frame is greatly reduced by sampling with a broad transmit beam. A large portion of the field of view is interrogated with each transmit pulse and thus few pulse/receive cycles (20 or less) are required to complete a frame acquisition (Fig. 9-24).

Following each transmitted pulse the echo-induced signals for every crystal element across the array are retained in a buffer (Fig. 9-25). Computer processing of the channel data by a method called iterative reconstruction allows the spatial registration of reflectors within the field of view. Essentially, an estimation of reflector positions and strengths is made initially and then their calculated echo pattern is compared with the measured echo signals. The differences prescribe adjustments to the 2D image and

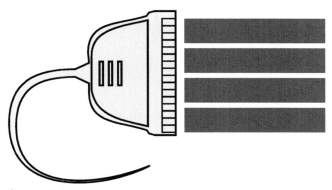

Figure 9-24 Zone sonography. Scanning across the entire field of view is accomplished by four wide transmit beams.

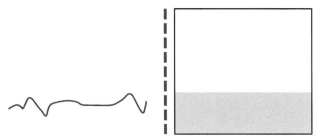

Figure 9-25 Each crystal detects and stores the echo wavetrain during the receive period for one transmit pulse. The time-varying signal for one channel is shown.

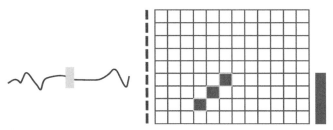

Figure 9-26 The composite signal at any point in time (gray area of channel signal) is a sum of echo signals originating at specific locations (red boxes) within the transmit beam (4 channels wide).

the process is repeated multiple times. At any time segment the net signal for a particular element is a combination of the echo-induced signals from well-defined locations (Fig. 9-26). Contributions are restricted to those locations in which the total path length for the transmit pulse and the returning echo are the same. Since crystals across the array make several measurements of the same spatial point during each transmission, a two-dimensional image of reflectors can be formed. The reconstruction time is short (5–10 milliseconds), and thus high frame rates are now possible (100 to 200 frames per second). Transmit focusing is not applied in zone sonography.

TISSUE HARMONIC IMAGING

Tissue harmonic imaging (THI) is an imaging technique that relies on the detection of the harmonic frequencies created by beam propagation through tissue. Even though

the detected signal is weaker than traditional echo ranging, contrast is often improved by the suppression of interfering signals from clutter (multiangle scattering).

Nonlinear Propagation

Under conditions of relatively high pressure amplitude, the speed of the sound wave (c) is not constant but varies over the propagation path (z):

$$9\text{-}1 \qquad c(z) = c_o + \left(1 + \frac{B}{2A}\right)u(z)$$

where c_o is the average acoustic velocity in the medium, $c(z)$ is the acoustic velocity at a point along the propagation path, $u(z)$ is the particle velocity at that point, and $(1 + B/2A)$ is the coefficient of nonlinearity. Equation 9-1 shows that the acoustic velocity at each point over the waveform is modulated by the particle velocity. Further, this contribution to wave velocity also depends on the medium via the ratio B/2A.

During the compressional phase particle velocity is positive, and the speed of sound increases during this portion of the wave cycle. However, particle velocity is negative during the rarefaction phase, and the speed of sound decreases (Fig. 9-27). Consequently, because the speed of sound is not constant during the wave cycle, the sinusoidal shape becomes distorted as the wave propagates through the medium (Fig. 9-28).

The distortion in the sound waveform at high intensity can be illustrated by a ball attached to a spring. If the ball is moved a small distance from the equilibrium position, the spring compresses. When released, the ball oscillates back and forth with relatively smooth sinusoidal motion (Fig. 9-29). If, on the other hand, the spring is compressed as much as possible before releasing the ball, the ball initially moves at very high velocity through the equilibrium position and then slows markedly as the spring is stretched. The sinusoidal motion becomes distorted (Fig. 9-30).

The change in shape from sinusoidal to saw-tooth corresponds to a change in frequency components of the sound wave. As shown in Fig. 9-31, energy is transferred from the fundamental frequency (f_o) to harmonic

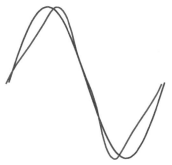

Figure 9-27 During nonlinear propagation particle velocity varies during compression (speeds up) and rarefaction (slows down) causing distortion of the particle density waveform (red line) compared with that from linear propagation (blue line).

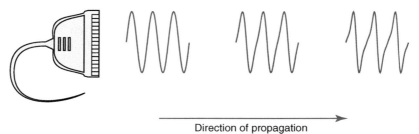

Figure 9-28 Nonlinear propagation distorts the sinusoidal waveform. The effect becomes more pronounced with depth.

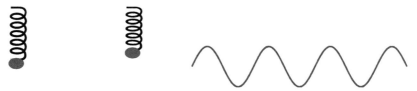

Figure 9-29 A ball connected to a spring exhibits smooth sinusoidal motion if the ball is displaced a small amount and released. The waveform shows the displacement of the ball versus time.

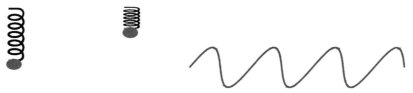

Figure 9-30 Example of nonlinear propagation. When the spring is compressed completely before the ball is released, the initial fast movement is slowed considerably as the spring is stretched. The waveform shows the displacement of the ball versus time.

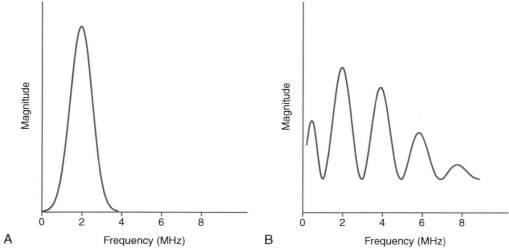

Figure 9-31 Frequency spectrum of the transmitted pulse at the transducer (**A**) and after a path length of a few centimeters (**B**).

frequencies (integral multiples of the fundamental frequency, such as $2f_o$, $3f_o$). If the fundamental frequency (also called first harmonic) is 2 MHz, then the next multiple or second harmonic is 4 MHz. As *the sound wave propagates through the medium, harmonic components intensify, and the waveform becomes more distorted.* Attenuation causes the fundamental frequency sound wave to lose pressure amplitude and revert to linear propagation. Energy is no longer transferred to the harmonic frequencies.

Meanwhile, the high-frequency harmonics are very rapidly attenuated in the medium (Figs. 9-32 and 9-33). Nonlinear propagation due to the high-frequency components exhibits more rapid pressure amplitude loss than predicted by the attenuation equation.

At present, the relatively weak amplitudes of the third and higher harmonics limit tissue harmonic imaging to the detection of the second harmonic. The amplitude of the second harmonic (p_2) depends on the acoustic pressure (p),

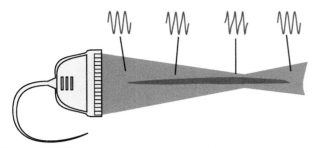

Figure 9-32 Harmonics are present in the central portion of the transmitted beam but offset from the transducer face.

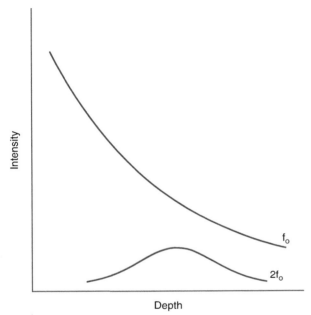

Figure 9-33 Relative intensity of the fundamental frequency and second harmonic frequency as a function of distance from the transducer.

frequency (f), nonlinearity coefficient, density of the medium (ρ), acoustic velocity (c), and the distance of propagation (z):

9-2
$$p^2 = \left(1 + \frac{B}{2A}\right)\left(\frac{\pi f}{\rho c^3}\right)zp^2$$

The sound wave must propagate a few centimeters in the medium before a transfer in energy to the second harmonic can occur. Little pulse distortion is present near the transducer, and this region is free of harmonics. A further increase in depth enhances harmonic production. High-intensity sound beams via the squared relation between acoustic pressure and second harmonic formation produce large harmonic components.

Two methods, harmonic band filtering and pulse phase inversion, are used in tissue harmonic imaging to isolate the second harmonic component and form the image. The intensity of the second harmonic is 10 to 20 dB lower than the fundamental. A low-noise, wide dynamic range receiver is necessary to preserve the relatively weak signal.

Harmonic Band Filtering

An object within the ultrasonic field where the second harmonic is present will be interrogated by both the fundamental frequency and the harmonic frequency. Harmonics are created as a result of propagation through tissue and are not produced upon reflection. (An exception to this statement is microbubble contrast agents, which scatter sound at harmonic frequencies.) The returning echo and thus the detected signals have a fundamental frequency component and a harmonic frequency component (Fig. 9-34). The propagation of echoes at relatively low intensity does not generate additional harmonic components. *A filter is applied to remove the fundamental echo signal, and only the tissue harmonic component is processed for image formation.*

The fundamental and harmonic bands should not overlap. The transmitted pulse must be carefully shaped and controlled to prevent high-frequency components within the harmonic region. If these high frequencies are present, they give rise to echoes of the same frequency (including noise and clutter), and the purity of the harmonic component generated from native tissue is corrupted. To separate the fundamental and harmonic bands, a narrow transmission bandwidth is formed by elongating the transmission pulse. This may degrade the axial resolution, but the increased detection frequency of the second harmonic compensates to some extent for the longer transmitted spatial pulse length.

Pulse Phase Inversion

A two-pulse sequence is transmitted along the same path in which the second pulse is shifted 180 degrees in phase. The echo-induced signal from the first pulse is stored until the signal from the second pulse is received. The received

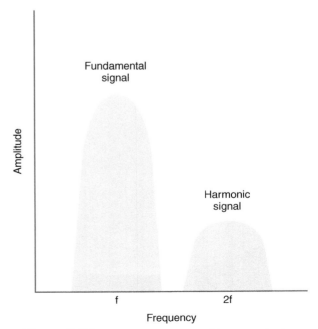

Figure 9-34 Frequency components of the received echo.

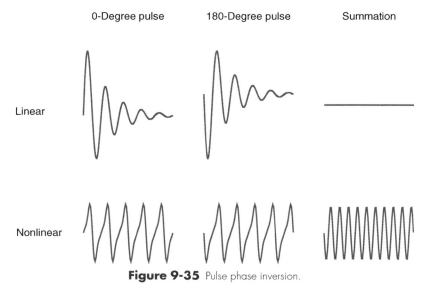

0-Degree pulse   180-Degree pulse   Summation

Linear

Nonlinear

Figure 9-35 Pulse phase inversion.

signals from each transmitted pulse are then summed. For linear propagation, the two received signals have the same amplitude but an 180-degree phase difference and cancel completely when summed. If nonlinear propagation occurs, harmonics are added in the same proportion to each waveform following transmission. The received signals are not identical in amplitude and produce the harmonic component when summed (Fig. 9-35). Note that the summed result has a frequency that is two times the fundamental frequency. Signal-to-noise ratio is thus increased, since the measurements of the harmonic signal are doubled. Because filtering is not used to isolate the harmonic frequencies, broadband transmitted pulses with short spatial pulse length preserve axial resolution. However, the multiple pulse technique requires longer sampling/processing time and is subject to motion artifacts.

Advantages of Tissue Harmonic Imaging

Clutter, grating lobes, and side lobes are generated at the fundamental frequency. Echoes from these sources are also at the fundamental frequency and are suppressed in the tissue harmonic image. Multiple scattering produces low amplitude sound waves, which do not form harmonics. Subcutaneous fat, particularly in large patients, defocuses the beam and masks the signals from deep-lying structures. The reduction of acoustic noise from these sources enhances contrast resolution and border delineation (Fig. 9-36). The detection and characterization of low-contrast solid lesions are improved. Acoustic enhancement and shadowing are more easily demonstrated. Liquid cavities are depicted with less fill-in.

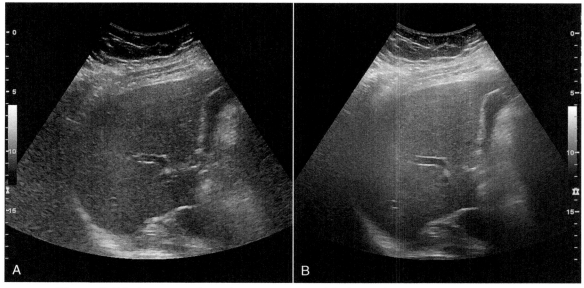

Figure 9-36 Comparison of tissue harmonic imaging with fundamental imaging. Sonograms of the liver obtained at 4 MHz. **A,** Fundamental. **B,** Harmonic. Note the improved image contrast with tissue harmonic imaging.

Reverberation artifacts are reduced. Echoes in general do not generate harmonics because of their low amplitude. The harmonic content of reverberation echoes is established by the transmission path to the target and is consequently much lower than that present in tissue echoes of equal transit time.

High acoustic pressure occurs near the main beam axis and within the focal zone. This is the source of harmonic production. The width of the harmonic beam is effectively narrower than the main beam at the fundamental frequency. Reduced beam width improves lateral resolution.

The overall penetration in tissue harmonic imaging is less than that obtainable in the conventional mode at the fundamental frequency because of higher attenuation rates for harmonics. The penalty is not as severe as anticipated, since harmonics travel only a portion of the total path length. Often, the fundamental frequency is lowered to image deep-lying structures. If visualized, these structures are depicted with greater contrast and spatial detail.

HIGH-FREQUENCY IMAGING

Transducers operating at a center frequency above 10 MHz are very desirable to improve spatial resolution. A 20-MHz transducer has achieved an axial resolution of 100 microns and a lateral resolution of 300 microns. The major concern is the ability to obtain good penetration, since beam intensity is rapidly reduced by attenuation. High sensitivity by suppressing noise and expanding the dynamic range is required. The maximum imaging frequency is limited by the digitization rate according to the Nyquist sampling theorem. The Nyquist limit for frequency is equal to half of the sampling rate. For a 20-MHz transducer the analog-to-digital converter must operate at 40 MHz.

High-frequency imaging at frequencies above 10 MHz is now routinely performed for superficial organs including muscles, tendons, breasts, thyroids, and testicles (Fig. 9-37). A scan range of several centimeters is possible. Applications in dermatology and ophthalmology, where

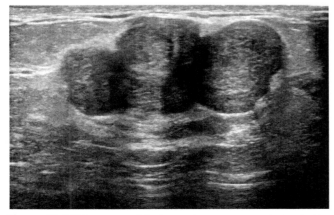

Figure 9-37 Sonogram of the breast showing a mass obtained with a center frequency of 15 MHz.

the scan range is a few millimeters, can be expanded to higher frequencies.

THREE-DIMENSIONAL IMAGING

In 3D imaging the spatial relationships of structures within a scanned volume are represented by an image or a set of images. Following data collection, echo information is processed for display as a static image. Real-time scanning of the tissue volume is called 4D imaging and is discussed in the following section.

Limitations of Real-Time Scanning

In 2D imaging, the sonographer must mentally form a 3D impression of the anatomy from a series of acquired B-mode images. This process is time consuming, subjective, and inconsistent. Depending on operator proficiency, spatial relationships are often distorted or misrepresented.

Patient management decisions often rely on measurements of organ or tumor volume. Real-time B-mode imaging provides an accurate measurement of area within the scan plane, but in order to project the structure into three dimensions for the calculation of volume, some idealized shape must be assumed. This technique is potentially inaccurate if the organ/tumor shape deviates from the projected outline. Also, monitoring of therapeutic regimens often requires repeated measurements, separated by long time intervals, of the same 2D image plane placed in the same location.

Acquisition Methods

Most 3D ultrasound systems acquire a series of 2D B-mode images throughout the volume of interest. The 2D images are most often arranged in a set of parallel slices. The position and orientation of the transducer for each 2D image must be accurately known to avoid geometric distortions in the 3D image. Mechanical and freehand scanning methods have been developed to sample the volume of interest. An alternative approach is to use a 2D array transducer, which acquires the 3D data set without moving the transducer.

The most common approach employs a phased array mounted in a mechanical assembly within the scan head that is translated linearly over the patient's surface. The 2D images are acquired parallel to one another and at well-defined intervals. Since the scanning geometry is known, short reconstruction time is possible. The mechanical translation of the crystals is along the elevation direction of the phased array.

In freehand scanning, the transducer is moved manually across the patient without any position sensing device. The transducer movement must be uniform and conform to the predefined scanning geometry. Deviations from the assumed scanning motion introduce geometric distortion in the reconstructed volume. This technique is limited to qualitative assessment, since measurements of distance, area, and volume are generally not accurate.

An alternative approach is to use a rectangular-array (2D or matrix) transducer. Ultrasound beam sampling direction is electronically controlled with the appropriate crystal-firing sequence. Parallel processing reduces sampling time. Matrix arrays offer the potential for data collection in orthogonal planes.

Image Reconstruction

The most common method to form the 3D volume data set is voxel-based reconstruction. A voxel is a 3D picture element with length, width, and thickness. The dimensions in each direction are not necessarily the same. Each pixel in the set of 2D images is placed at the proper location within the volume. If a voxel was not sampled by a 2D, the value for that voxel is calculated by interpolation using the values from neighboring voxels.

The original data set of 2D images is preserved. That is, if the appropriate plane in the 3D volume is selected, then the acquired 2D image can be displayed. Additionally, other views not present in the set of acquired 2D images can be displayed. Since these additional views depend on interpolation of the sampling data set, a distance greater than one half of the elevational thickness between 2D images degrades spatial resolution and misrepresents anatomy.

To adequately sample the tissue volume, large data files are generated. A single 3D scan of the liver may require 16 MB but may increase to as much as 512 MB for imaging the heart through the cardiac cycle. Other scanning modes such as power Doppler further enlarge the storage requirements.

Image Display

After reconstruction, the 3D volume is viewed interactively using computer graphics. The 3D volume contains massive quantities of data that cannot be viewed all at once. Information must be extracted from the volume data set and then displayed. The process of selecting and manipulating data for visualization is called rendering. Three types of rendering form 3D images for display: multiplanar formatting, surface rendering, and volume rendering.

Multiplanar Reformatting

The 3D data set is composed of voxels that are stacked together as a pile of bricks. Similar to isolating the bricks that comprise one layer, the operator can view a single plane in the 3D volume. Imagine that the pile of bricks can be cut in any orientation and a single layer of bricks extracted. Following their removal, another single layer of bricks with the same orientation but one layer offset from the first is extracted. The 3D volume can be rotated so that the operator can view its contents along any line of sight. Once the line of sight is established, the visualized

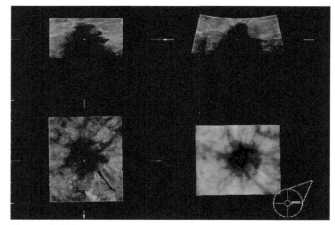

Figure 9-38 3D multiformat. Three orthogonal planes through the breast with a mass are displayed.

2D images are formed using one layer of voxels in the plane perpendicular to this line of sight. In this manner successive parallel plane images are generated at equal intervals along the operator's line of sight, and the operator can scroll through the set of 2D images. Typically, three orthogonal planes are displayed simultaneously with indicators regarding their orientation and intersection (Fig. 9-38).

In an alternative approach a polyhedron representing the boundaries of the reconstructed volume is displayed. Each face of the polyhedron depicts the 2D image for that plane. The polyhedron can be rotated to any desired orientation, and the plane of reference moved in or out. The 3D image set is then mapped to that face. The relative position of the reference plane with respect to other anatomy must be indicated.

Surface Rendering

Surface rendering depicts the surface of organs or other structures for display. The boundaries of the structure are identified by the operator or by computer contouring. The points within the boundary are interconnected by a wire mesh formed in triangular or polygonal segments. Once the surface is established, the texture and lighting are changed depending on the operator's viewing perspective (Fig. 9-39). Interactive display of the surface-rendered data is possible.

The surface-rendered image can contain artifacts and must be viewed in conjunction with the planar images. Spatial detail is lost unless a high-resolution mesh is used.

Volume Rendering

Multiformat planar and surface rendering form a 2D planar image that does not depend on information in the 3D data set outside of the 2D plane. Volume rendering, on the other hand, forms a 2D projection image based on data throughout the 3D volume set. Volume rendering is computationally intensive and may require dedicated hardware for interactive rendering.

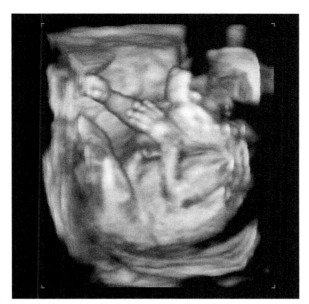

Figure 9-39 3D surface rendering of a fetal hand. (Courtesy of Yvette Ramos, RDMS, RVT.)

The viewing direction must first be established. Then, a set of parallel rays is cast through the 3D volume. Each ray corresponds to one pixel in the volume-rendered image. The voxels encountered along each ray are identified, the values are multiplied by factors, and their products are summed to obtain the final value for that ray (pixel). The array of pixels is configured in a 2D projection image.

One common approach is to generate a maximum intensity projection image. This type of volume rendering retains only the maximum voxel value along each ray. All other voxel values are excluded.

The translucent/opacity rendering technique weights the voxel values along each ray by opacity and color factors. The opacities, shades, and colors encountered along the ray are blended to produce the final pixel color and luminance in the 2D projection image. The opacity and color factors are adjustable to depict the desired anatomic structures. Volume rendering has been very successful in the display of fetal and vascular anatomy.

4D IMAGING

Display of a surface-rendered plane or multiple planes of the sampled volume in real time is called 4D ultrasound. The fourth dimension of time is combined with volumetric sampling to depict the dynamic spatial relationships of structures in three dimensions. Mechanically translated multiple element arrays and 2D array transducers have been developed to rapidly acquire volumetric data.

Multielement Arrays

The first approach mechanically sweeps a 1.5D crystal array back and forth across the beam port of the transducer. The direction of movement is perpendicular to the crystal rows. This is very similar to a mechanical sector scanner, except that the single crystal has now been replaced with a multiple-row crystal array. The crystal array allows electronic steering of the beam within the plane defined by the mechanical position of the crystal array. Instead of a single scan line directed from the crystal at each sampling position along the arc in a mechanical sector scanner, the phased array can direct the beam along multiple scan lines to acquire a plane at each sampling position along the arc. This interrogates a 3D volume. The crystal array is encased in fluid within the transducer housing to provide good energy transmission into tissue. Different transducer types including curvilinear, linear, and endocavity (end-fire and side-fire) are available.

A frame rate of five volumes per second is possible. Time constraints prohibit scan lines from being acquired plane by plane as the crystal array is swept across the volume. Rather, the beam is directed along selected lines of sight within a plane before the array is moved to the next position. Since fewer scan lines are acquired compared with 3D ultrasound, some loss in spatial resolution occurs in 4D ultrasound. Also, resolution deteriorates with distance from the transducer (lower scan line density).

2D Arrays

The alternative method to acquire volumetric data uses a 2D array transducer to electronically steer the beam throughout the volume without moving the transducer. As many as 9000 crystal elements comprise the 2D array. The field of view is smaller, but the frame rate is higher than that obtainable with the combination mechanical/electronic steering. The maximum frame rate is 20 volumes per second. To achieve this frame rate, the number of scan lines that compose the image are limited, and the sampling volume is restricted in size. Similar to other real-time systems, a trade-off exists between frame rate, scan lines, and sampling volume.

Limitations

A subtle difficulty is that the relationship between the echo-induced signal amplitude and the physical situation is not well defined by a single parameter. Unlike computed tomography, in which one physical characteristic (electron density) determines the measured value, in ultrasound many factors contribute to the reflectivity of an interface. The lack of a common unifying factor and small differences in signal levels makes some data manipulation techniques difficult to apply.

ELASTOGRAPHY

Elasticity imaging or elastography is a scanning technique that creates a visual display of information that would be obtained by manual palpation. A two-dimensional quantitative map of tissue stiffness throughout the region of interest is presented. Tissue changes shape or volume when a force is applied over a surface area. Stiffness is a measure of how likely it is that the tissue will maintain its shape when the force is applied.

This deforming force per area is called the stress. The relative displacement of tissue when subjected to stress is the strain. If the strain is proportional to the stress, then the material exhibits elastic behavior. The amount of stress required to cause a given displacement depends on the tissue type. The proportionality constant is called the elastic modulus of the material. Removal of the low-level stress restores the elastic material to the original shape and dimensions.

Tissue is considered elastic for the compression force applied during freehand scanning. However, at increased stress, tissue exhibits a nonlinear stress-strain relationship and changes stiffness as it is deformed. Elastic moduli of tissue types are not uniform in magnitude (fat < glandular tissue < carcinoma < fibrous tissue). That is, tissue types have different degrees of stiffness.

Elastography detects the relative tissue displacement between precompression (no stress) and compression (stress) measured by ultrasound. The radiofrequency signal for each line of sight is acquired before and after deformation. The A-line echo signal in each data set is divided into short segments (fraction of a millimeter), and each segment is sampled over time. The compression radiofrequency signal is then shifted in time to match the predeformation radiofrequency signal. The amount of time shift yields the displacement for that segment of tissue. Comparison with adjacent segments provides the rate of change of the displacement (also called the gradient), which is depicted in the strain image. In essence, the shift in position caused by overlying tissues is eliminated, and the displacement for the stress acting on each small tissue element is revealed.

Image contrast is based on the mechanical properties of the different tissue types and has the potential to produce high contrast when strain is being measured. Contrast is likely to change when elevated stress is applied, since the media are no longer elastic. Multiple A-lines and short radiofrequency segments allow two-dimensional tracking in the lateral and axial directions. This increases the contrast-to-noise ratio.

Acoustic Radiation Force

Palpation does not result in the application of force consistently by a single operator and is certainly even more variable among multiple users. To make elastography less dependent on the operator, the force to tissue is applied by an acoustic shear wave. A high-intensity single pulse is repeatedly focused to successive depths along one line of sight (force line). The combination of long pulse length and high pulse repetition frequency create a sonic shock wave that radiates perpendicular from the force line. The shear wave moves slowly (1–10 m/s) through tissue at a speed proportional to the elasticity of tissue. A wide beam at high pulse repetition frequency (5000 Hz) with dynamic receive focusing tracks the movement of the shear wave and assigns a stiffness value in pressure amplitude (kilopascals). Fluid produces a signal void.

Clinical Applications

Displays of elasticity and B-mode images are shown side by side in a split-screen format in real time. The operator denotes the region of interest for the strain images. The relative lesion size in B-mode versus elasticity images may allow tissue differentiation. Fibroadenomas and cysts are nearly equal in size in both image types (Fig. 9-40), whereas invasive ductal carcinomas are larger in the strain image compared with the B-mode image (Fig. 9-41). Quantification of stiffness may improve ultrasound's ability to identify lesions for biopsy. Elastography of the

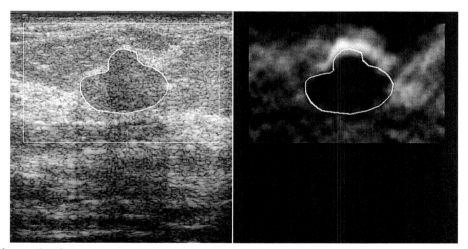

Figure 9-40 B-mode image *(left)* and elasticity image *(right)* of a fibroadenoma. The lesion is traced on the B-mode image, and that tracing is superimposed on the elasticity image. The size and shape of the lesion in the two images are very similar. (Courtesy of Timothy Hall, PhD, University of Wisconsin.)

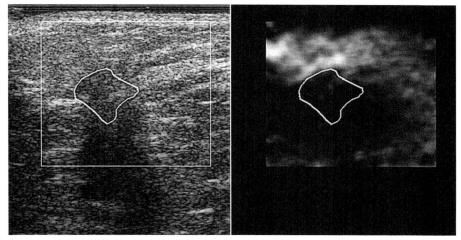

Figure 9-41 B-mode image *(left)* and elasticity image *(right)* of a scirrhous invasive ductal carcinoma. The lesion is traced on the B-mode image, and that tracing is superimposed on the elasticity image. The size of the lesion is larger on the strain image. (Courtesy of Timothy Hall, PhD, University of Wisconsin.)

breast has detected lesions less than 3 mm in diameter with a stiffness three times that of glandular breast tissue.

PORTABLE DEVICES

Portable ultrasound scanners are smaller and less expensive than conventional full-sized full-featured models. Often, the power source is an internal battery to broaden portability. Over 50 models from 20 manufacturers are now commercially available. Portable units are classified as laptop, handheld, USB-powered probe, and cart-based. High-end portable devices provide image quality and features that, in many ways, are comparable with full-size scanners including multiple transducers (linear, phased, vector, and curvilinear) and full compliment of operational modes (B-mode, M-mode, tissue harmonic imaging, 3D, 4D, pulsed-wave Doppler, continuous-wave Doppler, color flow imaging, and power Doppler). Applications include general imaging, obstetrics/gynecology, small parts, endocavitary, vascular, and cardiac.

The laptop is a size and shape descriptor rather than a computer by itself. The probes connect to the control panel and display. All scanning and processing functions are directed using the control panel. Handheld devices are designed to be held in one hand while scanning with the transducer in the other hand. The USB power probe contains the transducer and an electronics module, which is interfaced to a laptop computer. The computer becomes the operator control panel, display monitor for real-time images, archive for image storage, and means to process images. Cart-based or suitcase-style units are larger than laptop, handheld, and probe devices.

The miniaturization of electronics means some sacrifice in design capability is inherent in portable devices. The usual reduction in electronics is often extracted in the receive beam former. A major cost consideration is the piezoelectric elements in the transducer. Capacitive micromachined ultrasonic transducers (CMUTs) in portable scanners will probably be the first commercial application of this new technology.

SUMMARY

Ultrasound is one of the fastest-growing and most exciting areas of diagnostic imaging, and new operational modes are expanding its clinical utility. High sensitivity, improved image quality, and relatively low cost render ultrasound an attractive modality in health care reform. Design features including application presets, and calculation packages enhance the workflow. 3D imaging and 4D ultrasound provides tomographic presentation of the scanned volume with reduced examination time and lower likelihood of missed pathology. Broadband transducer technology and associated instrumentation are still evolving.

Digital Signal and Image Processing

10

Chapter Objectives

To identify types of signal and image processing available to the operator
To understand the function of the operator controls: gray-scale map, write zoom, persistence, dynamic range, edge enhancement, and panning
To describe the technique of logarithmic compression with relationship to dynamic range

Key terms

Bilinear interpolation
Cine loop
Compression
Contrast enhancement

Edge enhancement
Frame averaging (persistence)
Freeze frame

Panning
Read zoom
Smoothing
Write zoom

DIGITAL MODULAR DESIGN

Adaptation of the digital format for signal and image processing has resulted in substantial performance and cost advantages compared with specifically designed electronic analog components. Identical digital hardware can perform different tasks depending on the software. Essentially, if a processing technique can be described mathematically, then that algorithm can be implemented by a series of software instructions. This expands the processing options available. Often, upgrades for new and revised processing are instituted by changing software without a modification in hardware. Scan data can be stored and processed repeatedly by several pathways in parallel. Digital components are more reliable than analog devices and are not subject to electronic drift with temperature change. Additionally, digital hardware incorporates diagnostic testing of instrument condition to identify failed components and minimize downtime. Quantitative manipulation and analysis of the B-mode images in an expeditious fashion are possible using current computer technology.

CLASSIFICATION

With today's technology, the practical distinction between preprocessing and postprocessing functions has become blurred if not irrelevant in actual practice. In the past, postprocessing was applied after computer storage of the image, while preprocessing had to be performed during live scanning. Individual frames are now stored almost instantaneously and all types of processing functions can be performed while the system operates in live scanning mode. Furthermore, the newest machines now continually store raw scan data and allow the sonographer to retroactively alter many of the original acquisition settings that have traditionally been thought of as preprocessing functions, such as receiver gain, time gain compensation, compression, and magnification.

In this new classification signal processing is the manipulation of echo-induced radiofrequency signals before their input to the scan converter. The scan data are typically in analog format until after time gain compensation reduces the dynamic range of the signals. Digitalization and dynamic focusing occur in the receive beam former before signal level assignment. Additional signal processing subject to operator control (edge enhancement, compression, and weak-signal reject) are also applied before scan conversion. The incorporation of a digital scan converter in real-time instruments has facilitated processing of scan data in the matrix format (referred to as image processing). A large amount of information is presented in a compact and an easily recognizable form. Received echoes configured in a pictorial format, as light and dark regions on a display monitor, are readily comprehended and manipulated.

SIGNAL PROCESSING

Receiver gain, time gain compensation, reject, and edge enhancement are examples of signal processing techniques available to the sonographer. The scanner may employ additional signal processing based on the selected examination or preset application, which is transparent to the operator, including adaptive gain compensation and logarithmic compression. Signal processing is applied to echo wavetrains prior to positional assignment of signal level by the scan converter.

Receiver Gain

Receiver gain amplifies the echo-induced signals and provides the necessary signal strength for analog-to-digital conversion. The amount of amplification is quantified as the ratio of the output signal to the input signal. The application of gain is uniform throughout the scan range. *That is, all signals and noise are increased by the same factor.* The gain control is adjusted when an increase or decrease in the image brightness is desired. Within certain limitations (weak signals), the visual effect of increased gain is similar as an increase in the output power.

Time Gain Compensation

The attenuation of an ultrasound beam with depth causes equally reflective interfaces to produce different signal levels depending on their relative distances from the transducer. It is often advantageous to display reflectors of similar size, shape, and reflectivity with equal amplitude. Exponential amplification as a function of elapsed time referenced to the transmitted pulse corrects the received signals for attenuation; that is, the reduction in signal level caused by the increased depth at which echoes are generated is compensated by applying time-dependent amplification to the received signal. This processing technique is called time gain compensation. The initial application of time gain compensation is automated based on elapsed time only and does not require operator input. A manual adjustment of depth-dependent amplification is called selective enhancement or, more commonly, time gain compensation.

Selective Enhancement

Time gain compensation as an operator control enables the sonographer to selectively amplify signals from a particular depth of interest. Amplification of the received signals may be applied in a nonuniform manner to highlight echoes generated within a particular region of interest or to compensate for tissue differences along the scan path. This control is commonly configured as a series of slide keys, each key corresponding to a certain depth; the displacement of a key denotes the amount of amplification. Each slider may be individually adjusted as necessary to apply the appropriate amplification so that a uniformly bright image is produced. Time gain compensation adjustments are based on visual appearance of the image rather than on specific numeric values.

Adaptive Time Gain Compensation

Two weaknesses of time gain compensation are as follows: (1) the same initial variable depth gain is applied to each scan line without consideration of the nonuniformity of tissue along the path and (2) the operator must continually make manual adjustments as the scan plane is changed. Adaptive time gain compensation addresses these problems by calculating a unique gain function for each scan line and then automatically adjusting the amplification in real time. At all sampling points along a particular scan line, the locally applied gain at a specific depth is compared with the average gain from all scan lines at that same depth. For example, if the local gain function is greater than the global gain function, the local gain function is set equal to the global gain function. And if the local gain function is less than the global gain function, the local gain function is set to a weighted average of the two gain functions. Unique amplification is thus automatically applied to each depth component of the image.

Edge Enhancement

Ultrasound imaging is ideally suited to the detection of interfaces or boundaries between structures. Edge enhancement is a filtering technique that can be applied to the echo wavetrain to emphasize a change in signal levels across tissue boundaries. Suppose that eight points along one line of sight have the initial values shown in Table 10-1. The filtering process uses a kernel (i.e., a collection of weighting factors) applied to the original values. In this example the kernel is applied to three sequential points with weighting factors of -1, 3, and -1. To calculate the edge-enhanced value for point number 4, the kernel is centered on point number 4. The sum of each weighting factor times the respective original value of each point in the three-point

Table 10-1	Numerical Example of Edge Enhancement							
Point Number	**1**	**2**	**3**	**4**	**5**	**6**	**7**	**8**
Original value	200	200	200	200	100	100	100	100
Kernel			−1	3	−1			
Edge-enhanced value	200	200	200	300	0	100	100	100

sequence (point number 4 and the adjacent points) is calculated. This yields a new value of 300 for point 4. The edge-enhanced values for the remaining points in the original data set are determined in a similar manner by moving the center of the kernel to each point along the scan line. The kernel always operates on the original data; the edge-enhanced results must be maintained separately from the initial values. Changes in the magnitude or number of weighting factors in the filter modify the amount of edge enhancement. Sonograms with different edge enhancement settings are presented in Figure 10-1.

Rejection

Rejection, by passing only signals greater than a prescribed signal level, removes weak signals and noise. Noise reduction is desirable for improving image quality. However, weak signals corresponding to interfaces with low reflectivities or at deep depths may be lost. In some circumstances (e.g., an object with high reflectivity located off axis), the signal level exceeds the threshold value and will contribute to the final image.

Compression

Dynamic range is quantified as the ratio of the largest to the smallest signal a system or component can faithfully represent. The units of dynamic range are typically expressed in decibels. Alternatively, dynamic range is stated as the span of processed signals from lowest to highest. Each returning echo is converted to an electrical voltage waveform that must be categorized according to signal level and stored as a digital value in the scan converter. The stored pixel value must then be translated to a shade of gray for display. A second aspect of system response is how signals are partitioned into groups throughout the dynamic range.

The initial high information content of echo-induced signals cannot be maintained by succeeding system components. Consequently the dynamic range must be partitioned by a technique called compression; otherwise high (or low) signals beyond (or below) a certain value are no longer distinct. As an analogy, suppose that the height of individuals with a system dynamic range of 4 to 7 feet were recorded using a form that had three categories for height (4 to 5 feet, 5 to 6 feet, and 6 to 7 feet). Individuals greater than 7 feet or less than 4 feet in height would be lost in this census or inaccurately recorded in the wrong height classification. In order to expand the dynamic range, the height partitions could be arranged as 2 to 4 feet, 4 to 6 feet, and 6 to 8 feet. The total number of groups would be unchanged, but the ability to distinguish individuals of similar height would be sacrificed. This example demonstrates a linear compression throughout the dynamic range of 2 to 8 feet, since all height classifications are divided in equal increments of 2 feet. A logarithmic compression uses unequal increments, such as 2 to 3 feet, 3 to 5 feet, and 5 to 8 feet. Note that the dynamic range remains 2 to 8 feet.

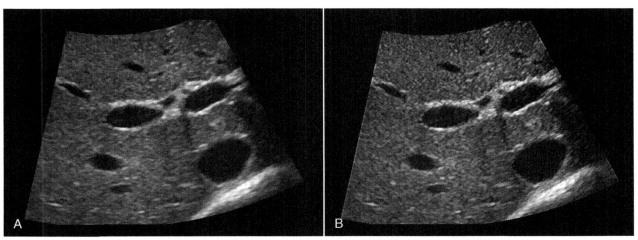

Figure 10-1 Edge enhancement. The original change in signal level detected along a particular line of sight is manipulated mathematically to produce a more dramatic difference at the boundary. **A,** Moderate edge enhancement. **B,** Extreme edge enhancement.

Because the latitude of analog signal levels (approximately 100,000:1 or more) exceeds the number of discrete digital values available in the scan converter matrix (usually 0–255), signal levels must be partitioned according to a logarithmic scale. The logarithmic translation is necessary since linear translation limits the signal variation by a factor of 255. Consequently, with linear processing, information content is lost and the entire dynamic range of signals from high to low cannot be retained. Logarithmic compression effectively increases the amplitudes of low signals and decreases the amplitudes of high signals so that all echo-induced signals are represented in the scan converter. A proportionally larger fraction of compressed signal range is devoted to low signal strengths. Increasing the digitization beyond 8 bits allows more numeric values to be stored, but the increased groups of signal levels are ultimately condensed by the display or recording device.

SCAN CONVERSION

The scanned area is probed by a series of ultrasound pulses directed along various scan lines. The beam orientation and depth information must be converted to the matrix format for display. By superimposing all the scan lines on the image matrix, it can be demonstrated that several pixels are not sampled by the ultrasound beam (Fig. 10-2). If these blank pixels were each displayed with a zero signal level, a disconcerting checkerboard image would result. Manufacturers avoid this by averaging the signals from nearby pixels that are sampled to generate a fill-in value for the blank pixel. The value for the blank pixel is thus inferred by examining the surrounding region.

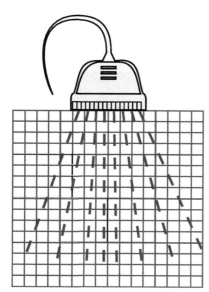

Figure 10-2 Lines of sight *(dotted)* superimposed on the matrix to demonstrate that not all pixels are sampled by the sound beam. The value assigned to the unsampled pixels is calculated by averaging signal amplitudes in the neighboring pixels.

Fill-in Interpolation

The most widely used scan conversion method is bilinear interpolation. Two algorithms, which can be executed in real time, have been developed to interpolate the scan data along the axial and angular directions. In the first technique, a synthesized scan line through the pixel of interest is generated by interpolating angularly between sampling points on adjacent scan lines (Fig. 10-3). Axial interpolation between two points on the synthesized scan line, which encompass the pixel, establishes the pixel value. In the alternative technique, additional axial values are calculated by interpolation along each scan line (Fig. 10-4). Angular interpolation between these new axial points establishes the pixel value.

IMAGE PROCESSING

Image processing techniques are applied after scan conversion; they include write zoom, panning, persistence, dynamic range, filtering, freeze frame, cine loop, and gray-scale mapping. The scanner may employ additional image processing based on the selected examination or preset application, which is transparent to the operator. These include image updating, image equalization, and adaptive frame averaging.

Image Updating

Because the ultrasound beam is repeatedly directed throughout the field of view, new information constantly becomes available. The most recent scan data are held in

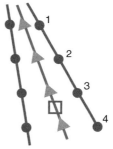

Figure 10-3 Fill-in interpolation. A synthetic scan line *(green)* through the pixel of interest is calculated by interpolating angularly between sampling points *(1, 2, 3, and 4)* on adjacent scan lines (blue). Axial interpolation along the synthetic scan line establishes the pixel value.

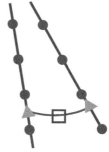

Figure 10-4 Fill-in interpolation. Additional axial values are calculated by interpolation along each scan line *(triangles)*. The pixel value is calculated by angular interpolation between these new axial points.

the buffer for updating the image data in the scan con-verter. Most simply, the old value at a particular location is replaced by the current value for that pixel location. This is referred to as last-value mode. The image data are updated continuously and rapidly with the newest echo data. Or, the new value is combined with the old value using various weighting factors. Other averaging options, which can be selected by the operator, include spatial compounding, frequency compounding, and frame averaging.

Gray-Scale Mapping

Each pixel is displayed uniformly as a particular shade of gray depending on the pixel value (Fig. 10-5). The trans-lation of the range of pixel values (stored signal levels in the scan converter) to brightness levels is called gray-scale mapping. A gray-scale map is selected by the operator and as such can alter the presentation of the displayed image. At this point, it is important to differentiate between the potential signal values that can be stored in the scan con-verter and the number of gray levels that can be displayed on the output device. The gray scale on most monitors consists of 16, 32, or 64 degrees of brightness. If the signal level is expressed as eight bits, obviously each signal level ranging from 0 to 255 cannot be represented as a separate and distinct shade of gray. A range of numeric values must be associated with each gray level. Figure 10-6 is a gray-scale map in which eight brightness levels are available. Pixels with values between 191 and 223 are all displayed as gray level 7.

Since the number of brightness levels is less than the nu-meric range of pixel values, multiple signal levels are dis-played with the same shade of gray. Pixels with similar values are displayed with either the same or different brightness levels depending on the gray-scale map. Alter-ing the gray-scale map does not change the stored value in the scan converter; rather, it modifies how that pixel is dis-played based on its stored value. Changing the shade of gray associated with various signal levels in accordance with well-defined processing techniques may enhance interpretation of the scan data.

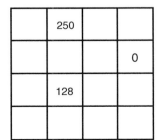
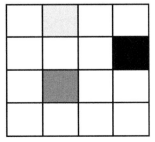

Figure 10-5 Display of pixels. Each pixel is assigned a value representing a signal level. Each pixel is depicted on the monitor as a uniform shade of gray based on the pixel value. Brightness levels for three pixels are shown.

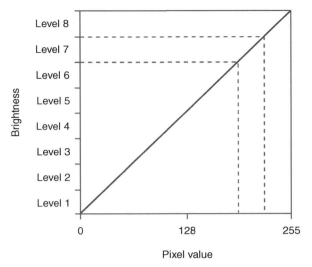

Figure 10-6 A gray-scale map provides the translation of stored pixel values to different brightness levels. For this system, eight brightness levels are possible. Usually level 1 is black and level 8 is white. Pixels with values from 191 to 223 are all displayed with brightness level 7 (near white).

The number of bits determines the available numeric values that can be used to quantify the signal level at any one pixel. If only one bit assigns signal levels, each pixel would be either "on" or "off" (0 or 1) and a bistable image would be created. A system that is two bits deep could represent four different values (four combinations of 1 s and 0 s—00, 01, 10, 11—equivalent to the decimal numbers 0, 1, 2, and 3). A two-bit system displays 0 as black, 1 as dark gray, 2 as light gray, and 3 as white. Sys-tems with more bits can exhibit more shades of gray. Most scan converters are eight bits deep, creating up to 256 nu-meric representations, and these stored values can be translated into various shades of gray to form the dis-played image.

Contrast Enhancement

Pixels with similar values over a narrow range can be dis-played with different degrees of brightness by changing the gray-scale map. This modification to emphasize a par-ticular range of signal levels is called contrast enhance-ment. For example, if the echo data range from 0 to 210 and the pixel values are visualized with eight shades of gray, every pixel with a value of 0 is depicted as black, and the signal levels above 0 are linearly distributed over the remaining seven shades of gray (Table 10-2). Each gray level is associated with specific values. Thus pixels with signal levels between 61 and 90 are each displayed with the same shade (gray level 3). Suppose that values less than 56 (weak echo signals) are not of interest and can be elim-inated for viewing purposes. By depicting these pixels as black and redistributing the gray scale over a new range of values (57 to 210), image contrast is enhanced. The range of pixel values associated with each gray level is then decreased from 30 to 22 following contrast enhancement,

Table 10-2	Change in Values Associated with Various Gray-Scale Levels Using Contrast Enhancement		
Original Values	**Gray Level**		**New Values**
181 to 210	7	white	189 to 210
151 to 180	6		167 to 188
121 to 150	5		145 to 166
91 to 120	4		123 to 144
61 to 90	3		101 to 122
31 to 60	2		79 to 100
1 to 30	1		57 to 78
0	0	black	0 to 56

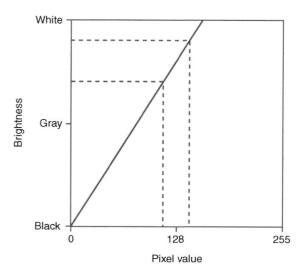

Figure 10-8 An enhanced gray-scale map in which pixel values near 128 are displayed as near white. The range of brightness levels for pixel values near 128 is wider than in Figure 10-7.

and pixels with similar values are more likely to be displayed at different gray levels. Whereas pixels with relative signal amplitudes of 65 and 85 were displayed as gray level 3 initially, they are presented as gray level 1 and gray level 2 after contrast enhancement and can now be distinguished in the image.

Contrast enhancement can also be illustrated with the aid of a graphic gray-scale map. Figure 10-7 is a gray-scale map that translates pixel values from 0 to 255 to the different brightness levels in a linear fashion. Pixels with values near 128 are displayed with intermediate shades of gray. If the gray-scale map is changed so that pixel values from 0 to 160 are distributed linearly over the various brightness levels and if values above 160 are displayed as white, pixels with values near 128 are now shown with very light shades of gray (Fig. 10-8). There are more brightness levels available to display a fixed range of values for the contrast-enhanced gray-scale map (e.g., see Fig. 10-8) than for the original gray-scale map (see Fig. 10-7). In other words, the distance along the vertical axis corresponding to a particular range of

pixel values is greater for the enhanced gray-scale map than for the initial map. The disadvantage is that contrast for high signal levels has been lost (all signal levels above 160 are displayed as white).

The gray-scale map is not restricted to a linear relationship. Logarithmic, inverse logarithmic, exponential, squared, and square root gray-scale maps are also available. The linear map distributes gray levels equally throughout the range of pixel values (echo strengths). The logarithmic map enhances the contrast of weak echoes. The threshold linear map eliminates the weak echoes and emphasizes variations in high-strength echoes. The exponential map enhances the contrast of strong echoes. Figure 10-9 is a sonogram of the liver displayed with different gray-scale maps.

Black and White Inversion

In black and white inversion, the brightness levels on a gray-scale map are inverted to extend from white (at the low signal amplitude) to black (at the high signal amplitude). A pixel value of 240, which is normally displayed as near white, is depicted as near black on the inverted image (Fig. 10-10).

Dynamic Range

Because the display monitor and other devices are unable to maintain the extremely wide range of signal levels with 256 partitions in the scan converter, further compression (reduction in the number of signal classifications) is necessary. The operator control that varies the displayed dynamic range is called dynamic range, compression, or log compression. Full contrast resolution of scan data is necessarily but selectively forfeited in the final displayed image. The dynamic range of the displayed image may equal the full dynamic range of the signals in the scan

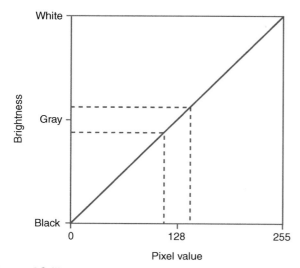

Figure 10-7 A linear gray-scale map in which pixel values near 128 (indicated by red dotted lines) are displayed as intermediate shades of gray.

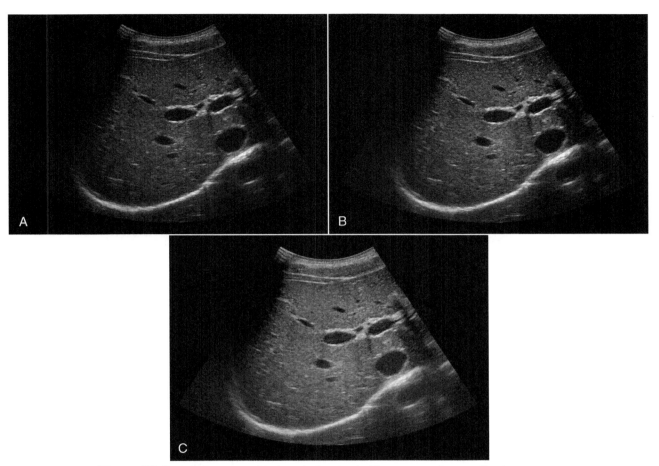

Figure 10-9 A-C, Sonogram of the liver displayed with different gray-scale maps. The data in image memory are unchanged, but the translation of pixel values to brightness levels is altered to produce radically different images.

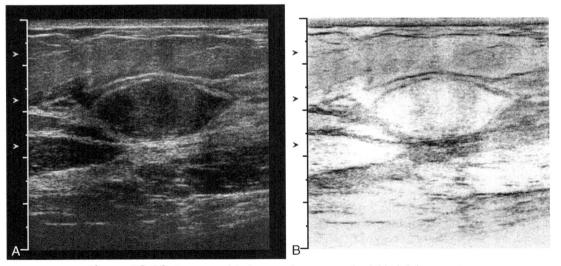

Figure 10-10 Sonogram of the breast with a mass, and with black/white inversion.

converter or may be more restricted by excluding some high or low signals. In the latter case the dynamic range of the displayed image is reduced. Low dynamic range improves image contrast but usually with a loss of weaker echoes. High dynamic range reduces image contrast but retains a broader extent of signal levels. However, most often differences in low signal levels are of interest clinically, and improper setting of compression can prevent the visualization of small, low-contrast structures. Sonograms with different dynamic range settings are presented in Figure 10-11.

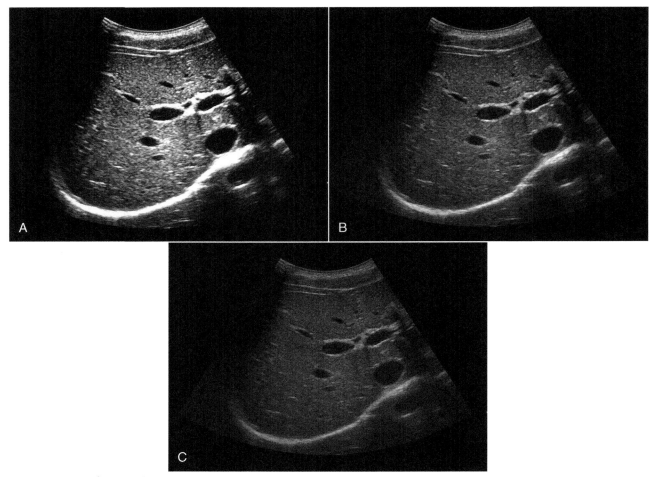

Figure 10-11 Sonograms of the liver with different levels of compression. **A,** 36 dB. **B,** 66 dB. **C,** 96 dB. Note the loss of weak scatterers when the dynamic range is reduced.

Frame Averaging or Persistence

Noise is the variation in signal level unrelated to the reflectivity of an object. In other words, multiple measurements of the echo from a particular reflector yield not the same but slightly different values. Thus a uniform reflector would be depicted by nonuniform pixel values throughout the image of the reflector.

Real-time scanners acquire images at a rate of 10 to 20 frames per second. Frame averaging (also called persistence) combines successive frames (as many as four or more) held in a buffer to increase the signal-to-noise ratio. Because noise is random while echoes from anatomic structures are consistent and repeatable, image quality can be improved by merging echo data from multiple scans of the field of view. However because, in effect, the sampling occurs over a longer time interval, temporal resolution is poorer. The rate of movement of the interfaces must be small; otherwise, anatomic landmarks in successive frames are not superimposed at the same location in the averaged image and blurring occurs. During imaging of the heart, high persistence is not appropriate, because the small, rapid motions of the valves cannot be perceived when several frames are added together. The technique of frame averaging does allow high-quality abdominal scans to be obtained.

Adaptive Frame Averaging

Frame averaging is designed to reduce noise, but it can create blurring of fast-moving structures. Adaptive frame averaging is a modification of this technique in which the image is subdivided into many small regions. The time variance of the pixel values in each of these small regions is assessed. More averaging is applied in regions with little change from frame to frame and less averaging is applied in regions with high variation. The amount of averaging with previous measurements for the respective interfaces is variable throughout the image. In this manner the signal-to-noise ratio for slow-moving structures is increased without the penalty of lag for the fast-moving structures.

Write Zoom

The most basic control to alter image size is the display depth. Depth control is used extensively and, when properly set, is an important component of image optimization. A decreased scan range for the purpose of image magnification is inappropriate in circumstances where the area of interest is not completely maintained within the field of view. If the area of interest occupies a portion of the field of view, then write zoom (also called magnification, regional expansion, reduced field of view, and zooming) can be applied to enhance spatial detail. The operator designates the region within the field of view to be magnified. A fraction of the scan converter matrix corresponding to the signals received only from this designated region is displayed on the monitor. *Because the physical dimensions of the zoomed region are much smaller than the original field of view and an equal number of display pixels compose the image, improved spatial resolution is now possible.*

The improvement in spatial resolution takes place because the monitor and scan converter are not matched in matrix size. Modern scan converters have more pixels than can be individually displayed on the monitor. For example, a 10 × 10 matrix in the scan converter stores an image that has physical dimensions of 1 × 1 cm. However, the display of the monitor only has 5 × 5 addressable locations (display pixels), which causes groups of four pixels in the scan converter to be combined for each display pixel. The entire field of view cannot be display with full spatial resolution. By designating the central region for expansion, the same 5 × 5 display now represents a portion of the field of view measuring 0.5 × 0.5 cm. The same number of display pixels is available in each case, but in magnified mode the display pixels are distributed over a smaller area. Write zoom decreases the physical size represented by a single display pixel from 0.2 × 0.2 cm to 0.1 × 0.1 cm. Spatial detail is thus enhanced with the application of regional expansion.

The disadvantage of write zoom is that the field of view is limited. The portraits of Abraham Lincoln displayed with the same number of pixels in normal and magnified modes demonstrate the effect of write zoom (Fig. 10-12). The normal and write-zoom views of the liver are shown in Fig. 10-13. In practice, the improvement in resolution is ultimately limited by the beam width and spatial pulse length.

Panning

Panning is an image-acquisition technique that allows the operator to shift the expanded region to a new anatomic location during scanning. The maximum field of view for a particular transducer is well defined. During panning, the sonographer can designate and move a small sampling area within the limits of the transducer field of view. In essence, panning provides a write-zoom image that can be translated vertically and horizontally under operator control to sample different locations.

Image Equalization

Image equalization is a method to automatically adjust brightness levels throughout the image to optimize contrast. Multiple techniques from different manufacturers have been employed for image equalization. Histogram analysis within a small region of interest examines the number of times pixels with certain values occur. Alternatively, statistical analysis of the distribution of pixel values is performed in real time to implement region-by-region adjustments to the acquisition parameters.

Freeze Frame

Freeze frame allows the operator to select an image of interest for prolonged viewing. The data collection of scan lines is suspended and the last frame acquired is displayed

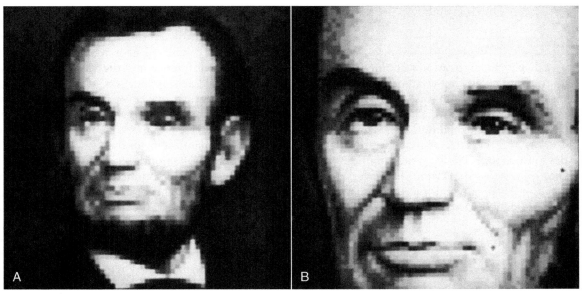

Figure 10-12 A, Portrait of Abraham Lincoln in normal mode. **B,** Write-zoom mode. The number of pixels in each matrix is identical, but in write-zoom mode spatial detail is improved.

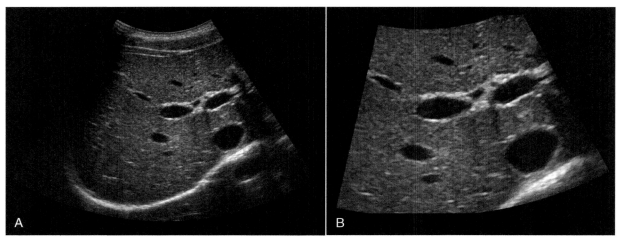

Figure 10-13 Sonogram of a liver. **A,** Normal mode. **B,** Write-zoom mode.

on the monitor. This enables the operator to analyze the image with various processing tools (annotation, region of interest, distance measurements, area measurements) or to record the image on a hard-copy device or to transfer the image to Picture Archiving and Communication System (PACS). With the freeze control, current scanners offer the ability to store and review still images and real-time video clips. After freezing the image, the sonographer can recall the most recently acquired frames from the system buffer (typically 100 to 200, but there can be several thousand frames). Activation of this viewing function is usually done simply by scrolling the trackball backward to display stored images frame by frame. Stored images can also be viewed in temporal sequence by using the cine loop function. Depending upon the scanner, cine acquisition may be retrospective or prospective with reference to the activation of this function. Certainly the ability to include frames obtained just prior to cine activation enables interesting findings seen in real-time to be included in the cine loop.

Read Zoom

Read zoom is a display magnification technique applied to the scan data to show pixels that compose the image in a larger format on the monitor; that is, the portion of the monitor screen associated with each pixel is enlarged. The number of pixels throughout the scanned area remains constant, and the area of tissue represented by each pixel does not change. Unlike write zoom, this technique does not improve spatial detail. However, technological advances—specifically the increased matrix size of scan converters—have essentially eliminated the option of read zoom.

Filtering

Digital filtering refers to the modification of a pixel value based on the values of surrounding pixels. Smoothing and edge enhancement are forms of digital filtering.

Smoothing is an image-processing technique for the reduction of noise. Noise is the variation in signal level associated with a particular interface. Electronic noise has no well-defined spatial pattern, which prohibits the use of a mathematical correction to eliminate its contribution in the image. Noise can be reduced, however, by averaging the values in nearby pixels if the pixels are representative of the same physical entity. This assumption fails at sharp boundaries, where a rapid change in pixel value occurs.

Smoothing is a two-dimensional spatial averaging technique whereby values in the surrounding pixels are used to calculate a new value for the pixel of interest. The most common smoothing operation employs a nine-point spread function, or kernel. A set of weighting factors is arranged in a 3 × 3 minimatrix, as shown:

1	2	1
2	4	2
1	2	1

The center of the kernel is superimposed on the pixel of interest in the raw data matrix. The smoothed value for that pixel is calculated as a weighted sum of the value of the pixel of interest and the values of the neighboring eight pixels. Each application of the kernel on the raw data matrix creates one new pixel value for the new matrix of smoothed values. All calculations are applied to the raw data, which requires that the smoothed matrix be generated separately from the raw data matrix.

The degree of smoothing is modified by changing the weighting factors or by increasing the size of the kernel (e.g., a 5 × 5 instead of a 3 × 3). Weighting factors of equal magnitude or those averaging a greater number of surrounding pixels produce a stronger smoothing effect.

The disadvantage of smoothing is that some spatial detail is lost, because the smoothed value represents the averaging over the nearby region. Compare, with the respective originals, the portrait of Abraham Lincoln and the sonogram of the liver after they have undergone the smoothing operation (Figs. 10-14 and 10-15).

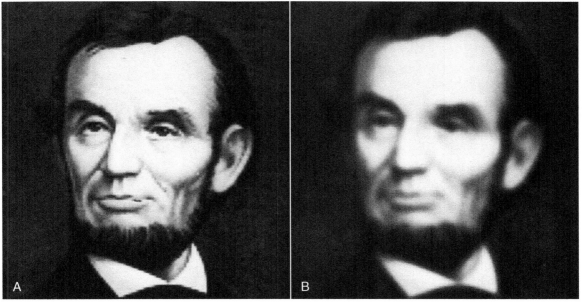

Figure 10-14 Digital filtering applied to the portrait of Abraham Lincoln. The smoothed image is on the right.

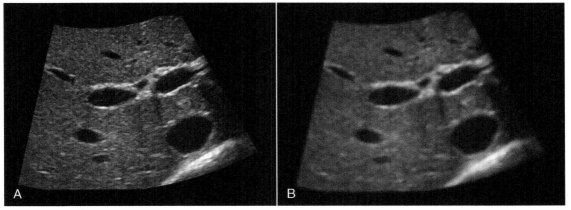

Figure 10-15 Digital filtering applied to the sonogram of a liver. **A,** None. **B,** Smooth.

Edge enhancement is a digital filtering technique used to emphasize a transition in signal level (border of a reflector) but with the disadvantage of increased noise content. As in smoothing, a two-dimensional spatial averaging technique is applied to pixels in the matrix. The amount of edge enhancement is modified by changing the magnitude or number of the weighting factors in the filter.

IMAGE ANALYSIS

Since the scan data were digitized to improve image acquisition and expand processing options, a secondary benefit is the ability to perform measurements of the structures depicted in the image. Average signal levels and physical dimensions can be assessed.

Region of Interest

Region-of-interest definition enables the operator to specify a portion of the image for analysis. The region of interest on the displayed image is denoted by defining the boundary of the desired area. This is accomplished by moving a visible cursor on the screen via a mouse or trackball. Pixels within the boundary are now designated for special consideration. For example, the average pixel value and the statistical variation within a particular area of the liver or gray-scale targets in a phantom (Fig. 10-16) can be determined.

Distance Measurement

Most ultrasound systems have two options for making measurements. The first utilizes a software calculation package, which is application-specific. The application

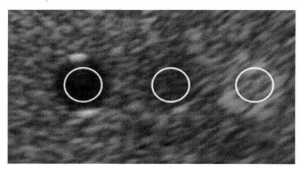

Figure 10-16 Region of interest. The boundary of the region of interest is marked with the cursor. Three areas corresponding to gray-scale targets in a phantom are shown. The mean pixel value in each area is determined.

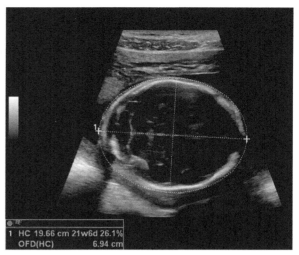

Figure 10-17 Distance measurements. An ellipse tool is used to measure head circumference.

preset determines, along with default settings for scanning, the appropriate calculation package. The measurement package guides the sonographer through the data acquisition process and ultimately creates a report of the results. The second option is a stand-alone measurement of linear distance, area, or circumference. These measurements are made by pressing the caliper button and positioning the on-screen cursor with the trackball. A "select" key activates each caliper alternately, so that the position of each caliper can be adjusted until the sonographer is satisfied with the position. Often, multiple sets of calipers can be displayed on the screen simultaneously.

The scan converter matrix is calibrated in terms of the physical size represented by the field of view. Pixel width corresponds to a known value (e.g., the physical dimension of a pixel corresponds to 0.2 mm), which is dictated by the transducer and the collection parameters. Therefore the distance between any two points of interest on the displayed image is readily calculated by the computer. The operator must identify the two locations, which is usually accomplished by moving a visible cursor on the screen via a trackball. Once the separation in number of pixels is determined, the actual distance is calculated by the computer using the product of the number of pixels and the calibration factor (0.2 mm per pixel). Distance measurements of femoral length, crown–rump length,

biparietal diameter, head circumference, and many others are routinely performed in the clinical environment (Fig. 10-17). The accuracy of distance measurements is compromised when a matrix with few pixels is used for imaging.

SUMMARY

The digitization of scan data provides a very complex environment in which the sonographer must obtain the optimal image. Multiple processing options to manipulate the image are available during as well as following data acquisition. The flexibility of numerous user-selectable protocols further complicates the practice of sonography. Many manufacturers have incorporated automated processing to facilitate the acquisition of images of reasonable quality. Examination-based calculation packages offer the advantage of quantitative analysis of sonographic data in very rapid fashion. The processing of images in a time-efficient manner to a form readily presentable for interpretation is the responsibility of the sonographer.

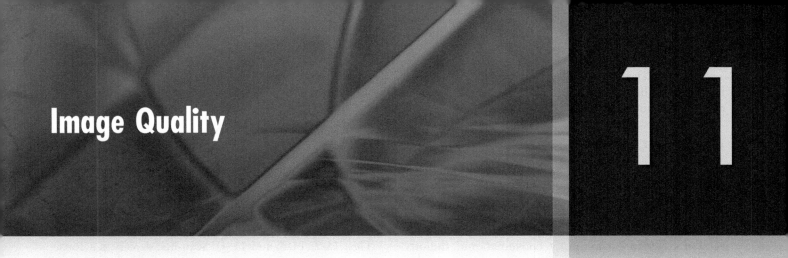

Image Quality

11

Chapter Objectives

To state the seven descriptors of image quality
To identify two sources of acoustic noise
To understand the effect of noise on low contrast resolution
To describe methods for speckle reduction

Key terms

Artifacts	Contrast resolution	Noise
Axial resolution	Geometric distortion	Speckle
Clutter	Lateral resolution	Temporal resolution

IMAGE COMPOSITION

The pattern of signals that form the image is a combination of reflected and scattered sound waves from structures interrogated by the ultrasound beam. Specular reflectors, such as fat—soft tissue at organ boundaries—produce high signals with little modulation. Scattering from organ parenchyma appears as a granular pattern with irregular bright and dark pixels. Image quality is a combination of many interrelated factors, which include axial resolution, lateral resolution, contrast resolution, artifacts, geometric distortion, noise, and temporal resolution. These components are interdependent; as a consequence, improvement in one to enhance image quality often means that another component is degraded. Also related to image quality is the concept of "dose," the amount of energy transmitted into the patient in order to perform the examination. Power can affect image quality, particularly in the presentation of weak echo-induced signals. Since the practice of ALARA (as low as reasonably achievable) is encouraged, the imaging should be conducted with the lowest power setting and examination time that yields the appropriate diagnostic information.

DESCRIPTORS OF IMAGE QUALITY

Axial resolution is the ability to resolve, as separate entities, reflectors located near each other along the axis of propagation. Alternative names for axial resolution include longitudinal, range, depth, and azimuthal resolution. The ability to resolve, as separate entities, reflectors located near each other along the direction perpendicular to the axis of propagation is described by the lateral resolution. Contrast resolution is the ability to discern reflectors that have different acoustic properties. Artifacts are structures in the image that do not represent the objects within the field of view with fidelity. (See Chapter 12 for a more complete discussion of image artifacts.) Geometric distortion describes the lack of adherence to true spatial relationships defined by the anatomic structures. Variations in signal independent of the echo-induced signal are generally classified as noise. Temporal resolution refers to the ability to accurately depict moving tissue along the path of motion.

AXIAL RESOLUTION

Axial resolution is determined primarily by the spatial pulse length, which depends on the center frequency and the bandwidth of the transducer (Fig. 11-1). Broad-bandwidth transducers operating at high frequency produce short transmission pulses, and the resultant short echo pulses can be faithfully converted into radiofrequency signals (good axial resolution). If the receiver bandwidth is less than that of the transmitted pulse, then the detected echo pulse length is elongated, resulting in a loss of axial resolution. Generally axial resolution is fairly constant with depth throughout the field of view.

The spatial pulse length defines the finite size of the detection sampling volume along the axial direction. By increasing transducer frequency and minimizing ringing, the spatial pulse length is shortened and the sampling volume is reduced in axial extent. At a fixed moment in time, all reflectors within the sampling volume are interrogated and generate echoes. The best possible axial resolution is considered to be half the spatial pulse length. The typical axial resolution of modern ultrasound systems is 0.25 to 2 mm. An object smaller than the resolution cell appears to be at least that size in the image (i.e., depicted with the incorrect size). Objects spaced closer together than the resolution cell merge together in the image (i.e., two objects appear as one).

Broad-bandwidth transducers require pulse shaping to maintain axial resolution throughout the scan range. As the pulsed beam propagates through tissue, high-frequency components of a broad-bandwidth spectrum are attenuated more rapidly than the low-frequency components. Consequently, the frequency composition of the detected echo shifts to lower frequency, with a subsequent loss in resolution as the depth of the reflector is increased. Pulse shaping minimizes the effect of this frequency shift so that axial resolution remains nearly constant at all depths.

LATERAL RESOLUTION

Consistent lateral resolution is desirable throughout the field of view. Lateral resolution is primarily determined by the beam width and scan-line density. Factors that affect in-plane beam width include focusing (transmit focusing, dynamic receive focusing, aperture, apodization, number and placement of focal zones) and frequency (Figs. 11-2, 11-3, and 11-4). Scan-line density is a consequence of the number of scan lines per frame, the width of the field of view, the scan format, and the number of elements in the array. The ability to observe small objects improves as the separation between scan lines decreases. Individual pixels and scan lines should not be discernible to the viewer. Interpolation attempts to mask the effect of the limited sampling by low scan-line density.

Unlike axial resolution, which remains fairly constant with depth, the lateral resolution, which depends on beam width, changes with depth. The in-plane beam width, and thus the lateral resolution, is best within the focal zone of the transducer. B-mode imaging systems can achieve a lateral resolution of 1 to 3 mm if dynamic focusing is used. However, the same problem arises as with axial resolution: A small object appears larger than it really is, and two objects separated by less than the beam width appear as one on the display. The limitation in resolution contributes to an incorrect representation of the size and shape of reflectors. Objects as small as 0.5 to 1 mm in diameter can be resolved by modern real-time units.

PARTIAL VOLUME

The finite beam width can create a partial volume artifact related to different tissue types within the sampling volume. The sampling volume has in-plane and out-of-plane components. For circular single-element crystals, annular

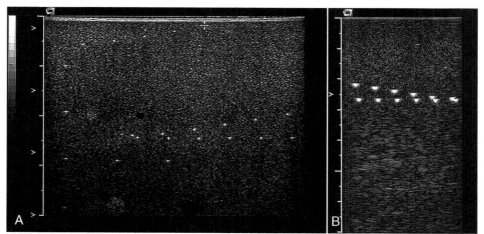

Figure 11-1 Frequency dependence of axial resolution. Image of a tissue-mimicking phantom obtained with a frequency of **(A)** 14 MHz and **(B)** 4 MHz.

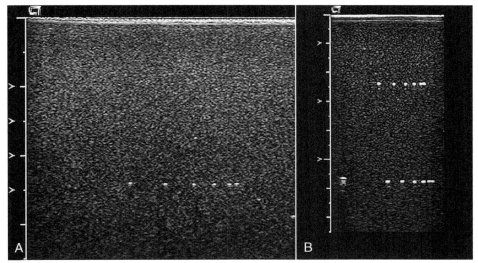

Figure 11-2 Effect of frequency on lateral resolution. Sonograms of a phantom with nylon rods. **A,** 14 MHz. **B,** 4 MHz. Note that the lateral extent of the rods is greater at lower frequency.

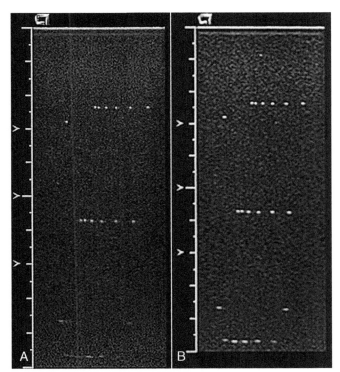

Figure 11-3 Effect of line density on lateral resolution. Sonograms of a phantom with nylon rods. **A,** High line density. **B,** Reduced line density. Note that the definition of the rods is improved at high line density.

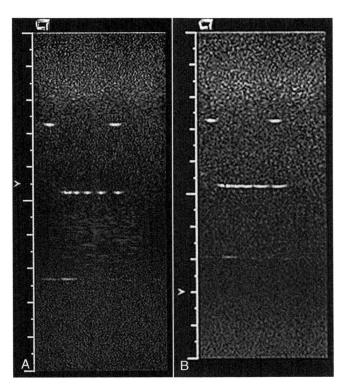

Figure 11-4 Effect of transmit focusing on lateral resolution. Sonograms of a phantom with nylon rods at a depth of 5 cm. **A,** Transmit focal zone corresponds to the depth of the rods. **B,** Transmit focal zone moved to a different depth. Note that the definition of the rods is improved with focusing.

arrays, and rectangular arrays, the beam shape is symmetrical (in-plane and out-of-plane dimensions are equal) at a given depth. Linear, phased, and curvilinear arrays produce a beam pattern that is mechanically focused in the elevation direction and electronically focused in the in-plane direction. The in-plane and out-of-plane dimensions of the beam are not symmetrical. Slice thickness (out-of-plane beam width) is generally not constant throughout the field of view. Fixed-focal-length mechanical focusing for multiple-element arrays establishes beam width in the elevation direction. The smallest slice thickness is within the fixed focal zone.

When the beam includes both a cystic structure (few scattering centers) and soft tissue, the scan line through that region is composed of echoes originating from both tissue types (Fig. 11-5). Thus the cyst would be misrepresented in the image as an object with immediate signal level. An accumulation of scan lines of this nature results

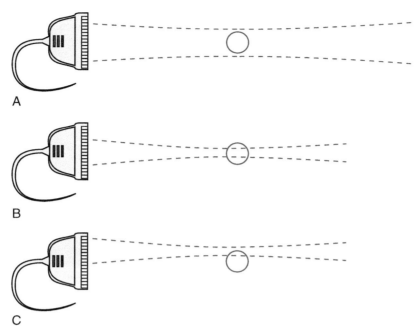

A

B

C

Figure 11-5 Partial volume effect. **A,** A large beam width extends beyond the boundary of the cyst, allowing echoes from surrounding tissue to contribute to the scan line. **B,** Reducing the beam width limits the sampling to the cyst through the central portion of the cyst. **C,** When sampling occurs at the edge of the cyst, a narrow beam may include echoes from surrounding tissue. This leads to fill-in near the border of the cystic structure in the image.

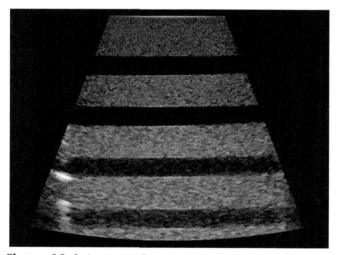

Figure 11-6 Sonogram of simulated cysts within a tissue-mimicking phantom. The scan plane is along the long axis of the cylindrical structures. The simulated cysts within the elevation focal zone exhibit high contrast. The increased beam width outside the focal zone causes fill-in of the hypoechogenic structures.

in fill-in of hypoechogenic structures (Fig. 11-6). If the beam width were small compared with the dimensions of the cyst, a more accurate portrayal would be possible.

CONTRAST RESOLUTION

Image contrast is the difference in brightness level (or optical density) between for the object and background in the displayed image on the monitor (or film). Often, the observer must make a decision as to whether or not a structure (called the target) is present within a generalized background. Low contrast resolution describes the ability to discern features with subtle differences in signal level and depends on the magnitude of the signal difference as well as the size of the object. Small reflectors with high signal levels are readily seen. A large reflector with a weak signal level may be visible, whereas a small structure at the same signal level is obscured by noise. Figure 11-7 demonstrates that

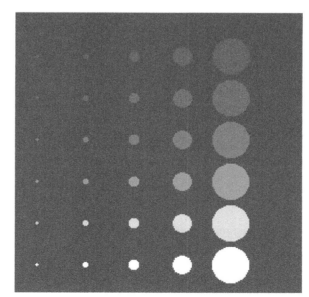

Figure 11-7 Low contrast resolution. Disks of varying size and intrinsic contrast are displayed on a uniform background. As object size decreases, more intrinsic contrast is needed to detect the object. (Courtesy of Mark Rzeszotarski, Ph.D., MetroHealth Medical Center, Cleveland, Ohio.)

progressingly smaller structures can be resolved as the relative signal levels between the target and background are increased.

Image contrast is made up of two components, intrinsic (detection) contrast and displayed contrast. Intrinsic contrast originates from physical differences between the detected reflectors (e.g., acoustic impedance mismatch), acquisition parameters (e.g., beam width, scan sequence, pulse shape), and processing (e.g., compression, edge enhancement). The stored pixel values in the scan converter represent intrinsic contrast. The displayed contrast translates pixel values to brightness levels on the monitor (or optical density on film) via the gray-scale map. Brightness also depends on proper monitor settings for contrast and brightness. The selected gray-scale map (e.g., logarithmic, linear, exponential) establishes the relationship between pixel value and brightness level (or optical density on film). Time gain compensation and dynamic range also affect the displayed image contrast.

The importance of matching the gray-scale map with the pixel values is illustrated by photographs of the Longaberger building in Newark, Ohio (Fig. 11-8). Intrinsic contrast in the three photographs is unchanged, and the translation of pixel values to brightness levels modifies the manner in which the data are displayed. Improper selection of gray-scale map alters image contrast and degrades image quality.

NOISE

The random variation in signal level contributed by noise causes brightness fluctuations in the image. Noise originates from both electrical sources (amplifiers, cabling, radiofrequency interference, and power line fluctuations) and acoustic sources (clutter and speckle). A common example of the effect of noise is snow in the television picture received from a distant station (now virtually nonexistent with the advent of cable transmission). Similarly, a scan of homogeneous tissue produces an image with variations in brightness. The preferred presentation would exhibit uniform brightness throughout the image of a uniform object. Weak echoes generate very low voltage signals, approaching the noise level of the electronics. Noise masks the signals from weak echoes and inhibits low contrast

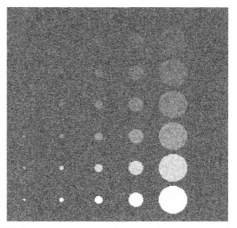

Figure 11-9 Low contrast resolution in the presence of noise. The introduction of noise to the image in Figure 11-7 inhibits our ability to discern low-contrast objects. (Courtesy of Mark Rzeszotarski, Ph.D., MetroHealth Medical Center, Cleveland, Ohio.)

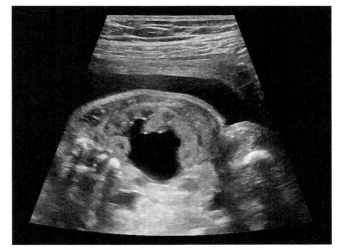

Figure 11-10 Sonogram of the fetal kidney.

resolution (Fig. 11-9). A low-noise sonogram is one in which liquid-filled structures exhibit very little signal (Fig. 11-10).

Acoustic noise is defined as echo-induced signals that do not correspond to structures along the sampling path

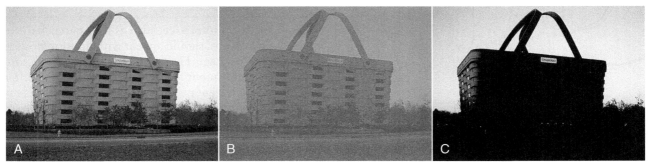

Figure 11-8 Effect of gray map on image contrast. **A,** Gray scale distributed across all pixel values. **B,** All pixel values mapped to narrow range of gray levels. **C,** Pixel values mapped as either black or white.

of the main beam. Clutter and speckle are often considered types of acoustic noise. Methods to reduce noise include rejection control, frame averaging, and adaptive frame averaging.

Clutter

The two-dimensional sonogram consists of multiple lines of sight acquired during a finite time interval. The data associated with a particular scan line, however, are not exclusively derived from structures located along that scan line. Clutter from scattering originating outside the main beam also contributes to the net induced signal (Fig. 11-11). This modulation of scan line data precludes the totally faithful portrayal of anatomic structures. Since clutter does not correspond to structures along the scan line, image contrast is degraded. Tissue harmonic imaging by tuning reception to twice the transmitted frequency improves image contrast by excluding clutter generated at the transmitted frequency.

Speckle

Numerous small scattering centers within the volume of tissue interrogated by the ultrasound beam produce multiple scattered echoes over a wide range of angles. Nonspecular reflections within soft tissue, blood, and other fluids scatter ultrasound energy, which ultimately returns toward the transducer along different pathways. Multiple wavefronts from these scattering events strike the transducer simultaneously (Fig. 11-12). The mottled or grainy appearance observed in the image is a result of the interference pattern from these numerous scattered echoes

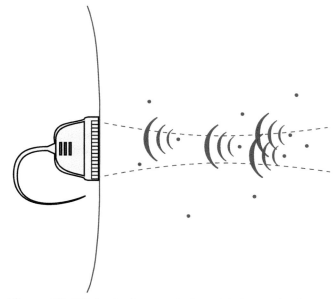

Figure 11-12 Small reflectors in the beam *(dots)* scatter the ultrasonic energy. The interference pattern produced at the transducer from numerous scatterers is called speckle.

incident on the transducer. The bright and dark variations in the image are responsible for the name speckle.

Speckle appearance depends on transducer position, beam dimensions, direction of propagation, and frequency. For a particular scan plane, the speckle pattern is constant with time. That is, if transducer position and other acquisition parameters are unchanged, successive images of stationary structures yield the same speckle pattern. Scattering is frequency-dependent; consequently the speckle pattern is altered if the transducer frequency is changed (Fig. 11-13).

Since speckle is a composite of numerous scattering events, the one-to-one correspondence between image brightness and physical structures is lost. Weak echoes from speckle are superimposed on other returning echoes. When echoes from specular reflectors are present, their signals dominate those from speckle; consequently speckle is masked in high-echogenic regions. Speckle is usually associated with regions devoid of strong reflectors (e.g., organ parenchyma).

Speckle Reduction

Ideally, uniform soft tissue, such as liver parenchal-free of vessels and lesions, should appear with uniform brightness in the B-mode image. However, on a cellular level, soft tissue is not uniform but rather composed of many different small structures that give rise to multiple points of scatter. The interference pattern at the transducer is expressed as speckle. Speckle inhibits the detection of low-contrast structures (i.e., objects with reflective properties similar to those of the surrounding tissue). Increasing ultrasound intensity does not suppress speckle. Very high frequency at 100 MHz would separate the interference from closely

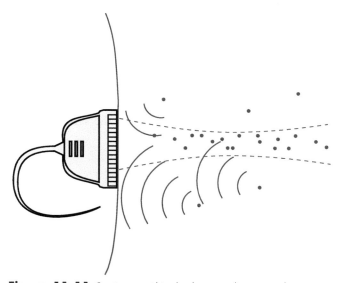

Figure 11-11 Scatterers within the beam redirect sound energy to structures outside the beam, where additional scattering events enable scattered sound energy to reach the transducer. The interference pattern produced by multiple path reflections is called clutter. Clutter suppresses contrast.

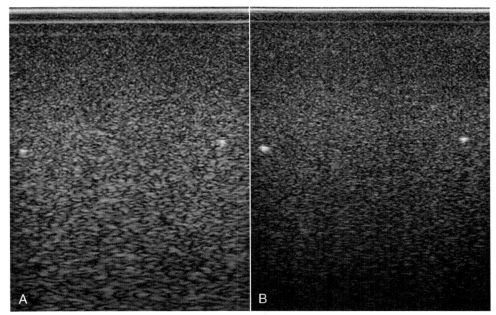

Figure 11-13 Frequency dependence of the speckle pattern. Sonograms of a tissue-mimicking phantom obtained with a frequency of **(A)** 5 MHz and **(B)** 11 MHz.

spaced reflectors; but because rapid attenuation dominates at this frequency, this approach is not practical. Methods to reduce speckle are classified in three general categories: averaging, filtering, and adaptive processing.

Frequency and spatial compounding enhances signals from tissue features while suppressing speckle. Multiple images of the same anatomic site are obtained under different conditions so that speckle patterns are not correlated. Speckle is partially canceled when the multiple images are added together. If the object is registered in the same location for each image, speckle is reduced without blurring the object. Limited spectral reduction is achieved by frame averaging, in which multiple frames separated in time are added together to cancel random variations (Fig. 11-14).

Frequency compounding acquires two images, each with a different frequency, and then sums these images. Since the speckle pattern is variable with frequency, speckle is diminished. A similar effect is achieved by extended signal processing. The received broadband radiofrequency signal is divided into two narrower bandwidth subsignals with different center frequencies, which are subsequently processed in parallel before they are recombined to form the composite signal.

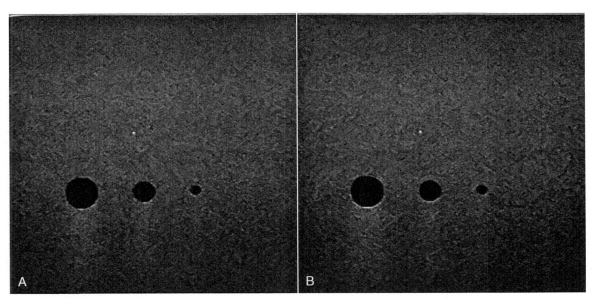

Figure 11-14 Sonograms of a tissue-equivalent phantom with a stimulated cysts. **A,** No frame averaging. **B,** Frame averaging. The borders of the cysts are more clearly defined with frame averaging.

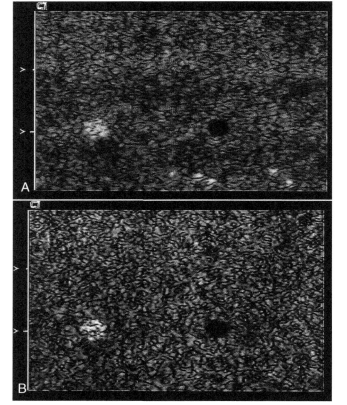

Figure 11-15 Sonograms of a tissue-equivalent phantom with a stimulated mass and cyst. **A,** No spatial compounding. **B,** Spatial compounding. The objects are more clearly defined with spatial compounding.

In spatial compounding, images are obtained with different beam angles and aperture locations; therefore, they exhibit different speckle patterns. The compound image has reduced speckle depending on the number of images added together and the independence of the sampling process. The improvement in contrast resolution by speckle reduction is illustrated in Fig. 11-15.

Processing the image with a two-dimensional filter averages the response of neighboring pixels to smooth the image, with a subsequent loss of spatial detail. Blurring is a major disadvantage of this technique.

Adaptive processing analyzes the neighboring pixels to determine if the changes in signal level are random or follow a trend. If the variations are random, then speckle associated with that variation is suppressed while local mean signal level is maintained. If the signal variation is interrelated, then these features are preserved with enhanced edges. The degree of speckle reduction can be adjusted to control the overall smooth appearance of the image (Fig. 11-16). No loss of spatial resolution is incurred with this method.

GEOMETRIC DISTORTION

The size, shape, and relative positions of objects within the scan plane should be accurately portrayed by corresponding structures in the image. The inaccurate presentation of spatial relationships causes geometric distortion. Spatial mapping of the echo-induced signals depends on scan-line density, beam width, number of sampling points along the scan line, interpolation during scan conversion, and spatial compounding. The acquisition parameter of pulse repetition frequency, variable tissue acoustic velocity, and refraction may also affect the spatial registration of the signals. An improperly calibrated PACS interface or image recording device may introduce geometric distortion.

ARTIFACTS

An ultrasound image is the portrayal of anatomy interrogated by an ultrasonic beam. An artifact is any structure in that image that does not correlate directly with actual tissue. Artifacts assume different forms—including perceived objects in the image that are not actually present, structures that should be represented in the image but are missing, and reflectors geometrically displaced from the true locations. These errors in acoustic presentation of the scanned subject are usually caused by technical

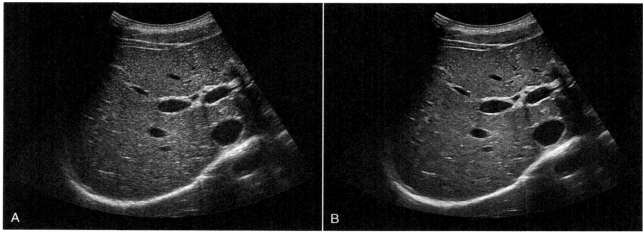

Figure 11-16 Sonograms of a liver. **A,** No speckle reduction. **B,** Adaptive speckle reduction.

limitations or anatomic factors, but occasionally equipment malfunction creates artifacts.

Miscalibration of ultrasound velocity, broken or deformed crystals, broken or improperly assembled backing or facing materials, faulty monitors, or defective recording devices can corrupt the imaging process. A defective recording device can introduce distortion, misrepresent the contrast scale, and cause a loss of image detail. An effective quality control program should identify malfunctions of the scanner and recording device.

Improper operation of equipment can also play a role in the production of artifacts. This is particularly true with poorly trained or inexperienced personnel. The sonographer may not properly set gain, time gain compensation, or other controls for sensitivity and uniformity. The wrong area may be scanned (not a true artifact), or the anatomy may be scanned too rapidly.

The acoustic properties of tissues and the propagation of ultrasound waves through them can create imaging artifacts. In addition, certain assumptions are necessary for the mapping of returning echoes into a composite picture; when these are erroneous, artifacts in the image result. A survey of image artifacts in real-time ultrasound is presented in Chapter 12.

TEMPORAL RESOLUTION

Sampling must occur at frequent intervals during the movement of an interface to accurately portray the motion. Abrupt changes would be missed or blurred if the sampling rate were not adequate. Thus the frame rate required to visualize a moving object without blurring depends on the speed of the object. *Temporal resolution* describes the ability of a series of several frames acquired sequentially in time to depict the movement of structures.

Methods to improve temporal resolution by operator controls include a decrease in scan range, scan-line density, persistence, or sector angle. Since frame rate, scan-line density, and scan range are interdependent, an increase in frame rate is usually accompanied by a reduction in scan-line density. The number of transmit focal zones also affects maximum frame rate. Some scanners allow direct adjustment of pulse repetition frequency so that the sonographer determines the trade-off between frame rate and lateral resolution. Acquisition techniques such as multiple beam formers, which obtain multiple scan lines per transmitted pulse, enable high frame rates with little loss in lateral resolution.

SUMMARY

Axial resolution, lateral resolution, contrast resolution, presence of artifacts, geometric distortion, noise, and temporal resolution each contribute to overall image quality. These factors are often interdependent. Adjustment in scan parameters to improve one of these factors causes degradation in another aspect. For example, increased scan-line density improves lateral resolution, but more time is required to compose the image with a reduction in maximum frame rate. In recent years manufacturers have developed processing techniques to reduce speckle. Even though their application presets establish initial scanning parameters, the sonographer, by adjusting operator controls, must optimize image quality for each examination to obtain the desired diagnostic information.

Image Artifacts

12

Chapter Objectives

To state the assumptions necessary to assign the spatial origin of the detected echo
To recognize common artifacts encountered in B-mode imaging
To describe the cause of enhancement, shadowing, reverberation, comet tail, mirror image, velocity error, and range ambiguity artifacts

Key terms

Banding
Comet tail
Defocusing (refraction)
Enhancement
Ghost image

Mirror image
Misregistration (refraction)
Partial volume
Range ambiguity
Reverberation

Shadowing
Velocity error (propagation error)

SOURCES OF ARTIFACTS

The complexity of ultrasound equipment sometimes makes it difficult to isolate and understand the causes of B-mode imaging artifacts. Limitations inherent in the ultrasound sampling process (i.e., the physical properties of ultrasound waves and their interactions with tissues) and equipment malfunction can contribute to the presence of artifacts. This chapter describes artifacts that can occur in real-time imaging.

ASSUMPTIONS FOR TWO-DIMENSIONAL ECHO MAPPING

Technical limitations (spatial pulse length, scan-line density, beam width, and pulse repetition frequency [PRF]) are inherent in the sampling process and restrict the fidelity of overall image quality. Certain assumptions are necessary for the spatial registration of returning echoes into a composite picture. When these assumptions, as listed below, are in error, image artifacts result.

- The transmitted wave travels along a straight-line path from the transducer to the reflector and back to the transducer.
- Attenuation of sound in tissue is uniform along the propagation path.
- Beam dimensions are small in both section thickness and lateral directions.
- All detected echoes originate from the axis of the main beam only.
- All received echoes are derived from the most recently transmitted pulse.
- The ultrasound wave travels at the rate of 1540 m/s in tissue; thus the distance to the interface is determined from the time of flight (1 cm corresponds to 13 µs).
- Each reflector contributes a single echo when it is interrogated along a single scan line.
- The induced echo signal is derived from a single object and is directly related to its reflective properties.

TYPES OF IMAGE ARTIFACTS

The reflector's size, shape, and location can be misrepresented. Small objects, in particular, may be unresolved or distorted. A single reflector can be replicated multiple times at various locations in the image. Brightness in the display does not always correspond with the reflectivity of the interface. Some artifacts (e.g., enhancement or shadowing distal to a structure) aid in the characterization of the structure with respect to content (fluid or solid). Artifacts must be recognized, because not doing so may result in an incorrect interpretation.

PARTIAL VOLUME

Finite beam width creates a partial volume artifact related to the simultaneous sampling of tissues with different acoustic properties. Recall that each pixel in the image is a depiction of three-dimensional volume encompassed by the ultrasound beam. Partial volume artifacts can occur in either the in-plane direction (lateral) or the out-of-plane direction (slice thickness).

For circular single-element transducers and annular arrays, the beam shape is symmetrical (lateral and elevation dimensions are equal) at a given depth. Linear, curvilinear, and phased arrays produce a beam pattern, which is mechanically focused in the elevation direction and electronically focused in the lateral direction. The in-plane and out-of-plane dimensions of the beam are not symmetrical. The in-plane beam width is most narrow within the transmit focal zone of the transducer. The out-of-plane beam width is most narrow within the fixed, mechanical focal zone of the transducer but results in variable slice thickness throughout the scan range.

An accumulation of scan lines in which the beam width is greater than the lateral dimension of the structure includes echoes from the surrounding tissue. This averaging of signal levels from multiple tissue types is most often observed for a fluid-filled structure in which signal from nearby tissue is superimposed on the hypoechoic fluid (Fig. 12-1). A false impression of object solidity is created. Partial volume artifacts have also occurred in the slice thickness direction and are most pronounced outside the mechanical focal zone. Improper machine settings (high receiver gain or time gain compensation) increase the visibility of this artifact.

ATTENUATION

The most easily recognizable and useful artifacts are related to attenuation of the ultrasound beam as it propagates through tissue. The rate of intensity loss may vary greatly among different types of tissue. *Enhancement and shadowing affect the brightness of the displayed echoes obtained along weakly or strongly attenuated beam paths.*

Cysts and other liquid-filled structures are normally less attenuating and are hypoechoic compared with surrounding

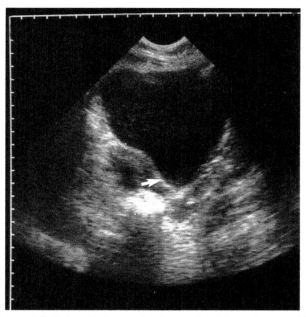

Figure 12-1 Partial volume artifact illustrated as debris at the base of the bladder *(arrow)*.

soft tissues. The region distal to them is interrogated with a beam having greater intensity than is obtained when the beam travels an equivalent distance in tissue. Thus, the region distal to a liquid-filled structure often produces stronger signal levels than are observed from similar, adjacent tissues at the same depth (Figs. 12-2 and 12-3).

Shadowing is the opposite effect; that is, calcifications, metal foreign bodies, and some solid masses are more attenuating than the surrounding soft tissues. The area distal to these structures is interrogated with a beam of decreased intensity; thus the displayed signal levels appear at reduced brightness compared with similar, adjacent tissue at the same depth (Figs. 12-4, 12-5, and 12-6).

Solid masses compared with fluid-filled structures are generally more attenuating and often more echoic, demonstrating internal structural detail that differs from the surrounding soft tissues. The ability of ultrasound imaging to distinguish cystic and solid structures noninvasively

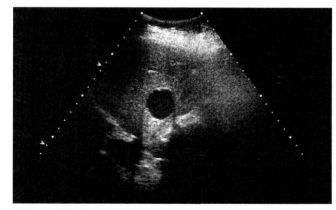

Figure 12-2 Attenuation artifact. Enhancement distal to a liver cyst.

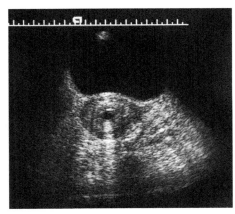

Figure 12-3 Attenuation artifact. Enhancement distal to nabothian cyst.

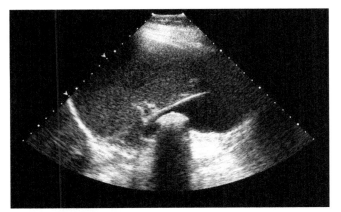

Figure 12-4 Attenuation artifact. Shadowing distal to stones in the gallbladder.

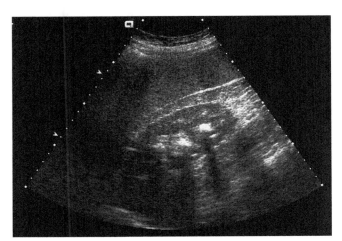

Figure 12-5 Attenuation artifact. Shadowing distal to kidney stones.

makes it a powerful diagnostic tool. However, hypoechoic masses that produce shadowing rather than enhancement do exist. Hyperechoic cysts, independent of partial volume effects, sometimes cannot be distinguished from solid masses. Scanning with different transducer orientation to alter the imaging plane may facilitate the presentation of these structures.

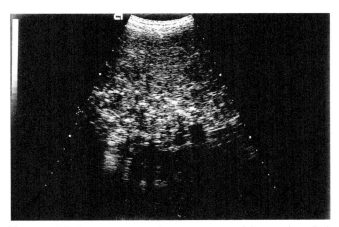

Figure 12-6 Attenuation artifact. Sonogram of liver with multiple calcifications.

BANDING

Focusing characteristics of the transducer may create a banding artifact (Fig. 12-7), which is a region of increased brightness caused by greater intensity within the focal zone. This is particularly noticeable with real-time systems that have fixed transmit focusing and dynamic receive focusing. Images obtained with multiple transmit focal zones are subject to banding when the amplitudes of signals from adjacent focal zones are mismatched. More commonly, banding is created by improper manual adjustment of the settings for time gain compensation.

REVERBERATION

When reverberations or multiple reflections from an interface are present, additional echoes from this interface are recorded in the image. The amount of sound energy

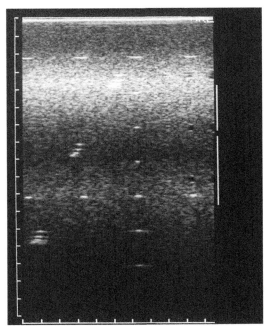

Figure 12-7 Focal zone banding artifact *(bright area on image).*

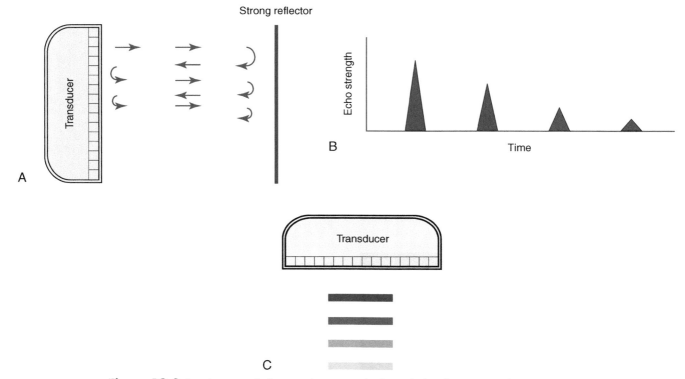

Figure 12-8 Reverberation. **A,** For a single transmitted pulse, multiple reflections occur between a strong reflector and the transducer. **B,** The echoes along one line of sight are separated equally in time. **C,** Two-dimensional mapping of a reverberation artifact.

reflected from an interface depends on the acoustic impedances of the two media. If the impedance mismatch is large (e.g., soft tissue-gas, fat-muscle, or liquid-gas) and the interface is oriented perpendicular to the direction of propagation, reverberations between the interface and the transducer can occur. A strong echo is initially created at the interface following the transmitted pulse. On return to the transducer, some of the echo energy is redirected into the patient, where it can undergo a second reflection at the same interface. The second echo returns to the transducer, and the sequence is repeated. Since each succeeding echo is displaced in time, a series of bright bands of decreasing intensity are registered equidistant from each other in the image (Fig. 12-8). The loss in intensity is caused by the multiple reflections that take place at the strong reflector and the transducer. A fraction of the incident energy is transmitted through an interface each time one is encountered. Attenuation by the elongated path length is balanced by time gain compensation.

The fat-muscle interface near the skin surface is often the source of reverberation artifacts. Reverberations can also occur between two strong reflectors along the path of the ultrasound beam; similarly, progressively weaker bands are depicted in the image. The spacing between bands is equal to the separation of the reflectors. Clinical examples of reverberation artifacts are shown in Figures 12-9 and 12-10.

Although anatomically related reverberation artifacts are commonly observed, defective equipment and improper technique can also produce them. Occasionally, an air

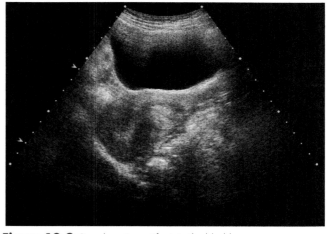

Figure 12-9 Reverberation artifacts in the bladder.

bubble is present within the fluid surrounding a mechanical sector crystal or is trapped in a fluid-filled condom encasing an endosonography probe. In either case a strongly reflecting interface located near the transducer inhibits proper sampling of the entire field of view.

COMET TAIL

Multiple internal reflections within a small but highly reflective object create a series of echoes. Compared with tissue, the object has high or low acoustic impedance. The acoustic impedance mismatch at the boundary of the

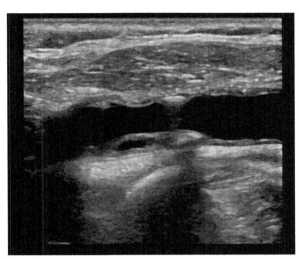

Figure 12-10 Reverberation artifacts in a vessel with ulcerated plaque. (Courtesy of Yvette Ramos, RDMS, RVT.)

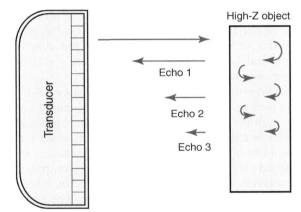

Figure 12-11 Comet-tail artifact. Internal reflections give rise to multiple echoes from an object.

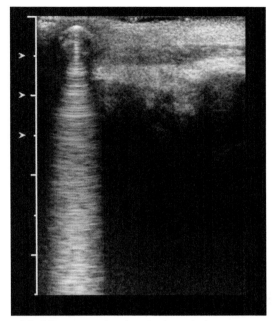

Figure 12-12 Comet tail artifact distal to a high acoustic impedance reflector (BB near the eye).

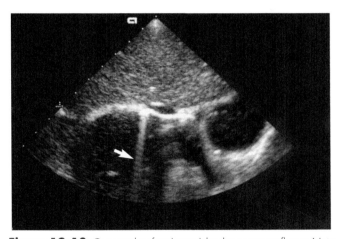

Figure 12-13 Comet tail artifact *(arrow)* distal to a strong reflector. Note the bands in the comet tail.

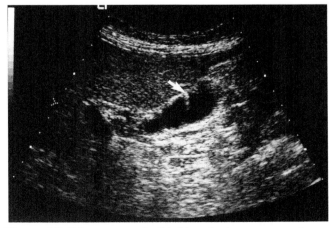

Figure 12-14 Sonogram of gallbladder with adenomyomatosis showing comet tail artifact *(arrow)*.

object forms two highly reflective opposing interfaces that produce short-path reverberations (Fig. 12-11). The time delay between echoes is short because the sound wave travels the distance across the object and back between echoes. The series of echoes is expressed as multiple small bands, called comet tails, distal to the object in the image. For very small path lengths, the bands may overlap. Comet tails are usually seen in relatively echo-free regions. The trail of echoes is usually short, less than 2 cm in length.

The possibility of creating a comet tail is enhanced by the increasing difference in acoustic impedances. The complexity of a comet-tail pattern depends on the shape, composition, and size of the object as well as on the scan orientation and the distance from the transducer face. Metallic objects such as clips, staples, and sutures are susceptible to comet tail artifacts (Fig. 12-12).

Comet tail artifacts typically arise from the near wall or lumen of the gallbladder when crystalline deposits of cholesterol are present (Figs. 12-13 and 12-14). Banding is rarely observed from the deep wall, not because crystals are preferentially formed in the near wall but because the hyperechoic background distal to the wall masks the comet tail.

RING DOWN

A closely related phenomenon, called a ring down artifact, occurs when a small gas bubble resonates, resulting in a continuous emission of ultrasound. The discrete banding associated with a comet tail is not seen. The track of ring down artifacts can be extensive, extending from the point of origin throughout the scan range (Figs. 12-15 and 12-16). Ring down artifacts produce additional echoes in the image and mask other, weaker echoes indicative of anatomic structures. Since the presentation is so similar to that from internal reflections, the terms *comet tail* and *ring down artifact* are often used interchangeably.

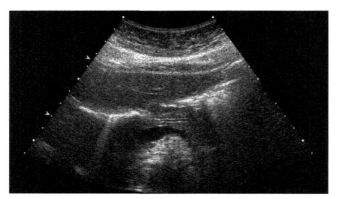

Figure 12-15 Ring down artifact from an air bubble introduced during amniocentesis.

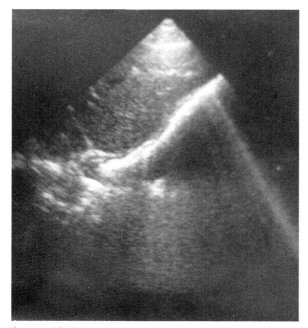

Figure 12-16 Ring down artifact caused by air in the stomach.

MULTIPLE PATH REFLECTIONS

Specular reflectors may direct the beam at an angle that may not intercept the transducer, resulting in a "missing" interface in the image. Nonspecular reflectors scatter ultrasound in all directions; therefore, they present a complex echo interference pattern to the transducer. Multiple path reflections cause an incorrect axial placement of an interface. The ultrasound beam strikes an interface at an angle and is subsequently reflected from a second (or third) interface before being directed toward the transducer. The detected echo does not travel in a straight-line path. A special case of multiple path reflection is the mirror image artifact.

Mirror Image

Mirror image artifacts are produced when an object is located directly in front of a highly reflective surface at which near-total reflection occurs. This artifact can also occur if the object is offset from a curved strong reflector or the object and strong reflector are oriented at an angle. Examples of strong reflectors include the diaphragm, pleura, and bowel. Human-made objects placed in the patient can also act as strong reflectors.

Consider the illustrative example in Figure 12-17. The object is imaged in the usual manner by scanning across it with multiple lines of sight. Along nearby scan lines (which normally would not interrogate the object), the ultrasound beam is reflected by the strong reflector toward the object. When the beam strikes the object, part of the energy is reflected back to the strong reflector, which then redirects the echo toward the transducer. The additional set of scan lines containing echoes from the object form a second image of the object located distal to the strong reflector. The time required for the sound wave to travel between the strong reflector and the object creates the mirroring effect, so that the true and false images are equidistant but on opposite sides from the strong reflector (Figs. 12-18 and 12-19).

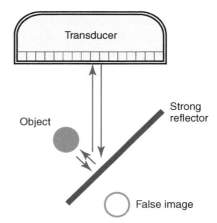

Figure 12-17 Mirror image artifact. A strong reflector allows sampling of the object along lines of sight, in which the sound beam does not follow a straight path.

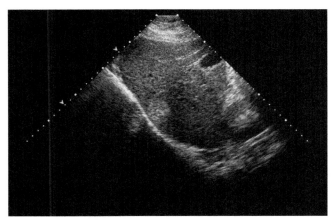

Figure 12-18 Mirror image artifact of liver with a mass. The diaphragm acts as a strong reflector. The mass is depicted improperly on each side of the diaphragm.

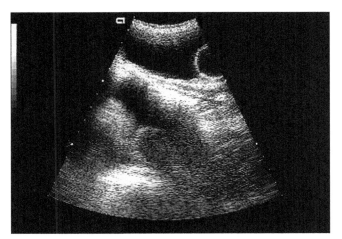

Figure 12-19 Mirror image artifact of a Foley catheter placed in the bladder.

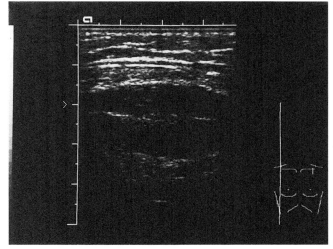

Figure 12-20 Sonogram showing fluid collection in the left thorax.

Clinical Example

An 85-year-old female presented with left thoracic pain following pacemaker insertion. Ultrasound examination with a 7-MHz linear array demonstrated a relatively large, subcutaneous, fluid-like structure in the anterior left thorax adjacent to the cardiac pacemaker (Fig. 12-20). The presence of a strong reflector and the symmetry of the echo pattern with respect to the strong reflector suggested that the distal portion of the fluid collection in the sonogram was a mirror-image artifact. Needle aspiration yielded a small quantity of blood, indicating that the mass was a hematoma. The strong reflector was identified as a pacemaker wire.

The fluid structure is imaged in the usual manner by scanning across it with multiple lines of sight. For each scan line in which the tissue-fluid interface is encountered, the following sequence of interactions occurs. When the ultrasound beam strikes the tissue-fluid interface, part of the energy is reflected back to the transducer (Fig. 12-21, *A*), and part of the energy is transmitted through the interface and strikes the pacemaker wire

(Fig. 12-21, *B,C*). The pacemaker wire reflects the sound energy back toward the transducer. At the tissue-fluid interface, part of the energy is transmitted to the transducer (Fig.12-21, *B*) and part is redirected toward the strong reflector, where once again total reflection occurs. The echo is then directed toward the transducer (Fig. 12-21, *C*). Multiple path reflections from the tissue-fluid interface form a second image of the object located behind the strong reflector (Fig.12-21, *D*). The additional time required for the sound wave to travel back and forth between the pacemaker wire and the tissue-fluid interface creates the mirroring effect, so that the true and false images are equidistant from the pacemaker wire.

REFRACTION

Refraction of the ultrasound beam at a boundary between two media with different acoustic velocities causes two types of refraction artifacts, misregistration and defocusing. In addition to improper placement, misregistration (refraction) may distort size and shape of the object. Defocusing (refraction) in this connotation describes a loss of multiple beam coherence.

Formation of the image is predicated on the assumption that the ultrasound beam always travels in a straight line through tissue. In Figure 12-22 an object appears at the wrong location in the image because the assignment of position is based on the projected straight-line path of the beam, whereas the true location of the object is actually offset from the assumed path. A similar effect caused by the refraction of light is seen when an object under water is viewed from above. If one reaches for the object through the water, the misregistration becomes immediately apparent.

As predicted by Snell's law, the amount of deviation from the expected straight-line path changes with the angle of incidence and the velocities in the associated media. Although refraction is not a major problem in diagnostic ultrasound, under certain conditions the bending of the

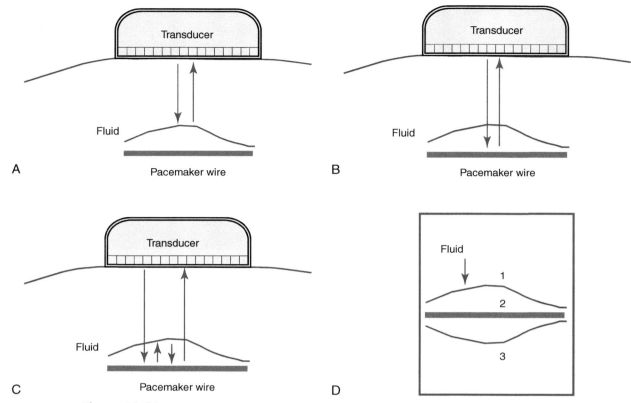

Figure 12-21 Sampling of the tissue-fluid interface. The arrows are shown left to right to indicate the sequence of events. Only one line of sight is sampled for the events depicted. **A,** Proper placement of the tissue-fluid interface, labeled 1 in **(D)**. **B,** Proper placement of the strong reflector, labeled 2 in **(D)**. **C,** Improper placement of tissue-fluid interface by multiple path reflections, labeled 3 in **(D)**. **D,** Illustration of mirror image artifact.

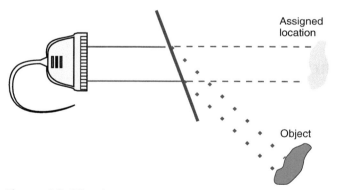

Figure 12-22 Refraction along the beam path causes the object to be mispositioned in the image.

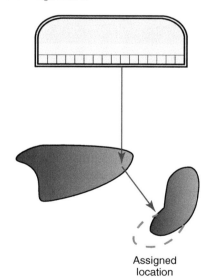

Figure 12-23 Refraction. Bending of the sound beam by the liver causes the spatial assignment for the pole of the kidney (dashed line) to be in error.

sound beam can cause artifacts. In Figure 12-23 the fat layer surrounding the liver bends the beam from the straight-line path (velocity in fat is less than velocity in soft tissue). This causes the pole of the kidney located laterally to the assumed direction of sampling to be placed incorrectly along the scan line. The kidney is properly represented by other beam paths that do not traverse the liver. Consequently, the kidney appears elongated, since the pole of the kidney is duplicated in the image (Fig. 12-24). This artifact is avoided by scanning with a posterior approach or along a pathway that is completely covered by the liver.

A similar effect is sometimes seen in examining the heart with a phased array placed in a subxiphoid location to image the left ventricle in the short axis (Fig. 12-25). Duplication of the moving ventricular wall is depicted, which disappears during part of the respiration cycle (attributed to the changing position of the liver).

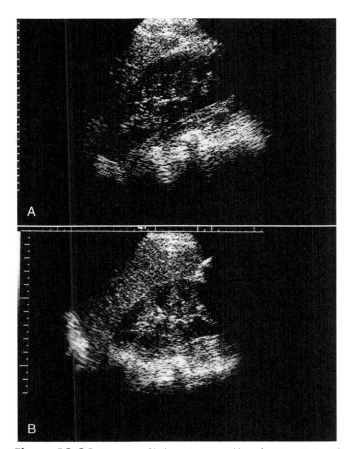

Figure 12-24 Distortion of kidney size caused by refraction. **A,** Partial coverage by liver in which refraction depicts the kidney with increased size. **B,** Complete coverage by liver (no distortion in size).

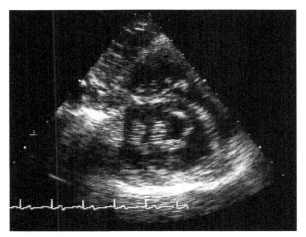

Figure 12-25 Refraction artifact shows a duplication of the inferior base and inferolateral basal segments. (Courtesy David A. Foley, M.D.)

Defocusing

Refraction also produces shadowing at the edges of large (compared with the width of the ultrasound beam) curved structures. The amount of bending varies along the curve surface, resulting in a loss of scan-line coherence. After passing through such structures, the beams from multiple scan lines diverge or converge depending on the velocity within the structure. For a cyst, the velocity is typically

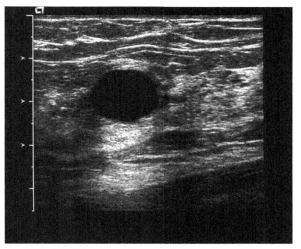

Figure 12-26 Refraction (defocusing) artifact at the edge of a cystic structure, illustrating shadowing.

lower than in the surrounding tissue, and a narrow-angle shadow projection is created (Fig. 12-26). A wide-angle shadow projection occurs when a relatively high-velocity structure, such as bone, is encountered. The shadowing is in part caused by the increased attenuation as the beam is bent along the walls of these structures (effectively creating a longer path through the wall).

GHOST IMAGE

A special case of refraction misregistration artifact, called the ghost image, is caused by altered paths of the sound beam as it passes through the overlying rectus abdominis muscles. The rectus muscles act as lenses, causing refraction of the ultrasound beam and leading to duplication of a small object distal to the muscles. The multiple sampling of small objects by the redirected sound beams results in the duplication or triplication of these objects. Recognition of this artifact is critical, since a single gestational sac may appear multiple times (Fig. 12-27). One common

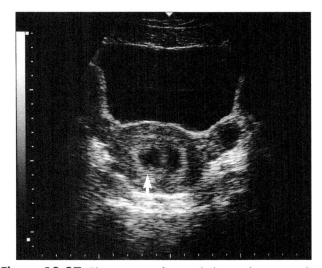

Figure 12-27 Ghost image artifact in which a single gestational sac (arrow) is duplicated in the image.

indication of ghost imaging is when the movement in unison of the displayed fetuses actually turns out to be motion of one that is mirrored. The ghosting can be removed by scanning from different angles or directions. Changing to an endosonography probe eliminates the artifact.

SIDE LOBES

Side lobes, which are present with all transducers, result from interference phenomena attributed to nonthickness mode vibrations and multiple-source beam formation. The regular periodic spacing of elements within a multiple-element array causes one type, the grating lobe. Side lobes are typically of low intensity compared with the main beam (less than 10% of the main beam intensity) and are generated at various angles with respect to the main beam.

Side lobes and grating lobes cause misplaced reflectors. These off-axis lobes interrogate structures outside the main beam. If a highly reflective interface is encountered, it will be incorrectly positioned in the image along the path of the main beam (Fig. 12-28). This artifact is sometimes observed during needle biopsy with ultrasound guidance (Fig. 12-29). Gas in the bowel or another strong reflector can contribute a side lobe artifact in the scan of the abdomen (Figs.12-30 and 12-31).

The highly reflective structure may lie outside the scan plane and may not be readily identified as a source of additional echoes. In this case reorientation of the scan plane is required. Linear and curvilinear arrays are most likely to produce off-axis lobe artifacts.

RANGE AMBIGUITY

When the area of interest is limited in depth by high PRF, structures beyond the indicated scan range may be depicted in the image. This range ambiguity in depth

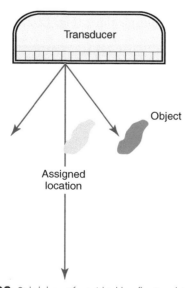

Figure 12-28 Side lobe artifact. A highly reflective object along the path of a secondary lobe *(small arrows)* produces an echo that is incorrectly assigned a location in the direction of the main beam *(large arrow).*

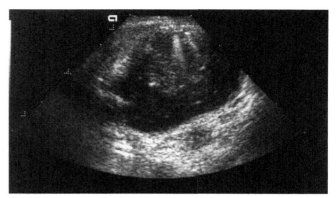

Figure 12-29 Sonogram of a thyroid during needle biopsy. A single needle is shown at two different locations in the image.

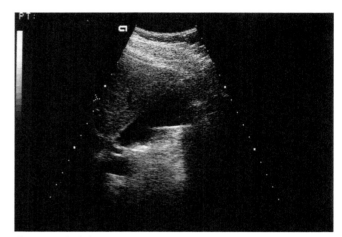

Figure 12-30 Sonogram of a gallbladder. Gas in the duodenum located outside the scan plane produces a side lobe artifact.

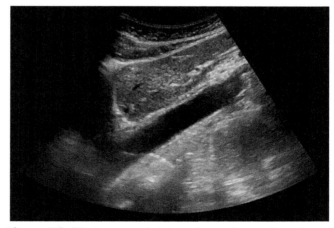

Figure 12-31 Sonogram of abdominal aorta. Strong reflector located outside the scan plane produces a side lobe artifact.

placement occurs because the time between the transmitted pulse and the detected echo is not measured properly. Real-time image formation assumes that all received echoes are formed from the most recent transmitted pulse. Normally, a short pulse of ultrasound is sent out from the transducer and the transducer is silent for a time to listen for returning echoes. All echoes received during this sampling period are assigned a depth based on the time interval between the transmitted pulse and the detected echo. A second pulse is then sent out, and the transducer again is silent to listen for returning echoes. At high PRFs, echoes from deep structures interrogated by the first pulse arrive at the transducer after the second pulse has been transmitted. These echoes are interpreted as having originated from the most recent (second) transmitted pulse and are incorrectly placed near the transducer in the image (Figs. 12-32 and 12-33).

VELOCITY ERROR

Axial placement of interfaces in the image is based on the echo ranging principle, in which the velocity of ultrasound is assumed to be 1540 m/s. Errors in device calibration of the velocity or scanning through tissues (bone, lens of the eye, cartilage, fluid, silicone, and fat) that have different acoustic velocities can cause incorrect spatial registration, an artifact called a velocity error or propagation error. In these circumstances the actual acoustic velocity in the medium deviates from the calibrated velocity and the measured elapsed time is not accurately converted to depth.

Propagation speed error causes an axial displacement of the interface in the image. If a structure having low acoustic velocity is encountered along the scan line path to a more distant object, the echo is delayed in time and the object is misrepresented at an increased depth. If a structure with high acoustic velocity is encountered along the scan line

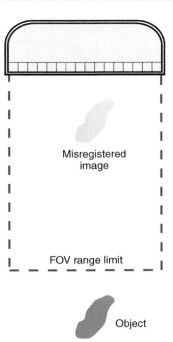

Figure 12-33 Depth assignment ambiguity. When the range of scanning is limited by a high pulse repetition frequency, deep-lying structures are incorrectly placed near the transducer in the image.

path to a more distant object, the elapsed time for echo detection is reduced and the object is misrepresented at a more shallow depth (Figs. 12-34, 12-35, and 12-36).

Measurements of distances, areas, and volumes are of particular importance in diagnostic ultrasound. For small objects, a large velocity difference is necessary to observe a significant error. For large objects, however, a small deviation in velocity can introduce a large error in distance measurements, leading to an incorrect conclusion.

An interface is displaced toward the transducer and the size of the object is reduced if the actual acoustic velocity along the propagation path is greater than the calibrated value. For example, consider a mass 10 cm in diameter in which the front face is 5 cm from the transducer and the velocity of ultrasound is 2000 m/s. The front interface of the mass is properly located in the image because the velocity in the overlying tissue is correct; however, the back of the mass is displayed at a depth of 12.7 cm (rather than the actual 15 cm). The calculation is illustrated in Example 12-1.

Example 12-1

The acoustic velocity of the mass (c_m) is 2000 m/s. Determine the time to travel the path length (d) through the 10-cm mass (actual distance is 20 cm or 0.2 m because of the 10 cm down and 10 cm back).

$$d = c_m t$$
$$0.2 \text{ m} = (2000 \text{ m/s})(t)$$
$$t = \frac{0.2 \text{ m}}{2000 \text{ m/s}}$$
$$t = 1 \times 10^{-4} \text{ s}$$

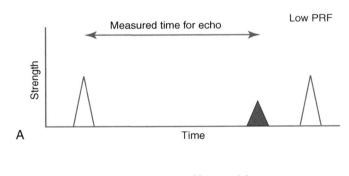

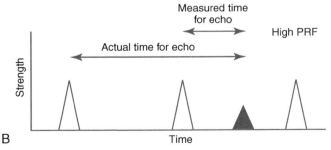

Figure 12-32 Timing between the transmitted pulse *(clear area)* and the echo *(shaded area)*. **A,** At low pulse repetition frequencies (PRFs) the measured time for the echo is proper. **B,** At high PRFs the time between the most recently transmitted pulse and the echo does not correspond to the actual depth.

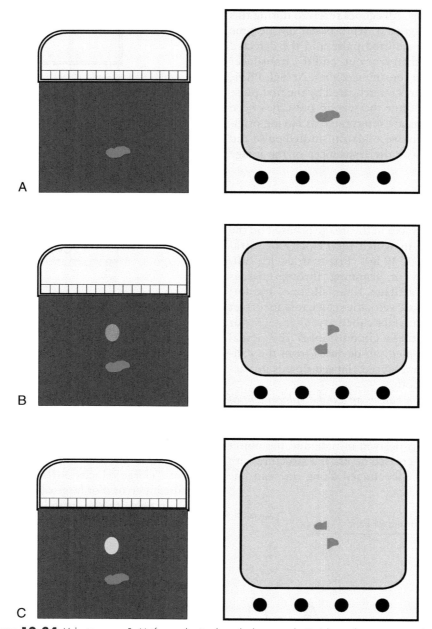

Figure 12-34 Velocity error. **A,** Uniform velocity along the beam path. **B,** A low-velocity structure along the beam path causes the interface to be displaced distal to the true location. **C,** A high-velocity structure along the beam path causes the interface to be displaced proximal to the true location.

Convert this time to the axial length in tissue (z), assuming the unit is calibrated for 1540 m/s.

$$z = 0.5(1540 \text{ m/s})(1 \times 10^{-4} \text{ s})$$
$$z = 0.077 \text{ m or } 7.7 \text{ cm}$$

The actual diameter displayed is 7.7 cm, rather than the true 10 cm. Of course, the opposite effect (reflector position depicted farther away from the transducer and the object magnified) occurs if the actual velocity is less than the calibrated velocity. Another scenario that produces similar results occurs when the actual velocity in tissue is 1540 m/s but the unit is calibrated for a different value.

DISTANCE MEASUREMENT

The measurement of distance is usually more accurate along the direction of propagation than along the direction perpendicular to the beam path. Axial mapping, even with the changes in velocity for different types of soft tissue, has a misregistration error less than the lateral smearing of objects caused by beam width.

ENVIRONMENTAL INTERFERENCE

Instrument noise, induced by environmental electrical or radiofrequency interference from other electronic devices in the vicinity, can cause artifacts in the image. Normally,

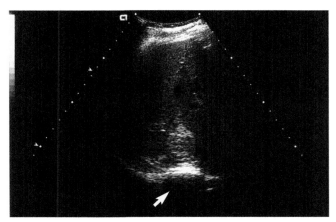

Figure 12-35 Velocity error artifact. Sonogram of the liver with a hyperechoic mass causing a disjointed image of the diaphragm *(arrow)*.

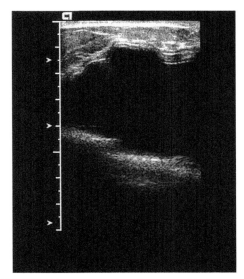

Figure 12-36 Velocity error artifact. Sonogram of the breast with a silicon implant causing a disjointed image of the fibrous capsule surrounding the implant.

though not always, a repetitive pattern of stripes or flashes occurs across the screen of the monitor. Although these artifacts are usually easily recognizable, their actual source may be difficult to determine. If severe enough, they can cause the unit to be unusable where these spurious electrical signals are present. Manufacturers have improved the shielding design to reduce environmental interference; thus these site-specific problems are rarely encountered.

SUMMARY

In addition to operator error and machine malfunction, violations of the assumptions with regard to image formation create potential artifacts. Some types of artifacts are

inherent from technical limitations in the imaging process and cannot be totally eliminated. Propagation properties of ultrasound in tissues, side lobes, high PRFs, and finite beam size can contribute to the improper spatial mapping of detected echoes. This can result in missing interfaces, wrongly placed interfaces, interfaces with misrepresented size or shape, interfaces with improper brightness, and false interfaces. A summary of different types of artifacts, including cause and effect, is presented in Table 12-1. Sonographers must be aware that if not correctly identified, artifacts can lead to errors in the interpretation of the B-mode image.

Table 12-1	**Classification of Artifacts**	
Type	**Effect**	**Cause**
Partial volume	Fill-in	Beam width extends over different tissue types
Attenuation	Shadowing	Absorption greater than adjacent paths
Attenuation	Enhancement	Absorption less than adjacent paths
Reverberation	Equally spaced banding	Multiple echoes from single reflector
Comet tail	Closely spaced bands	Multiple internal echoes from single reflector
Ring down	Continuous band extending through field of view	Gas-bubble resonance
Mirror image	Structures duplicated	Presence of strong reflector near the object
Side lobe	Misregistration (lateral)	Strong reflector interrogated by a secondary lobe
Refraction	Misregistration (lateral)	Bending of the sound waves along the beam path
Refraction (defocusing)	Edge shadowing	Bending of the sound waves by a curved surface
Range ambiguity	Misregistration (axial)	Echo not generated by most recent transmitted pulse
Velocity error	Misregistration (axial)	Velocity not constant along beam path

Doppler Physics and Instrumentation

13

Chapter Objectives

- To state the Doppler effect
- To calculate the Doppler shift frequency for moving reflectors
- To recognize the limitations of discrete sampling in the assessment of motion
- To categorize the advantages and disadvantages of continuous-wave operation mode
- To categorize the advantages and disadvantages of pulsed-wave operation mode

Key terms

Aliasing	Doppler effect	Quadrature phase
Beat frequency	Doppler shift frequency	detection
Doppler angle	Nyquist limit	Wall filter

DOPPLER MEASUREMENTS

Doppler ultrasound can detect the presence, direction, velocity, and time variation of blood flow in vessels. Several types of Doppler devices are available. Although each relies on the Doppler effect to detect motion, the manner in which each acquires, processes, and displays velocity information distinguishes one type of instrument from another. Continuous-wave (CW) Doppler and pulsed-wave (PW) Doppler are introduced in this chapter.

DOPPLER EFFECT

The Doppler effect is a phenomenon in which an apparent change from the transmitted frequency is observed if there is relative motion between the source of the sound and the receiver. An analogy involving waves striking a boat on the water illustrates the Doppler effect. Assume that the wind is blowing at a constant rate from the west and that there is the same distance between the peaks of all the waves (same wavelength). By remaining stationary in the water, the boat encounters the same number of wave crests each second (constant frequency) as are produced by the wind. If the boat travels westward, the wave crests are encountered more frequently. A person standing on board sees an increase in the wave frequency, although the waves are actually created at the same rate. If the boat reverses its direction and travels eastward (away from the source of the waves), fewer crests are seen. The observed frequency decreases. As the boat moves faster in either direction, the difference between the created and observed frequencies becomes more pronounced. The only circumstance in which these frequencies coincide is when the boat is stationary.

A sound source produces a series of concentric pressure wavefronts radiating outward from the point of origin. The same effect (in two dimensions) is seen when a stone is dropped into a pond. Concentric rings form, the most peripheral being the oldest and the most central being the newest. The source sets the frequency of the waves while the medium dictates the speed of propagation, both of which together define the wavelength (or separation between successive wavefronts).

A stationary receiver views the same number of pressure waves as are emitted by the stationary source (Fig. 13-1). Relative motion between the source and receiver distorts the pattern of symmetrical wavefronts and alters the observed frequency. The change in frequency between the transmitted frequency and the received frequency caused by the motion is the Doppler shift frequency (often abbreviated as Doppler shift).

The Doppler effect is experienced in daily life when an ambulance approaches with its siren sounding (the siren produces sound of constant frequency) and the sound appears to increase in pitch. As the ambulance moves past the listener, an apparent decrease in pitch is heard, although the siren is still producing sound at the same constant frequency.

Doppler Shift Equation

The Doppler shift frequency depends on how rapidly the sound source, receiver, or both are moving; that is, an increase in the relative velocity between source and receiver causes a greater deviation from the transmitted frequency. The velocity of sound in the medium (c) and the transmitted frequency (f) also affect the Doppler shift frequency. The Doppler shift frequency (f_D) produced by a moving reflector is calculated from the 11th essential equation of sonography:

13-1
$$f_D = \frac{2vf}{c} \cos \theta$$

where v is the velocity of the interface and θ is the angle between direction of movement and direction of beam propagation (called the Doppler angle), as illustrated in Fig. 13-2. Equation 13-1 is in reality an approximation based on the assumption that the speed of the interfaces for biological systems is relatively small (0.5 to 2000 cm/s) compared with the velocity of sound in tissue (1540 m/s).

Example 13-1

Calculate the Doppler shift frequency (f_D) produced by scanning an interface moving toward the transducer at a velocity of 15 cm/s if the angle of insonation is 45 degrees. The transmitted frequency is 5 MHz.

$$f_D = \frac{2vf}{c} \cos \theta$$

$$f_D = \frac{2 \, (15 \, cm/s)(5 \times 10^6 \, Hz)}{154,000 \, cm/s} \cos 45°$$

$$f_D = 689 \, Hz$$

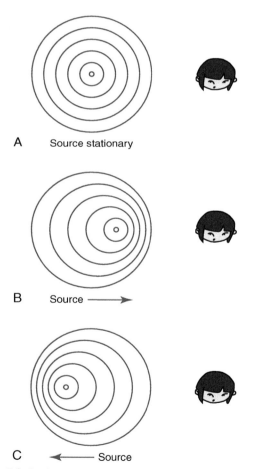

A   Source stationary

B   Source ⟶

C   ⟵ Source

Figure 13-1 The Doppler effect. **A,** Stationary sound source and receiver, showing a constant observed frequency equal to the frequency of the sound source. **B,** Sound source moving toward the receiver, showing an increase in the observed frequency compared with the actual frequency emitted by the sound source. **C,** Sound source moving away from the receiver, showing a decrease in the observed frequency compared with the actual frequency emitted by the sound source.

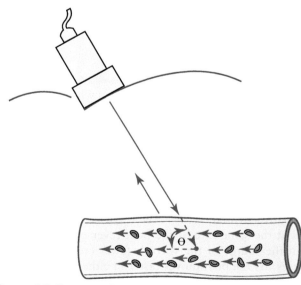

Figure 13-2 Motion of red blood cells through the vessel, which is not parallel with the direction of travel of the sound beam. The observed frequency differs from the transmit frequency. The angle θ is the Doppler angle.

The observed frequency is 5,000,689 Hz or a Doppler shift frequency of 689 Hz above the original 5-MHz transmitted frequency. If the object is moving away from the transducer at 15 cm/s along the same path, the observed frequency will be 4,999,311 Hz or 689 Hz below the original transmitted frequency. The combination of v and cos θ in Equation 13-1 gives the component of the velocity along the direction of propagation for the ultrasound beam. If the Doppler angle is decreased from 45 to 0 degrees, the Doppler shift frequency is 974 Hz for parallel incidence instead of the 689 Hz obtained with the angle to flow. *For a given reflector velocity, the Doppler shift frequency decreases as the Doppler angle is increased.*

Actual determination of the Doppler angle may be difficult. Minimal frequency shift occurs at a 90-degree angle of incidence because the cosine of 90 degrees is zero. In practice, the signal never disappears completely, because beam width or beam divergence causes some portion of the beam to sample at an angle that is not perpendicular to the motion.

Velocity Determination

The velocity of the sound wave in a medium remains constant. The observed change in frequency occurs because relative motion is present between the source and the detector. The Doppler equation predicts that an increase in velocity of the interface results in a greater Doppler shift frequency. *If the frequency shift can be measured, the velocity of the moving reflectors can be determined.*

The velocity of a moving interface is calculated from measurements of the Doppler shift frequency and Doppler angle by rearranging Equation 13-1.

$$13\text{-}2 \qquad v = \frac{cf_D}{2f \cos \theta}$$

The absolute determination of reflector velocity requires that the Doppler angle be included in this calculation. Ignoring the contribution of the Doppler angle causes an underestimation of the true velocity.

Uncertainty in measuring the Doppler angle, particularly at large angles, introduces error in the velocity computation. A 5-degree error for a 70-degree Doppler angle causes the velocity estimation to deviate by 24% (Table 13-1). A decrease in the Doppler angle to 40 degrees reduces this deviation to 8% for the same uncertainty of 5 degrees in angle measurement. When the beam is near parallel to flow, this 5-degree inaccuracy in the angle estimation results in a 1% error in the calculation of flow velocity. As a general guideline, Doppler signals from superficial blood vessels (e.g., the carotids) should never be acquired at angles greater than 60 degrees. For cardiac applications, Doppler angle is generally ignored because Doppler measurements are performed with the sound beam nearly parallel to the flow direction.

Table 13-1	Percent Error in Velocity Measurements for a 5-Degree Angle Error
True Angle (Degrees)	**Percent Error**
0	0.5
10	2
20	3.5
30	5
40	8
50	10
60	15
70	24
80	50

Scattering from Blood

For monitoring flow in vessels, red blood cells (RBCs) act as scattering centers. Because the RBC, with a diameter of 7 microns, is much smaller than the wavelength of the sound wave (usually 0.2 to 0.5 mm), Rayleigh scattering occurs. Rayleigh scattering exhibits a very strong frequency dependence (proportional to the fourth power of the frequency). Scattering from a group of small moving targets creates multiple wavefronts that form a fluctuating interference echo pattern in time and space.

The intensity of the scattered sound depends on the number of RBCs and thus the quantity of blood in the sample volume. The scattering from blood, however, is small compared with echoes produced by soft tissue interfaces. The echo-free appearance of blood-filled vessels on the B-mode image demonstrates this relatively weak generation of echo from blood. To increase the magnitude of scattering, a high-frequency transducer should be used; but as frequency is increased, the rate of absorption of the sound beam by the intervening tissues is also increased. These two effects must be balanced by matching the transducer frequency with the depth of the region of interest.

Doppler transducers usually operate in the frequency range of 2 to 10 MHz because other constraints are placed on the system: a single transducer with dual imaging and Doppler functions, a desired frequency range for Doppler shift frequency, and the problem of aliasing (discussed later in this chapter). High transmit frequencies, typically 5 to 7 MHz, are employed for peripheral vascular Doppler examinations, whereas examinations of deep-seated vessels are performed at frequencies near 2 MHz.

Doppler Display

Doppler units are designed to extract the Doppler shift frequencies from received signals. This change in frequency is in the audible range (typically between 200 and 15,000 Hz), which enables loudspeakers to be used as output devices. For visual display the preferred format is to convert the measured Doppler shift frequency to velocity, which is independent of instrument parameters. Doppler shift frequencies expressed in kilohertz from repeated examinations, different instruments, or various hospitals are not readily comparable.

CONTINUOUS-WAVE DOPPLER

The CW Doppler transducer contains two crystals: one to transmit the sound waves of constant frequency continuously and one to receive the echoes continuously (Fig. 13-3). A single crystal cannot send and receive at the same time because an ultrahigh dynamic range receiver circuit would be required to detect the small echo signals superimposed on the transmitting signal. Since the transmitted sound wave is not pulsed, broad-bandwidth transducers are not used or even appropriate (wide frequency range yields multiple Doppler shifts for a reflector moving at constant velocity).

The sampling volume is restricted by the transmitted ultrasonic field and by the geometric arrangement of the crystals. The two elements are tilted slightly to allow overlap between their respective fields of view (transmission and reception). For detection of a moving reflector located along the path of the transmitted beam, the resulting echo must strike the receiving crystal. The sensitive volume is defined by the intersection of the ultrasound field and the reception zone. In essence, each two-element transducer is focused to a particular depth. Depending on the clinical application, the sonographer selects a CW transducer with the appropriate operating frequency and depth of focus.

Doppler Measurement

The transmitted sound wave interacts with various reflectors, some of which are stationary and others moving. A fraction of the incident sound intensity is reflected at each interface. If the reflector is stationary, the frequency of the reflected sound wave is the same as the transmitted frequency; consequently, no Doppler shift frequency is observed. A moving interface initially acts as a "receiver" of the ultrasound beam and causes the frequency of the echo to shift up or down depending on whether the movement is toward or away from the sound source. The second crystal in the transducer is the receiver for the returning echoes. Although the receiving crystal is stationary, another change in frequency occurs because the moving interface that generated the echo is now acting as a sound source. This sequence of two occurrences of the Doppler effect is responsible for factor 2 in the Doppler shift frequency equation.

The method used to measure the Doppler shift frequency is based on the principle of wave interference. The reflected wave received from a moving interface varies slightly in frequency from the original transmitted wave because of the Doppler effect. Waves with slightly different frequencies algebraically add together, yielding a slowly oscillating broad pattern of peaks and valleys called the beat frequency (Fig. 13-4). The beat frequency equals the difference in frequency between the combined waves and thus corresponds to the Doppler shift frequency.

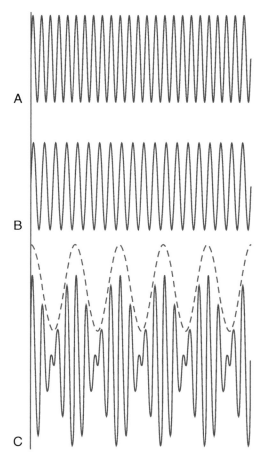

Figure 13-4 Beat frequency. **A,** Continuous transmitted wave of constant frequency (25 cycles are shown). **B,** Continuous reflected wave of constant frequency (20 cycles are shown). **C,** Addition of the transmitted and received sound waves in **(A)** and **(B)** produces a complex waveform. The beat frequency (5 cycles are shown) is illustrated as the outer envelope *(red dotted line)* of this complex waveform.

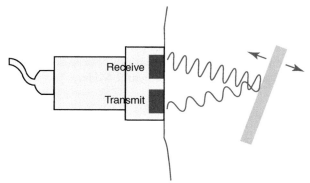

Figure 13-3 Continuous-wave Doppler transducer. One crystal acts as the transmitter, the other as the receiver. The continuous sound wave is reflected from the moving interface (green).

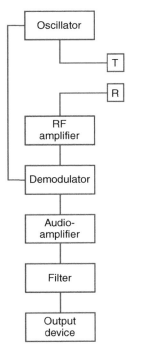

Figure 13-5 Continuous-wave Doppler unit. T, Transmitter; R, receiver.

Figure 13-5 illustrates the steps necessary to generate the Doppler signal. An oscillator regulates the transmitter to emit a continuous single-frequency sound wave. The returning echo incident on the receiving crystal is converted to a radiofrequency signal. An amplifier increases the echo-induced signal level. The reference waveform from the oscillator (mimicking the transmitted wave) is then combined with the received signal, which creates a complex resultant wave by the process of wave interference. This resultant wave is demodulated to remove the rapid oscillating components but retains the overall beat pattern. Isolation of the beat frequency forms the Doppler signal, which has a frequency equal to the Doppler shift frequency.

Complex Doppler Signal

The signal processing illustrated by Figure 13-4 yielded a single beat frequency, which denoted reflectors moving at a single constant velocity. RBCs within a vessel have a range of velocities, depending on the flow pattern. Each velocity associated with moving reflectors corresponds to a characteristic beat frequency upon echo detection and processing. Multiple beat frequencies, representing all detected motion, comprise the Doppler signal. A complex Doppler signal is formed by the summation of all the Doppler shift frequencies present after demodulation.

The CW Doppler unit as described in Figure 13-5 detects only speed of movement. It must be modified to determine the actual direction of movement (i.e., whether toward or away from the transducer). Various directional methods are discussed later.

Signal Processing

After demodulation, the Doppler signal is sent to an audio-amplifier, filtered to remove unwanted low-frequency components, and routed to a loudspeaker for audible "display." The pitch of the audio output corresponds to the frequency shift between the transmitted and received sound waves and indicates the flow velocity within the vessel. As flow velocity becomes greater, a higher pitch is heard.

Large, slow-moving specular reflectors in the body (e.g., vessel walls) generate strong echoes with low-frequency Doppler shifts. The distracting thumping sound produced in the unfiltered output is called "wall thump." High-pass filtering removes these low frequencies, which are normally not of major interest and could mask other signals. The wall filter (high-pass filter) accepts all frequencies above a threshold value and rejects all frequencies below the threshold value. The threshold is usually set to remove frequencies below 100 Hz, although on some units the cutoff frequency is adjustable to between 40 and 1000 Hz. Most units automatically set the threshold value based on study type. Because the high-pass filter removes all frequencies below the cutoff value, Doppler shifts from slow-moving flow may be eliminated from the final output. The high-pass filter should be set at the lowest possible value to remove wall thump while not distorting the blood-flow components of the Doppler signal.

Because the Doppler shift corresponding to motion along the direction of sound propagation within a reception zone is detected, no scanning arm is necessary to denote the position of the transducer. The observed Doppler signal can be extremely complex, however, because the sum of Doppler shifts generated by all the moving interfaces within the sensitive volume is represented. If the sampling volume includes multiple vessels, the superposition of resulting Doppler shifts becomes especially problematic.

Extensive flow volumes (e.g., those encountered in the left ventricle) cannot be accurately assessed with CW Doppler methods. CW Doppler units operate at low acoustic power levels but provide no depth information, and since the time between transmitted sound wave and detected echo is unknown, time gain compensation cannot be applied. Consequently, provided that they are of similar acoustic properties, superficial moving structures produce stronger signals than deep moving structures do.

Operator Controls

Most CW Doppler units have operator controls for power, gain, audio volume, and wall filter. Transmit power adjusts the intensity of the ultrasound beam transmitted into the patient. Increased transmitted intensity enhances sensitivity (detection of low-volume flow). Receiver gain modifies the amplification of echo-induced signals before demodulation. This can also affect the sensitivity. The volume control for the audio amplifier regulates loudness for

Doppler signal output to speakers. Wall filter sets the low-frequency threshold for display.

Characteristics

CW Doppler has high sensitivity to detect slow flow with small Doppler shift frequencies and further can discriminate small differences in flow velocity (Fig. 13-6). The long sampling time of CW Doppler enables this modality to identify small changes in frequency corresponding to slow flow. At the other extreme, high-velocity flow is accurately measured with no limitation in velocity range. Depth discrimination is not feasible with CW Doppler and must be achieved by pulsing the transmitted ultrasound wave.

PULSED-WAVE DOPPLER

PW Doppler via the echo-ranging principle provides quantitative depth information of the moving reflectors. The transducer is electrically stimulated to produce a short burst of ultrasound and then is silent to listen for echoes before another burst is generated. Doppler shift frequency determination requires a longer pulse duration than is used in B-mode imaging. The necessity for increased pulse duration lies in the desire to detect received frequencies associated with slow flow that are almost the same as the transmitted frequency. Imagine that the sampling were confined to the first four cycles in Figure 13-6. Certainly, the ability to distinguish small changes compared with the transmitted frequency would be reduced as sampling time was decreased.

The received signals are electronically gated for processing, so only the echoes that are detected in a narrow time interval after transmission, corresponding to a specific depth, contribute to the Doppler signal. The delay time before the gate is turned on determines the depth of the sample volume; the amount of time the gate is activated establishes the axial length of the sample volume (Fig. 13-7). Gate parameters are selected by the sonographer; thus the axial size

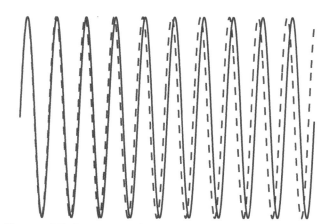

Figure 13-6 Sensitivity of continuous-wave Doppler. The received frequency from a slow-moving reflector *(red dotted line)* is only perceived as different from the transmitted frequency *(blue solid line)* after the buildup of several cycles.

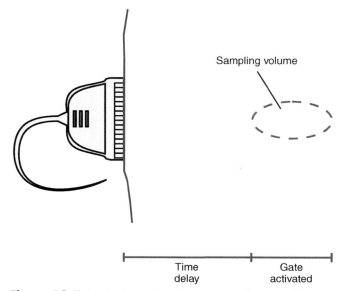

Sampling volume

Time delay   Gate activated

Figure 13-7 In pulsed-wave Doppler, activation of the gate determines the depth and axial length of the sampling volume.

of the sensitive volume can be adjusted. The axial sample length is as small as 1 mm. The remaining dimensions of the sampling volume are dictated by the beam width in the in-plane direction and beam width in elevation direction, which are influenced by the transducer frequency and focusing characteristics.

Multiple echoes from a moving reflector separated in time must be accrued to detect the motion. In order to achieve this, transmitted pulses are repeatedly directed along the same scan line to interrogate the sampling volume. Suppose Ansel Adams took a single stop-action photograph (with an extremely short shutter time) of a car traveling west at 60 miles per hour on Highway 66. If you were shown that photograph, you would be unable to tell if the car was moving or not. And certainly the direction of travel and speed would not be discernible. However, if a series of stop-action photographs were acquired and then shown rapidly one after the other, the motion of the car would be clearly depicted.

In PW Doppler, the basic CW design is modified to accommodate gating and collect successive processed echoes in a sample and hold circuit (Fig. 13-8). Time registration is essential. The time between consecutive echoes from a reflector is set by the pulse repetition period and gating is based on elapsed time following the transmitted pulse. Some units allow the sonographer to adjust the pulse repetition frequency (PRF) manually, whereas others vary the PRF automatically in response to the sampling depth. A single gate limits the interrogation to one depth along the line of sight.

Signal Processing

The received echo must be evaluated to determine whether the reflector is moving. This is accomplished by comparing the phase of the echo with a reference waveform for

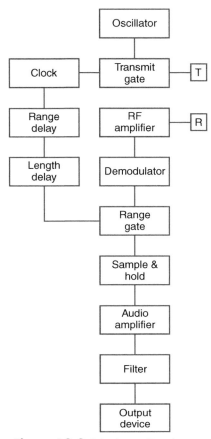

Figure 13-8 Pulsed-wave Doppler unit.

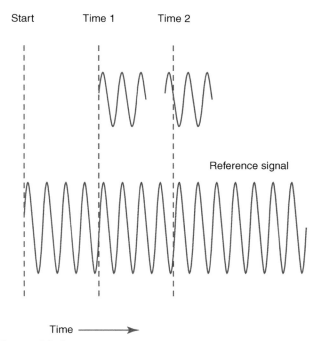

Figure 13-9 The echo from a stationary reflector received at time 1 is in phase with the reference signal. The echo from a moving reflector received at time 2 is not in phase with the reference signal.

which phase is synchronized with the transmitted pulse. Two waves are described as being in phase if their maximum, minimum, and zero points occur concurrently. The echo from a stationary reflector has the same phase as the reference waveform, whereas the echo from a moving structure undergoes a phase shift via the Doppler effect. The phase relation between detected echoes and the reference waveform is depicted in Fig. 13-9.

The echoes from different reflectors, one moving and the other stationary, are received after different time intervals (time 1 and time 2) following the transmitted pulse. The reference waveform has the same frequency and phase as the transmitted pulse but is extended over time so that the received signals can be compared with the original transmitted waveform. The dotted lines in Figure 13-9 place the detected echoes on the same time scale as the reference waveform. The phase is unchanged for the stationary reflector, whose echo is received at time 1. The shift in phase at time 2 indicates that the reflector at a specific depth is moving.

Sample and Hold

For a single reflector moving at constant velocity within the sampling volume, a series of echoes from successive transmitted pulses are obtained over time in a sample and hold circuit. The depth-specific echo from each transmitted pulse when processed provides one instantaneous value of the Doppler signal. The sample-and-hold circuit assembles the measured values obtained from multiple transmitted pulses to form the Doppler shift frequency. In essence the transmitted pulse rate indicates how often the Doppler signal is sampled. Typically, a sequence of 64 to 128 pulses is transmitted along the scan line to interrogate the sample volume. The total observation time is usually 10 ms or less.

A description of the sample and hold circuit function follows. Each echo-induced signal is combined with the reference waveform (same frequency as the transmitted pulse) to generate one point in the sample and hold data set. The relative phase between the echo signal and the reference waveform determines the magnitude of the sample-and-hold signal, which is plotted as a function of time. The time axis is defined by the time during which the sequence of transmission pulses is directed along the line of sight to the sampling volume. Multiple measurements create an oscillatory pattern from which the beat frequency is inferred (Fig. 13-10).

The beat frequency is not as well defined as with CW Doppler because the pulsed echoes are equivalent to sampling the demodulated signal at discrete intervals (Fig. 13-11). The oscillatory pattern can be more clearly delineated if the sampling rate is high, which requires a high PRF. Multiple reflectors moving with a range of velocities within the sample volume give rise to a complex Doppler signal consisting of many different Doppler shift frequencies.

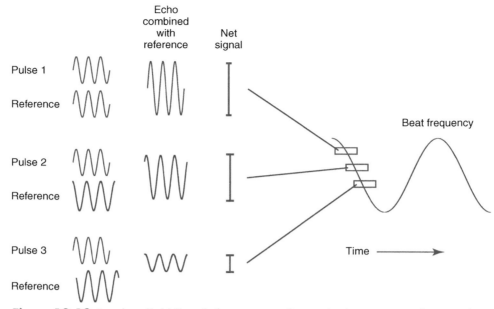

Figure 13-10 Sample and hold. The echo from a moving reflector within the range gate undergoes a phase shift, which in combination with the reference signal yields the net signal. Multiple echoes are acquired from the same reflector at a time interval equal to the pulse repetition period. Successive echoes from the moving reflector have varying phase shifts. The net signal is reduced in magnitude as the phase shift is increased. The beat frequency is formed by plotting the net signal from the series of echoes as a function of time.

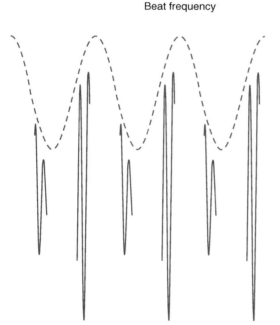

Figure 13-11 The addition of pulsed sound waves to the reference signal yields the interpreted beat frequency (red dotted line).

Velocity Detection Limit

At a minimum, two pulses are required per beat cycle to define the beat frequency unambiguously. This creates a very important limitation in PW Doppler. The maximum Doppler shift, $f_D(max)$, that can be detected is related to the sampling rate or PRF:

13-3
$$f_D(max) = \frac{PRF}{2}$$

To accurately measure a fast-moving reflector producing high Doppler shift frequency, a high sampling rate is necessary; however, a high PRF limits the depth that can be interrogated because a certain time is required to collect the echoes arising from that depth before the next transmit pulse is sent out. The problem becomes more complex when it is realized that the Doppler shift frequency depends on transducer frequency. Nevertheless, the relation between depth of interest (R), transducer frequency (f), Doppler angle (θ), velocity of sound in tissue (c), and maximum reflector velocity (V_{max}) is described by a single equation (the 12th essential equation of sonography):

13-4
$$V_{max} = \frac{c^2}{8fR \cos \theta}$$

The ramifications on velocity determination are threefold (Table 13-2). First, as the depth of interest is increased, the maximum reflector velocity that can be measured is decreased. Second, a low-frequency transducer allows greater velocities to be detected. Third, a larger Doppler angle extends the maximum velocity limit. These limitations occur, because the motion of the reflector is sampled at discrete intervals and not continuously, as with CW Doppler ultrasound. Unless low-pass filtering is applied to eliminate high-frequency noise components, CW Doppler has no maximum velocity limit.

Table 13-2	Dependence of Maximum Velocity Limit on Transducer Frequency and Depth of the Moving Reflector in Pulsed-Wave Doppler		
	Maximum Velocity Limit^a (cm/s)		
Depth (cm)	**2 MHz**	**5 MHz**	**10 MHz**
1	1480	590	295
5	295	120	60
10	150	60	30
15	100	40	20
20	75	30	15

^{a}The Doppler angle is 0 degrees.

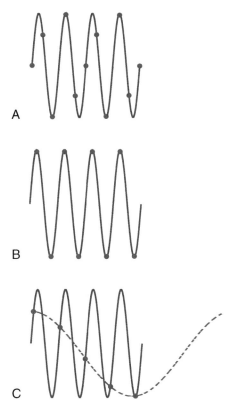

Figure 13-12 Intermittent sampling of the beat frequency (*solid line*). **A,** Multiple measurements during four cycles allow accurate assessment of the beat frequency. **B,** A minimum of two measurements per cycle also provides accurate interpretation of the beat frequency. **C,** When the sampling rate is not adequate, the true beat frequency (*solid line*) is interpreted incorrectly as a lower frequency (*dotted line*).

The following numerical example illustrates a practicable application of the maximum velocity limit in the clinical environment. The maximum PRF for a 10-cm depth is approximately 7700 pulses per second. Using a 3.5-MHz transducer with a Doppler angle of 30 degrees, the maximum Doppler shift frequency is 3850 Hz, which corresponds to a velocity of 98 cm/s. If the transducer frequency were lowered to 2 MHz, the maximum detectable velocity would increase to 171 cm/s. Changing the depth of interest to 15 cm while maintaining the transducer frequency at 3.5 MHz reduces the measurable maximum velocity to 65 cm/s. Fortunately these conditions are such that the physiologic velocities of moving structures (except the heart) usually occur within the detectable range of PW Doppler units.

Aliasing

Because beat frequency is sampled intermittently, it must be inferred from the limited data available. If the sampling rate is not adequate for a high-frequency Doppler shift frequency, an artifactual lower-frequency Doppler shift frequency is recorded. When the sampling occurs less than twice during a beat cycle, the data are misinterpreted as being at a lower frequency than the actual beat frequency. The requirement that the sampling rate must be at least twice the maximum frequency present in the Doppler signal is referred to as the Nyquist criterion. Half of the PRF is the Nyquist limit as defined by Equation 13-3; Doppler shifts above the Nyquist limit are falsely depicted as low-frequency shifts corresponding to slow-moving reflectors. Imagine that a measurement is taken of the amplitude of the beat frequency at various points and that a new waveform is constructed from this collection of amplitude measurements (Fig. 13-12). The actual beat frequency is misinterpreted as a waveform with a lower frequency because sampling occurred only five times over four cycles. This is called aliasing, and it also is not present in CW Doppler.

The motion picture industry provides a visual example of aliasing. In movies of the old West, a buckboard is often pulled across the prairie by a team of horses. You undoubtedly recall how the wheels on the buckboard appeared to be going backward, which was visually inconsistent with the movement of other objects depicted in the scene. In making the movie, a series of stop-action photographs was taken and shown one after another to give the appearance of motion. There was a time delay between frames, however, which meant that the recording system was sampling the motion at discrete intervals. If the motion became very rapid, as with the rotating wheel on the buckboard, the sampling could not properly represent the motion. (The spokes of the wheel move too large a distance between successive photographs.) To solve this problem, the time between frames could be decreased (i.e., more photos taken) so the wheel moved a shorter distance between photographs. More frequent sampling allows the recording system to reproduce the motion accurately. Note that in the movie, only objects moving at high velocity were affected by the noncontinuous sampling; the motion of slower-moving objects was correctly reproduced. In ultrasound the boundary for the correct interpretation of object velocity is given by the Nyquist limit, which depends on the PRF.

Example 13-2

Calculate the minimum PRF necessary to prevent aliasing if the velocity of the moving reflector is 15 cm/s. The angle of insonation is 40 degrees, and the transducer frequency is 2 MHz.

$$f_D = \frac{2vf}{c} \cos \theta$$

$$f_D = \frac{2(15 \text{ cm/s})\left(2 \times 10^6 \text{ Hz}\right) \cos 40°}{(154,000 \text{ cm/s})}$$

$$f_D = 298 \text{ Hz}$$

The minimum PRF is equal to two times the Doppler shift.

$$PRF = 2f_D = 2(298 \text{ Hz}) = 596 \text{ Hz}$$

If reflectors are moving at velocities above those imposed by the Nyquist limit, the sonographer has several options to remove the aliasing artifact:

1. An increase in the PRF raises the Nyquist limit, possibly to a level that is sufficient to measure reflector velocity accurately. The maximum PRF is usually set by the pulse transit time to the depth of interest. If a PRF corresponding to this transit time limit does not remove the aliasing artifact, then adjusting the PRF even higher may do so. An ambiguity in sampling location, however, is created by ignoring the transit time limitation. In effect, echoes are now obtained simultaneously from two sampling volumes. Strategic positioning of one sampling location where no flow is present removes the ambiguity.
2. If reverse flow is not of concern, the baseline can be adjusted to devote the entire range of velocity detection to a single direction of flow. This technique doubles the maximum velocity that can be measured without aliasing but assumes that no flow in the opposite direction is present.
3. Examination of Equation 13-4 reveals that the Doppler angle and transducer frequency also affect the maximum velocity limit. By increasing the Doppler angle or lowering the transducer frequency, aliasing may be eliminated.
4. Finally, switching from PW to CW modes enables the fastest motion to be observed without an aliasing artifact (although depth information is then sacrificed in the CW mode).

Pulsed-Wave Bandwidth

The PW Doppler transducer does not produce a single-frequency sound wave. Because the pulsed ultrasound beam is of short duration, each transmitted pulsed wave consists of a range of frequencies characterized by the bandwidth. As with imaging transducers, a very short pulse creates a spectral distribution of frequencies with a wide bandwidth. Hence, some frequencies expected in the returning echoes from moving reflectors are initially present at transmission. In addition, the multiple frequency

components cause frequency variations in the observed Doppler shifts and a reduction in the signal level. Decreasing the bandwidth by lengthening the pulse improves the system's ability to detect slow flow (small Doppler shifts) and small differences in flow velocity, but longer spatial pulse length degrades the spatial resolution. Note that several cycles were required in Figure 13-6 to observe a difference between the transmitted wave and the received wave. The same principle applies in PW Doppler. The reflectivity of blood is less than soft tissue and results in a detected Doppler signal with a low signal-to-noise level. Manufacturers compensate for the poor Doppler signal level by increasing the acoustic power.

The spectral distribution of frequencies poses two additional problems. First, the preferential attenuation of high-frequency components as the beam penetrates tissue causes a downward distortion in the frequency distribution, which is interpreted incorrectly as a Doppler shift. This attenuation effect varies with the depth of the moving reflectors. Second, the frequency dependence of scattering enhances the high-frequency components in the echo and thus tends to counteract the effect of attenuation.

DIRECTIONAL METHODS

The received echo from a moving reflector is shifted in frequency above or below the reference signal depending on whether the motion is toward or away from the transducer. Demodulation indicates that a frequency shift has occurred, but it cannot identify whether the shift is positive or negative. Three processing methods—including single sideband, heterodyne, and quadrature phase detection—have been developed to distinguish between motion toward and motion away from the transducer.

Single-Sideband Detector

The received signal consists of reflected echoes from both stationary and moving structures. The reflections from stationary structures are equal in frequency to the transmitted beam, whereas those from moving structures are offset in frequency.

The signal from the radiofrequency amplifier is split into two components and then filtered. One filter is designed to pass all frequencies above the transmitted frequency (forward motion) and the other to pass all frequencies below the transmitted frequency (reverse motion). The output of each filter is mixed with the reference waveform and then processed with a sideband filter to isolate the Doppler shift frequencies. This results in two separate output signals corresponding to the forward and reverse motions.

Heterodyne Detector

In a heterodyne detector the offset signal is combined with the reference waveform before being added to the received signal and subsequent demodulation. This technique

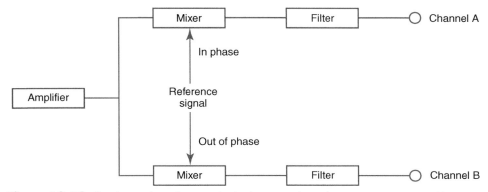

Figure 13-13 Quadrature phase detection divides the received signal into two components and then mixes these with a varying phase reference signal.

displaces the Doppler shift frequency to a new frequency range. Forward and reverse motions are differentiated by comparison with the offset frequency. For example, an offset frequency of 5 kHz allows reverse motion to be displayed as frequencies below 5 kHz and forward motion to be displayed as frequencies above 5 kHz.

Quadrature Phase Detector

Figure 13-13 illustrates quadrature phase detection, the most commonly used directional technique. The signal from the amplifier is split into two components and each is mixed with the reference waveform (one channel 90 degrees out of phase with the other). After filtering, the output from each channel contains a mixture of forward and reverse flow signals. The presence of flow in one direction only causes each channel to exhibit the same voltage variation as a function of time, although the pattern is shifted in time. If flow is in the forward direction, the output from channel A shows the leading edge of the pattern first. Flow in the opposite direction causes the output from channel B to precede the output from channel A. The outputs from both channels are analyzed simultaneously by comparing their relative phase to determine whether flow is in the forward or reverse direction. Quadrature phase detection does not work properly, however, if forward and reverse flow signals occur concurrently.

A technique called frequency domain processing is applied after quadrature phase detection to generate two output signals, each associated with a particular direction of flow. These signals can be routed to headphones in which the sounds in one ear represent motion toward the transducer and those in the other ear correspond to motion away from the transducer. Figure 13-14 demonstrates the operation of the frequency domain detector. A pilot signal within the audible frequency range is mixed with the channel output signals from the quadrature phase detector (channels A and B). The mixed signal from channel A is added with the unmixed quadrature signal from channel B to produce the reverse flow channel. Similarly, the mixed signal from channel B is added with the unmixed quadrature signal from channel A to produce the forward flow channel.

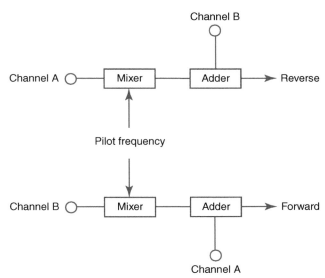

Figure 13-14 Frequency domain processing. A pilot signal is applied to each channel output from a quadrature phase detector. Each mixed signal is then added with the unmixed opposite quadrature channel output, and the frequency components of the output are separated into the forward and reverse flow signals.

DUPLEX SCANNERS

Duplex Doppler units combine real-time imaging with CW or PW Doppler detection. The B-mode image depicts stationary reflectors (e.g., plaques inside the vessel and other anatomic structures), whereas the Doppler mode provides flow information for the designated region. The display of anatomic structures aids in selecting the line of sight for CW Doppler or placement of the sample volume for PW Doppler. Markers for the sampling region are superimposed on the real-time image. The Doppler angle can be ascertained from the B-mode image. The assessment of angle assumes that flow is parallel to the vessel wall and that the vessel does not curve within the scan plane. While these assumptions may not be entirely correct, the errors introduced are generally small, so that reasonable estimates of velocity can be obtained. Visualization of the physical size and shape of plaque with real-time scanning aids in the diagnosis of vascular disease.

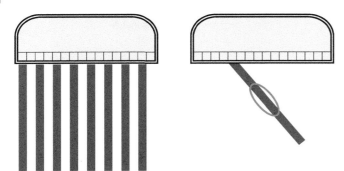

Figure 13-15 Duplex scanning with a linear array transducer. The B-mode image is obtained with parallel scan lines across the length of the array. The beam is then electronically steered along the line of sight designated for Doppler acquisition. By gating the signals from received echoes from this line of sight, the sampling volume is established *(ellipse)*.

Table 13-3	Pulsed-Wave Duplex Scanning	
Advantages	**Disadvantages**	
Simultaneous display of B-mode and Doppler	Small sample volume	
Ability to define Doppler angle	No global presentation of flow	
Measurement of flow velocity	Manual adjustment of Doppler angle	
Identification of complex flow components	Reduced frame rates	
Real-time flow information		

The duplex scanner must perform both imaging and Doppler functions with near simultaneity (Fig. 13-15). Because the optimal design specifications for each of these functions are not the same, various transducer configurations have been developed. Today, multiple-element-array transducers are generally used so that the beam can be steered along the operator-designated Doppler sampling direction. Real-time imaging is interrupted while the flow information is acquired, usually over a period of several milliseconds. The ultrasound beam must be repeatedly directed along one line of sight in the Doppler mode. Multiple echoes from the same reflector are necessary for determining the beat frequency. The electronic interleaving of Doppler pulses between imaging pulses in duplex scanning permits real-time imaging, though at a reduced frame rate. A single broadband transducer operating at low frequency in the Doppler mode and high frequency in the imaging mode is common.

In duplex scanning, the flow information is acquired for a highly restricted region and displayed in real time. *The global pattern of flow must be ascertained by sampling multiple regions one after the other throughout the field of view.* Isolated flow disturbances may go undetected. The characteristics of PW duplex scanning are presented in Table 13-3.

SUMMARY

Doppler instrumentation detects the presence of motion, primarily blood flow. The Doppler shift frequency is extracted by combining the detected echoes with the reference waveform followed by demodulation. PW Doppler allows the depth of the moving reflector to be determined, but with a maximum velocity detection limit imposed by the intermittent sampling. Aliasing occurs if reflector velocity exceeds the Nyquist limit. CW Doppler does not produce aliasing artifacts, although spatial information is lost. A comparison between CW and PW Doppler modes is shown in Table 13-4. Two essential equations of sonography (Doppler shift frequency and maximum velocity limit for PW Doppler) were introduced.

Table 13-4	Comparison of Doppler Instruments
Continuous-Wave Doppler	**Pulsed-Wave Doppler**
No range resolution	Depth information
Narrow bandwidth	Wide bandwidth
No velocity limit	Maximum velocity limit
High sensitivity to slow flow	Low sensitivity to slow flow
No aliasing	Aliasing

Doppler Spectral Analysis

14

Chapter Objectives

- To identify the components of the pulsed-wave Doppler spectral waveform
- To understand the function of pulsed-wave Doppler controls
- To describe scanning techniques that may eliminate aliasing
- To recognize the characteristics of the pulsed-wave Doppler spectral waveform depicting turbulent flow

Key terms

Baseline
Doppler cursor
Doppler gain
Doppler output power
Doppler reject
Doppler spectral
 waveform
Fast Fourier transform (FFT)

Flow disturbance
High-PRF mode
Maximum Doppler shift
Maximum velocity
 waveform
Power spectrum
Range gate
Sample volume

Spectral analysis
Spectral invert
Sweep speed
Transit time broadening
Turbulence
Velocity scale
Wall filter

DOPPLER SIGNAL

In the cross section of a vessel, red blood cells (RBCs) at various radii from the center are moving at different velocities, resulting in an overall Doppler signal that is a combination of multiple Doppler shift frequencies. The process of determining the individual frequency components that are present in this composite Doppler signal and the relative importance of each is called spectral analysis. Spectral analysis, when repeated rapidly in time, characterizes the flow in vessels.

FAST FOURIER TRANSFORM

The analysis of the composite Doppler signal is accomplished with a mathematical algorithm called the fast Fourier transform (FFT). Fourier analysis separates a complex waveform into a series of single-frequency, sine waves. When algebraically combined, these single-frequency components yield the original complex waveform. Several examples follow to illustrate the principle of spectral analysis applied to blood flow.

Figure 14-1 is a cross-sectional view of a vessel lumen. In regions 1, 2, and 3, RBCs move at different velocities ($v_3 > v_2 > v_1$) through the vessel. For simplicity, the same total number of RBCs is assumed to pass through each region and to flow at a continuous (nonpulsatile) rate. If the ultrasound beam is made very small, so that each of these regions is sampled individually, a characteristic Doppler shift frequency is obtained for each region (Fig. 14-2). Three distinct Doppler shift frequencies are

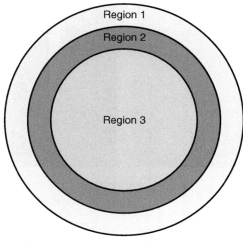

Figure 14-1 Regions of red blood cell velocity across a vessel lumen.

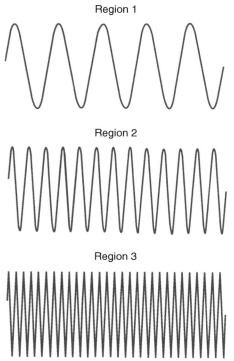

Figure 14-2 Beat frequencies of regions 1, 2, and 3 in Figure 14-1. Note that they increase with increasing velocity of the red blood cells.

observed (f_1, f_2, and f_3) associated with the respective regions. The Doppler shift frequency is largest for region 3, because RBCs in this region are moving at the greatest velocity. Since an equal number of RBCs is present in each region, the amplitudes (signal levels) of all Doppler shift frequencies are equal. This is represented by the heights of the individual waveforms in Figure 14-2, which are identical.

If all three regions are sampled simultaneously by the ultrasound beam, a complex Doppler signal is obtained, as shown in Fig. 14-3, which is an algebraic sum of the three single-frequency waveforms in Figure 14-2. This

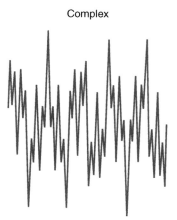

Figure 14-3 This complex Doppler signal is the sum of the waves in Figure 14-2.

detected Doppler signal must be simplified to associate groups of RBCs with the corresponding Doppler shift frequency and thus with flow velocity. Spectral analysis separates the composite signal into its individual frequency components and determines the relative importance of each; that is, the waveform in Figure 14-3, the detected Doppler signal, is mathematically converted into the various individual Doppler shift frequencies shown in Figure 14-2. *The determination of the frequency shifts present in the Doppler signal is performed without prior knowledge of these frequency components.* All Doppler shift frequencies present in the Doppler signal are isolated by spectral analysis.

POWER SPECTRUM

An alternative but informationally equivalent method to display the spectral analysis is in the form of a power spectrum, in which the magnitude of each individual frequency component is plotted with respect to frequency (Fig. 14-4). This graphic presentation converts the complex Doppler signal from the time domain into the frequency domain.

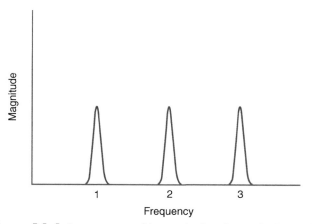

Figure 14-4 Power spectrum of the complex Doppler signal in Figure 14-3. Each flow velocity is depicted as a peak. The three flow velocity peaks corresponding to different regions are the same height.

The power spectrum is an extremely useful analysis technique because the desired flow information, the distribution of Doppler shift frequencies, is displayed directly. The magnitude is determined by the amplitude of the respective waveform corresponding to a particular frequency and represents the relative importance of each frequency (i.e., the number of RBCs moving at the velocity given by the frequency shift). In this case the height for each observed frequency is the same since the initial assumption was that an equal number of RBCs is flowing through each region.

Suppose, for example, that the number of RBCs moving through region 1 were doubled. The amplitude of the beat frequency corresponding to this region would also be doubled and result in an altered complex Doppler signal, as shown in Figure 14-5. The Doppler shift frequency for region 1 remains the same because the velocity of the RBCs has not changed. The spectral analysis presented by the power spectrum in Figure 14-6 depicts the increased importance of the lowest frequency by the increased height of the peak corresponding to this frequency. The display of the complex Doppler signal in the time domain does not allow the sonographer to readily ascertain this increase in flow volume through region 1, but it can be easily interpreted from the power spectrum.

The relationship between the frequency domain display and the velocity of RBCs is further illustrated by the power

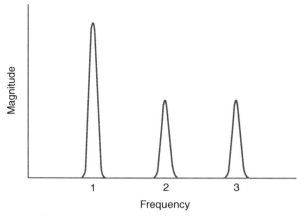

Figure 14-6 Power spectrum of the complex Doppler signal in Figure 14-5.

spectrum associated with plug flow. Plug flow is blood moving at a single velocity. Suppose that essentially all the RBCs throughout the vessel were moving slowly at a constant velocity; thus the power spectrum would contain a single peak at low frequency. If the velocity of the RBCs increased, the power spectrum would once again show a single peak but at a higher frequency.

Laminar flow consisting of many components is often encountered in the vascular system. Laminar flow with a velocity profile ranging from zero near the vessel wall to a maximum in the central portion of the vessel yields a continuous power spectrum, as shown in Figure 14-7.

INFLUENCE OF BEAM SHAPE

In the previous examples of power spectra associated with different velocity distributions, the magnitude of the frequency component indicated the volume of blood moving at the velocity given by that particular frequency. The ultrasound beam is assumed to be large enough to insonate all RBCs within the vessel uniformly. Pulsed-wave (PW) Doppler scanners are designed to generate highly directional beams that restrict sampling to small volumes. Beam shape, as characterized by cross-sectional uniformity and sample axial length, has a major effect on the detected Doppler signal.

Consider once more the situation of laminar flow in which the velocity profile varies from zero near the vessel wall to a maximum in the central portion of the vessel. The effect of sampling volume on the power spectrum is shown in Figure 14-8. If the ultrasound beam encompasses the entire vessel uniformly, a power spectrum depicting all velocity components is obtained. When the vessel is insonated nonuniformly, the contribution to the power spectrum by the slowly flowing RBCs near the wall is diminished. If the beam were restricted to the central portion of the vessel, only the most rapidly moving RBCs contribute to the Doppler signal. In each case the conditions of blood flow would not change, but the measurement process would yield very different results depending on the relative dimensions of the vessel and the ultrasound beam.

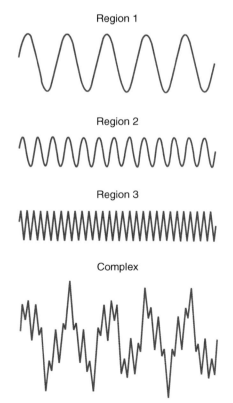

Figure 14-5 Beat frequencies for regions 1, 2, and 3. Region 1 contains twice as many red blood cells (RBCs) as the other regions, and changes in the complex Doppler signal occur from doubling the number of RBCs in that region.

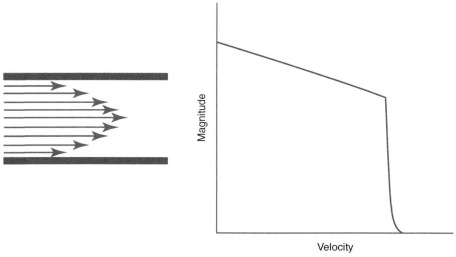

Figure 14-7 Power spectrum of red blood cells (RBCs) moving with laminar flow.

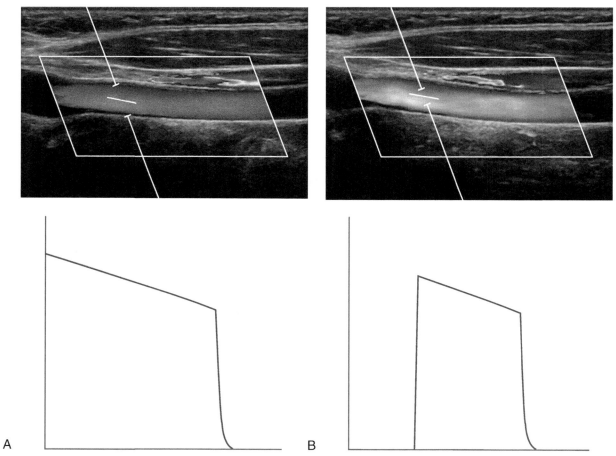

Figure 14-8 Effect of sample size on the laminar flow power spectrum. The parallel lines along the cursor indicate the sampled region in each case. **A,** sampling of the entire vessel lumen with uniform intensity. **B,** sampling with decreased intensity at the vessel wall.

continued

TIME DISPLAY OF THE POWER SPECTRUM

In vessels the velocity distribution is not constant with time; rather, cyclic pressure variations give rise to pulsatile flow. Consequently, it is desirable to display the changing flow patterns depicted by the power spectrum as a function of time (called Doppler spectral waveform). Three variables (frequency, magnitude, and time) must be included in this two-dimensional display. The magnitude in the power spectrum is now represented by varying

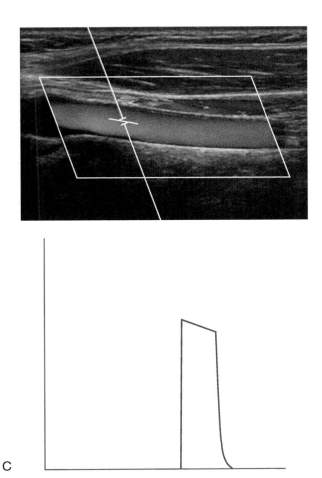

Figure 14-8—cont'd C, sampling restricted to the central portion of the lumen.

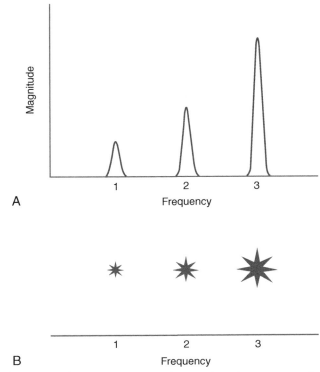

Figure 14-9 A, Power spectrum depicting three discrete groups of red blood cells in which the signal decreases in importance from high frequency to low frequency. **B,** Brightness-modulated power spectrum, which has the same information content as **(A)**.

the brightness level to indicate the relative importance of each frequency. Consider the power spectrum in Figure 14-9, *A,* in which the high-velocity group of RBCs produces twice the signal as the middle-velocity group, which in turn produces twice the signal as the low-velocity group. This information is converted to points of differing brightness along a straight line, representing the frequency axis (Fig. 14-9, *B*). Increased distance along the axis denotes higher frequency. Note that, in this example, the high frequency is brighter than the middle frequency, which is brighter than the low frequency.

Flow hemodynamics is not constant throughout the cardiac cycle. Peak flow velocities typically occur at peak systole. Good temporal resolution is necessary for the interpretation of flow patterns. The dimension of time is obtained by sampling the Doppler signal repeatedly in small increments of a few milliseconds. An FFT frequency analysis is then applied to each short time segment of the Doppler signal. High-speed digital-integrated circuits perform the necessary calculations on the most recently collected data while the Doppler signal for the following time segment is acquired. FFT processing allows a series

of power spectra to be analyzed in real-time. The display of these multiple analyses consists of a vertical axis corresponding to frequency and a horizontal axis corresponding to time. At each frequency point along the vertical axis, the strength of the signal is encoded with varying brightness levels. Each analysis of a short time segment of the Doppler signal is presented as a single vertical line. By placing succeeding frequency analyses side by side, a fixed distance apart, the vertical lines scroll left to right with time to build up a pattern (Fig. 14-10).

A more useful presentation is to convert the frequency distribution to a velocity distribution using the Doppler shift equation with values for transmitted frequency, acoustic velocity in tissue, and Doppler angle. The display of quickly changing velocities within the sampled region thereby becomes possible (Fig. 14-11). The normal internal carotid artery Doppler spectral waveform (Fig. 14-12) demonstrates a maximum peak velocity during systole with a narrow distribution of velocities. Time-varying physiologic signals (e.g., an electrocardiogram) can be displayed in conjunction with the brightness-modulated power spectra.

B-mode images and Doppler spectral waveforms must be interpreted based on a knowledge of anatomy, hemodynamics, disease processes, instrumentation, and physics. Time-varying Doppler spectral analysis yields waveforms that are characteristic of flow within the respective arteries. Although ultrasonographic examination of vascular

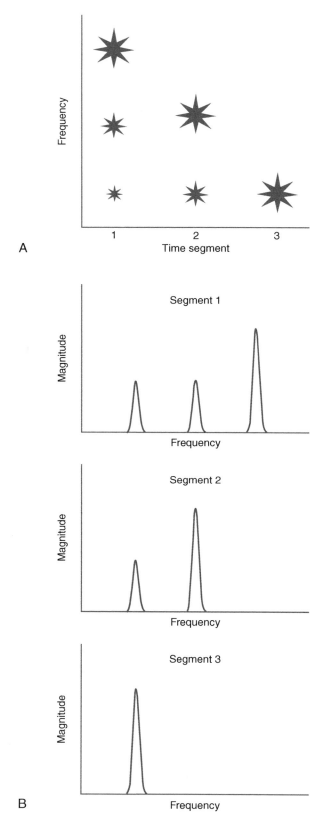

A

B

Figure 14-10 A, Time sequence of the brightness-modulated power spectra shown in **(B)**. **B,** Power spectra corresponding to the three time segments in **(A)**.

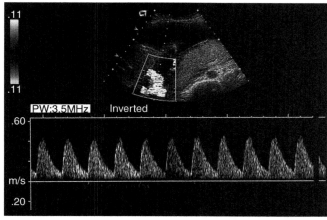

Figure 14-11 Doppler spectral waveform obtained for the umbilical cord.

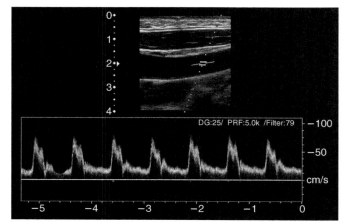

Figure 14-12 Doppler spectral waveform obtained for the carotid artery. The sample volume was positioned to encompass the central portion of the vessel.

anatomy has become a well-accepted clinical diagnostic procedure, limitations do exist. Improper Doppler angle or incorrect designation of the direction of flow introduces error in the Doppler measurements. Attenuation artifacts from calcifications may obscure a segment of the vessel.

OPERATOR CONTROLS

The Doppler cursor is a line superimposed on the B-mode image that indicates the path of the sound beam when operated in Doppler mode. The angle and left-right position of the cursor may be controlled in a variety of ways, depending on the manufacturer and model of the machine. The Doppler cursor appears when pulsed-wave (PW) or continuous-wave (CW) Doppler mode is selected.

The PW Doppler sample volume defines the three-dimensional region from which Doppler information is obtained and displayed. The sample volume is determined by the beam width as well as by the size and position of the range gate. The range gate is displayed on screen as a small box or double set of lines located along the Doppler cursor

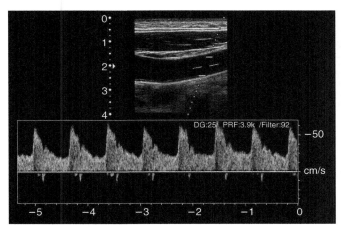

Figure 14-13 Doppler spectral waveform obtained for the carotid artery. The sample volume was positioned to encompass the full width of the vessel. Compare this waveform with that in Figure 14-12.

line. The gate depth is usually controlled with the trackball and must be positioned so the sample volume is located within the area of flow to be interrogated (Fig. 14-13).

The Doppler angle is defined as the angle of the beam axis with respect to the direction of the moving reflector, in this case RBCs. The direction of the Doppler sound beam is indicated by the Doppler cursor. The Doppler angle to flow may be estimated by determining the angle between the Doppler cursor and a line parallel to the vessel walls or to the projected direction of flow within the heart. The sonographer must specify the angle by adjusting an angle-correct pointer on the screen to be parallel with the direction of flow. Because of the angular dependence of the cosine function, the consideration of Doppler angle to flow in vascular and cardiac applications is fundamentally different. In vascular applications, a Doppler angle of 30 to 60 degrees is readily obtained, whereas an angle of zero degrees is not. However, in working with angles in the 60-degree range, an accurate estimation of the Doppler angle is critical and the angle-correct pointer must be adjusted accordingly. Conversely, the majority of Doppler measurements in cardiac applications are performed with the sound beam parallel to the flow direction. The Doppler angle is assumed to be 0 degrees or close to 0 degrees, where the induced error in velocity measurement

from variations in Doppler angle is small. Therefore cardiac sonographers rarely if ever use angle correction.

Doppler gain amplifies the received Doppler signal. Raising the Doppler gain increases both the brightness of the Doppler spectral waveform and the volume of the audio signal. Doppler gain must be balanced with Doppler output power. Output power set too low results in the gain setting near maximum with high noise content present in the display.

The Doppler output power control (not available on some scanners) also affects the brightness of the Doppler spectral waveform and the volume of the audio signal. However, this is accomplished by increasing excitation voltage to the transducer rather than by amplifying the received signal. Doppler output power should be kept to a moderate level if possible, both from the standpoint of spectral quality (output power at maximum is usually unnecessary and may introduce noise) and from the consideration of patient exposure.

The velocity scale denotes maximum velocity in both the positive and negative directions that can be displayed without aliasing. If flow exceeds the maximum velocity, aliasing occurs (Fig. 14-14). On most current machines, the Doppler PRF is coupled to the maximum displayed velocity. The upper limit of the velocity scale (in both positive and negative directions) is established by the Nyquist limit, which is equal to half the Doppler PRF. The velocity scale may be increased by changing the PRF to accommodate higher flow velocities until the maximum velocity limit is reached (Fig. 14-15). The maximum velocity limit corresponds to the highest Doppler PRF that can be used without spatial misregistration when sampling at the gate depth.

The spectral Doppler display shows flow velocities towards and away from the transducer simultaneously. Often, the baseline is positioned in the center of the display to partition maximum velocity equally in both positive and negative flow directions. The baseline control may be adjusted up or down, positioning the baseline off center, in order to expand the displayed maximum velocity in one direction with subsequent reduction in the other direction (Fig. 14-16).

Depending on the application and the anatomy being examined, the spectral Doppler waveform may be displayed primarily above the baseline (flow toward the

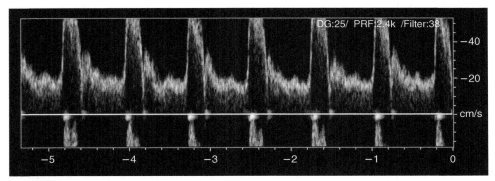

Figure 14-14 Aliasing artifact in which high-velocity components demonstrate wraparound. The velocity range on the vertical scale is −20 to 55 cm/s.

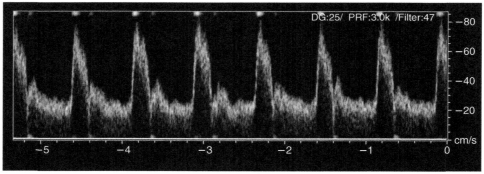

Figure 14-15 Doppler spectral waveform obtained for the carotid artery in which the maximum velocity scale was raised to 85 cm/s from 55 cm/s in Figure 14-12.

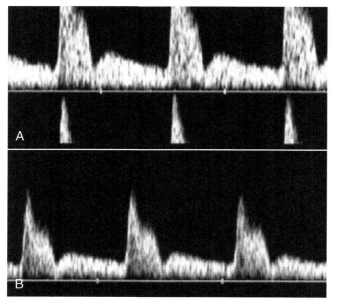

Figure 14-16 Adjusting the baseline to remove the aliasing artifact. **A,** Baseline is in the center to show forward and reverse flow. **B,** The velocity range is expanded to show flow in the forward direction only.

transducer) or below (flow away from the transducer). In some circumstances, the spectral display is inverted to show an otherwise negative or "upside down" waveform as "right side up." Traditionally, cardiac Doppler signals have been displayed in the direction in which they occur without inversion of the waveforms. In vascular applications, such as carotid artery scanning, common practice is to display all normal waveforms above the baseline. If the waveform appears upside-down because of the Doppler angle to flow, the spectral invert control "flips" the waveform for the right-side-up display. The notation for positive/negative axes on the spectral display is also simultaneously inverted, so that the waveform is still depicted with the correct flow direction (Fig. 14-17).

The sweep speed of the spectral display may be adjusted to show more detail in each waveform (increased sweep speed) or multiple waveform cycles in each sweep (decreased sweep speed). For example, in a venous duplex exam of the lower extremity, a slow sweep speed is desirable because the venous response to several manual limb compressions can be recorded in a single sweep.

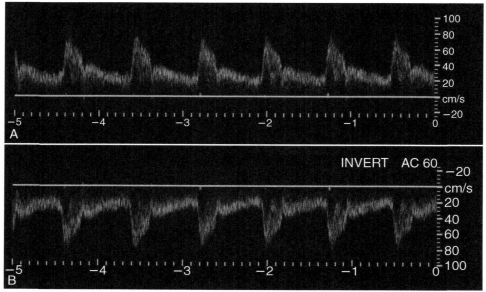

Figure 14-17 Spectral invert. **A,** Forward flow is shown above the baseline. **B,** By activating the invert control, forward flow is shown below the baseline.

Conversely, in a carotid artery exam or an aortic valve evaluation in an echocardiogram, each waveform is expanded using high sweep speed for improved analysis of the individual cycle characteristics and more accurate measurements.

A wall filter applied to the Doppler signal removes spectral data below a specific frequency from the display. The purpose of the wall filter is to eliminate the distracting low-frequency movement of the vessel wall, but it may remove low-velocity blood flow components in the power spectrum as well. Wall thump and other slow-motion Doppler artifacts are typically generated at frequencies below 100 Hz. Therefore, a wall filter setting of 100 Hz often eliminates these unwanted artifacts. However, at too high a setting of the wall filter, low-velocity flow information is also removed from the low-frequency portion of the waveform (Fig. 14-18). Under these conditions the velocity distribution becomes distorted by the application of the wall filter. This is usually an undesirable consequence and requires that the wall filter be reduced to a lower frequency.

The Doppler reject control eliminates low-amplitude signals to suppress noise in the spectral display. The threshold for rejection is based on signal level rather than on frequency.

SPECTRAL MIRROR ARTIFACT

Another improper presentation of the power spectra, called the spectral mirror artifact, occurs when weak Doppler signals are detected with high power and gain settings (Fig. 14-19). The quadrature phase detector becomes saturated and cannot process all incoming Doppler signals, resulting in a loss of directional discrimination. Forward and reverse spectra emulate each other.

FAST FOURIER TRANSFORM FREQUENCY RESOLUTION

For the spectral display to respond to rapid changes in the velocity distribution, short sampling times are desirable. The duration of the analyzed segment, however,

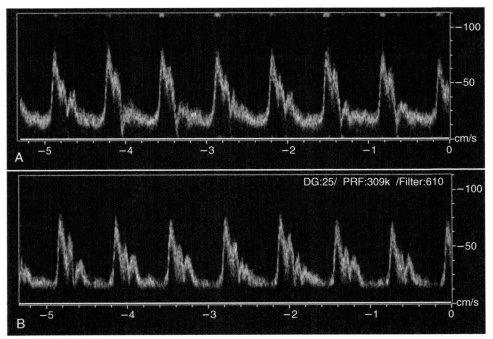

Figure 14-18 Wall filter. **A,** Low frequency setting. **B,** High frequency setting, which removes low-velocity components present in A.

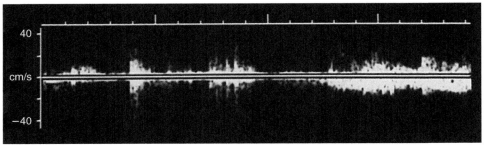

Figure 14-19 Pulsed-wave Doppler spectral waveform showing spectral mirror artifact.

determines the frequency resolution. Each brightness-modulated dot in the power spectrum represents a range of Doppler shift frequencies equal to the inverse of the sampling time. A time segment of 5 ms yields a frequency resolution of 200 Hz; a longer time segment, 10 ms, improves the frequency resolution to 100 Hz.

SPECTRAL BROADENING

A single-frequency Doppler shift for a reflector moving at constant velocity is obtained only for a very large-plane target insonated by a large acoustic field. A reflector only contributes to the backscattered signal during movement within a finite-width beam. The fluctuation of the detected signal as RBCs move in and out of the sampling volume causes the beat frequency to vary in amplitude, which is interpreted as additional frequency components above and below the idealized Doppler shift frequency. This broadening of the spectrum is called transit time broadening and creates difficulties in spectral interpretation. A spectrum produced by scatterers moving at different velocities is the same as that observed when scatterers are moving at constant velocity with transit time broadening. The overall effect of transit time broadening is to smear the single Doppler shift frequency associated with a single velocity over a wider range of frequencies.

Narrowing the beam width and shortening the receiver gate in PW mode accentuate the broadening effect. The simultaneous measurement of reflector position and velocity in PW Doppler limits the ability of these systems to determine high-velocity flow in small, localized regions. Long axial gate and wide beam width with a corresponding loss in positional information are necessary to assess high-velocity flow accurately.

The transmitted pulse consists of multiple frequencies, which introduces variations into the received frequency and contributes to spectral broadening. Also, the physical size of the beam aperture creates a range of angles that intercept the vessel (Fig. 14-20). Even if all RBCs were moving at the same velocity, a range of Doppler shifts would be detected, because the angle of insonation is not uniform across the beam width.

MAXIMUM VELOCITY DESCRIPTOR

Maximum frequency is a descriptor of the power spectrum that helps characterize Doppler signals. The maximum Doppler shift (f_{max}) corresponds to the fastest-moving RBCs within the sample volume at the time of measurement. Each FFT segment is analyzed for the maximum Doppler shift frequency, which is then presented as a time-varying trace on the display. Usually a 1% to 5% upper cutoff limit is applied to prevent the maximum Doppler shift from being associated with high-frequency noise. The cutoff limit indicates the portion of the power spectrum that is above the calculated maximum frequency. Perhaps the alternative description is easier to conceptualize: 100 minus the cutoff limit gives the percentage of total Doppler signal that lies below the calculated maximum frequency. Figure 14-21 illustrates the relation between FFT analysis and maximum frequency. If the power spectrum demonstrates a relatively steep falloff in magnitude for the high-frequency components, f_{max} is a good approximation of the true maximum frequency.

The maximum Doppler shift in each time segment is commonly converted to velocity using transducer frequency and Doppler angle. This trace is referred to as the maximum velocity waveform (Fig. 14-22). An electrocardiographic tracing may be included in the display to associate events with the cardiac cycle.

ALIASING

Aliasing is characterized by wraparound, whereby the high-velocity flow above the Nyquist limit in one direction appears as low-velocity flow in the opposite direction. The

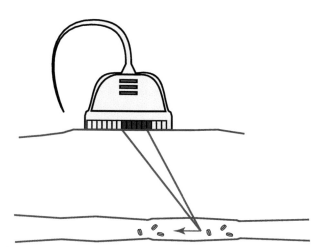

Figure 14-20 The physical dimensions of the active aperture create multiple insonation angles for a steered beam.

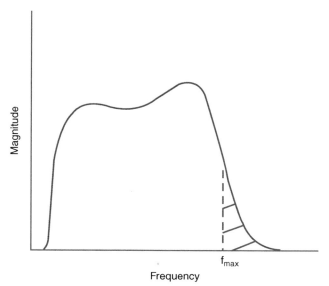

Figure 14-21 Maximum frequency derived from the power spectrum with a cutoff limit of 5%.

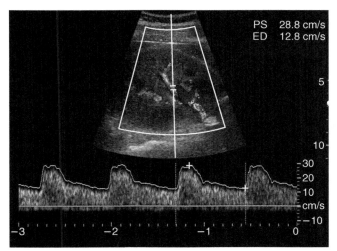

Figure 14-22 Maximum-velocity waveform.

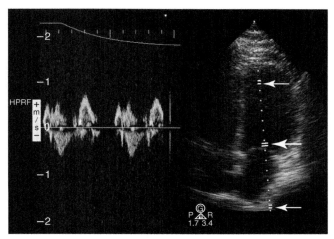

Figure 14-23 Apical four-chamber view in high pulse repetition frequency (PRF) mode. Note the primary sample volume *(large arrow)* and two secondary sample volumes *(small arrows).* The Doppler waveform of the mitral valve *(left side of image)* was obtained from the primary sample. Note that the shallow secondary sample is positioned in the ventricular apex, where little flow is present; the deeper secondary sample is outside the heart altogether.

aliasing artifact is removed by changing the velocity scale or adjusting the baseline. An increase in the pulse repetition frequency extends the maximum velocity according to the Nyquist criterion, which is expressed as the upper range limit on the velocity scale. The velocity range for reverse flow can be set to a lower value than that for forward flow (zero if reverse flow is not a concern). Adjustment of baseline can double the maximum velocity in one direction, but directional discrimination is lost.

The maximum Doppler PRF allowed at a given depth, and thus the Nyquist limit, is governed by the transit time required by each ultrasound pulse. As the depth of the sample volume is increased, the maximum Doppler PRF is reduced. Aliasing is far more likely when high-velocity flow at deep depths is encountered. An innovative method, called high-PRF mode, increases the Doppler PRF above the echo-ranging constraint to reduce the possibility of aliasing in this situation. High-PRF violates the basic tenet of range-resolution: that an ultrasound pulse is not transmitted until the echoes generated by the previous pulse have returned from the entire scan range. At high Doppler PRF (e.g., twice the maximum Doppler PRF based on echo ranging), pulse transmission occurs before all the echoes have been received. Range ambiguity is introduced and multiple sampling areas appear on the screen (Fig. 14-23). In most cases, by examining the positions of the two sample volumes compared with the anatomy on the screen, one is able to identify the origin of the high-velocity flow.

Other techniques to eliminate the aliasing artifact are to increase the angle of insonation, decrease the depth to the sample volume by rocking the transducer heel to toe, switch to a lower transmitted frequency, or switch to CW Doppler.

In summary, aliasing can be eliminated by the following techniques:
- Increase velocity scale (PRF)
- Adjust baseline
- Increase angle of insonation

- Decrease depth to sample volume
- Switch to High-PRF mode
- Switch to lower transmitted frequency
- Switch to CW Doppler

DISTURBED FLOW

Flow disturbance is generally accepted to mean a deviation from purely laminar flow, but without the energy losses seen with turbulence. Eddy currents and helical flow are often present. Disturbed flow usually reverts readily back to laminar flow as the area causing the disturbance is passed. Turbulence is complete loss of flow coherence and represents a state in which movement of blood cells is often at right angles or even 180 degrees to the axis of the vessel (reversed).

Arterial obstruction is usually a locally formed atherosclerotic plaque. A plaque presents a mechanical obstruction within the vessel, causing an effective narrowing of the vessel lumen. Stenosis occurs when the vessel lumen is narrowed to the point where blood flow is affected. Mild plaque initially results in disturbed flow with some characteristics of laminar flow still maintained. As the plaque continues to develop, with more pronounced luminal narrowing, blood flow velocity through the area of obstruction becomes steadily higher until turbulence occurs. At near total blockage, flow volume and consequently flow velocity are greatly reduced.

For a vessel with a nearly uniform velocity distribution, the spectral display, particularly during systole, shows a characteristic window appearance (Fig. 14-24, *A*). The window is an area between the high-velocity components and the baseline that is relatively signal-free. Doppler shifts are confined to a relatively narrow velocity range. Stenosis, which causes a 75% reduction in a cross-sectional

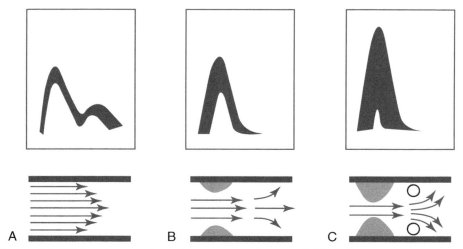

Figure 14-24 Doppler spectral waveforms. **A,** Normal. **B,** Partially blocked lumen. **C,** Severe stenosis.

area (or, equivalently, a 50% reduction in luminal diameter), disrupts the normal flow patterns. High-velocity jets are formed in the region of maximum narrowing. Sampling within the stenotic jet produces high-velocity uniform flow with a clear spectral window. The peak velocity in particular increases as luminal size decreases and is used as an indicator of severity of the stenosis. Immediately distal to the stenosis the flow velocities become less uniform and are distributed over a wider range. Spectral analysis detects this change as a continued high-velocity peak (although usually less than the stenotic jet) and a fill-in of the window (Fig. 14-24, B). The window is reduced and is not as distinct. The high-speed components and lack of window become more pronounced as the blockage becomes more severe (Fig. 14-24, C). A severely blocked lumen creates high-speed jets with rotating flow elements. Arterial regions with eddy flow exhibit time-dependent behavior in which the velocity distribution reverts to laminar flow during periods of reduced pressure. The Doppler spectral waveform changes shape to reflect a loss in pulsatility. Turbulence is often observed distal to severe stenosis before the normal flow pattern is reestablished (Fig. 14-25).

In summary, a hemodynamically significant stenosis alters the flow characteristics within the vessel (1) proximal to, or upstream from the stenosis, (2) at the point of

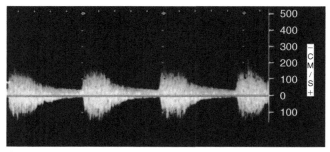

Figure 14-25 Doppler spectral waveform for the internal carotid artery, in which turbulence is present.

maximum stenosis, (3) immediately distal to or at the exit of the stenosis, (4) distal to the stenosis, and (5) further downstream from the stenosis (Fig. 14-26).

- Proximal to or upstream from the stenosis (region 1): laminar flow and evidence of increased downstream resistance (decreased or absent diastolic flow).
- At the point of maximum stenosis (region 2) abrupt increase in maximum velocity and formation of jets through stenosis itself.
- At the exit of the stenosis (region 3): abrupt decrease in velocity (except in the path of the jet) and loss of laminar flow with eddy currents.

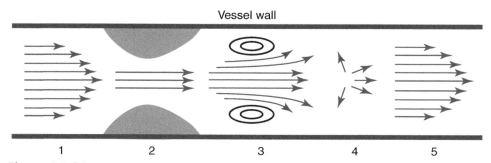

Figure 14-26 Disruption of flow caused by stenosis *(shaded regions)*. Velocity profiles include (1) laminar, (2) jet, (3) flow reversal, (4) turbulence, and (5) laminar.

- Distal to the stenosis (region 4): abrupt decrease in velocity and the presence of turbulence with a total loss of laminar flow, which may extend far downstream.
- Downstream from the stenosis (region 5): eventually flow returns to laminar with a permanent energy loss (pressure drop).

SUMMARY

Doppler techniques are an important tool for the investigation of blood flow dynamics, including the presence of flow, flow direction, and other physiologic aspects of flow (pulsatility, high-velocity jets, and turbulence). The Doppler signal obtained from RBCs is analyzed for frequency (and hence velocity) components using the FFT. The power spectrum shows the relative contribution of each velocity component. Velocity profile across the vessel lumen and sampling conditions affect the power spectrum. Time-dependent flow velocities within a vessel are depicted by brightness-modulated power spectra acquired successively in short time segments.

The information content of the brightness-modulated power spectra is simplified by displaying the maximum velocity waveform. This time-varying trace corresponds to the maximum Doppler shift frequency and thus the fastest-moving RBCs within each FFT segment.

B-mode imaging and PW Doppler spectral analysis are both necessary for evaluations of the vascular system. Vessel size and surrounding anatomy are shown in the gray-scale image, and clots and plaques, when present, are often visualized. The B-mode image acts as a road map for placement of the directional cursor for CW Doppler or the sample volume for PW Doppler. The time-dependent spectral Doppler spectral waveform indicates the velocity components in a small segment of the vessel. However, multiple samplings from different locations must be obtained before a global picture of flow can be formulated.

Color Doppler Imaging

15

Chapter Objectives

To identify the two major types of color Doppler imaging
To state the rationale for autocorrelation signal processing in color Doppler imaging
To understand the function of color Doppler imaging controls
To recognize artifacts unique to color Doppler imaging, including color aliasing, color bleed, and color noise

Key Terms

Asynchronous scanners	Color line density	Combined Doppler mode
Autocorrelation	Color map	Dwell time
Color baseline control	Color-map invert	Mean frequency
Color box	Color persistence	Packet size (ensemble
Color flow imaging	Color reject	length)
Color gain	Color velocity scale	Power Doppler imaging
Color gate	Color wall filter	Variance

COLOR FLOW MEASUREMENTS

Color Doppler imaging (also called color flow imaging, color flow Doppler, color Doppler, color velocity imaging, energy Doppler, and power Doppler) is a scanning mode that combines gray-scale imaging with two-dimensional color mapping of flow information in real time. Maximum frame rates are slower than those achieved by real-time B-mode scanning (considerably more computational analysis is required), although a frame rate of 20 frames per second is not uncommon. The gray-scale component of the image is designated as real-time, gray-scale, two-dimensional (2D), or B-mode. Motion is depicted throughout the scan plane by superimposing different colors on the two-dimensional gray-scale image. Color encoding is based on a single parameter related to velocity (color flow imaging) or Doppler signal level (power Doppler imaging).

COLOR FLOW IMAGE FORMAT

In color flow imaging both stationary and moving structures are detected by analyzing the received echoes with respect to amplitude, phase, and frequency (Fig. 15-1). Stationary structures are assigned a gray-scale brightness level based on signal strength as previously shown for B-mode scanners. Moving reflectors cause a phase shift in the received echo signals that indicates the presence and direction of motion (toward or away from the transducer). Doppler signal processing measures the mean Doppler shift frequency, which yields the relative velocity of the moving reflectors via the Doppler shift equation (not corrected for Doppler angle). *At each sampling site*

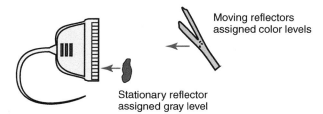

Figure 15-1 Doppler imaging. Echoes from stationary and moving reflectors are detected and processed to depict flow and anatomy.

where motion is detected, a single representative velocity (usually the mean) is color encoded by hue, saturation, or brightness and superimposed on the gray-scale image. The highest priority in color flow imaging is the observation of motion. If certain criteria are met, the assignment of color takes precedence over gray-scale associated with stationary structures.

Classification of scanners is based on how the color flow image is formed. Asynchronous scanners collect gray-scale and flow data at different times, whereas synchronous systems collect the two data sets simultaneously. In the latter case the field of view for imaging and color coincide, whereas in the former a color box defines a subdivision of the gray-scale field of view for color analysis. Color display does not encompass the entire screen but is restricted to a small region so that frame rate can be maintained. Asynchronous scanners dominate the marketplace.

COLOR ENCODING

A color map assigns various shades or brightness of color to depict different velocities while maintaining directional information (either toward or away from the transducer). The "blue away, red toward" (BART) and "red away, blue toward" (RABT) formats use color saturation to code for velocity. Color coding with saturation adds white light to a color to decrease the purity of the light. In the BART format, red indicates motion in one direction (toward the transducer), and blue indicates motion in the opposite direction. Regions with high-velocity flow are displayed by increased color saturation (increased whiteness). Fast-moving reflectors are represented in light shades of red or blue and slow-moving reflectors in dark shades. The association of color with a particular direction of flow is interchangeable, however. The importance of the two-color scheme is not to code for arterial and venous flow but rather to simultaneously depict flow in opposite directions on the real-time image.

Alternative color maps use colors of the rainbow (violet, blue, green, yellow, orange, and red) to encode velocity information. Each color signifies a specific velocity range. Red progressing to yellow (toward) and purple to blue (away) allows rapid flow in opposite directions to be more easily differentiated. In color flow imaging numerous color maps are available for selection by the operator. Compare color flow images of the liver, which use three

different color maps to display the same scan plane (Fig. 15-2). The information content is the same, although the translation from velocity to color is different.

COLOR VELOCITY SCALE

The color velocity scale is incorporated into the color flow display and is shown as the color-scale bar with the maximum velocity indicated (usually, in centimeters per second). Velocities less than the maximum velocity are shown without color aliasing. The velocity range is set by the sonographer depending on clinical application. Increasing the velocity scale enhances the ability to display fast-moving reflectors, while decreasing the velocity scale improves the partition of slower flow.

SPATIAL FLOW PATTERNS

The major disadvantage of duplex scanning is that flow is not evaluated throughout the field of view concurrently but rather is sampled at one particular location as selected by the sonographer. To establish the regional flow pattern, the spectral analysis must be performed at multiple sites throughout the vessel, which requires repeated repositioning of the sampling volume. Focal regions of abnormal flow are sometimes overlooked. Also, the repetition of sampling is a time-consuming process. *By displaying the two-dimensional spatial distribution of flow velocities and the temporal changes in these velocity patterns, color flow imaging overcomes these difficulties and enables regions of flow disturbance to be more easily visualized.*

RANGE-GATED PULSED-WAVE VELOCITY DETECTION

To assess motion, multiple echoes from the same reflector must be collected using a series of transmitted pulses. Recall the analogy in which a series of stop-action photographs of a moving car allows its velocity to be determined, but a single photograph in the series does not indicate whether motion is present. Color flow imaging requires positional information as well as the velocity of the moving reflector. Spatial origin of the echoes along the Doppler line of sight is obtained by the principle of echo ranging, in which the induced signals from echoes are time-gated. For each Doppler line of sight, multiple transmitted pulses contribute to Doppler signal formation. Different sampling paths compose the color field of view by electronic steering of the beam.

Velocity information must be obtained for a large number of sample volumes throughout the field of view in a very limited amount of time. Range-gated pulsed-wave (PW) Doppler spectral analysis requires a relatively long sampling time for each line of sight (typically about 10 ms). The sampling time or dwell time is the product of the pulse repetition period and the number of pulses used to interrogate the moving reflectors along one line

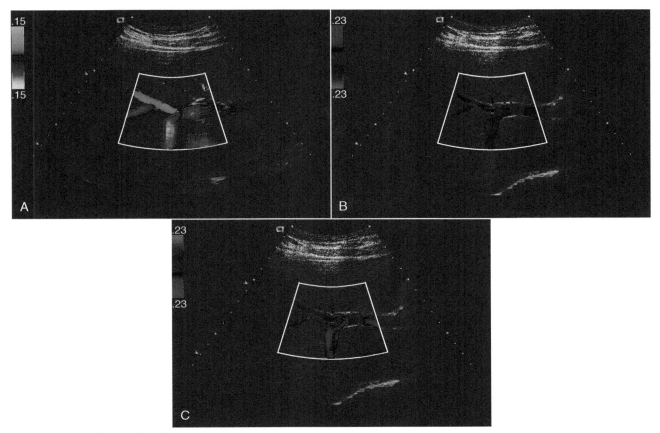

Figure 15-2 Doppler imaging of the portal vein. **A,** Flow in the anterior right portal vein and the posterior right portal vein is shown using a rainbow color map. **B,** BART color map shows the flow toward the transducer in red. **C,** RABT color map shows the flow toward the transducer in blue.

of sight. Hundreds of gates, to acquire the Doppler signals partitioned by depth along the entire scan line, are necessary. Parallel processing of a multigated system allows several locations along the scan line to be examined with no increase in sampling time. The gates are activated sequentially following the excitation pulse. Each gate corresponds to one pixel.

The most important consideration is the time constraint imposed by the requirement that the image must be updated every 0.05 to 0.1 second (corresponding to a frame rate of 10 to 20 images per second). Range-gated PW Doppler spectral detection does not satisfy this condition because the time necessary to form an image is on the order of seconds. Each image consists of 100 to 200 scan lines, and each scan line requires a dwell time of 10 ms. A faster method to detect Doppler signals is needed.

AUTOCORRELATION

Spectral analysis has a high informational content in that the individual frequency components of the Doppler signal are identified. By characterizing the Doppler signal with a single parameter (usually the mean frequency), informational content (spectral distribution of the Doppler shift frequencies) is sacrificed, but the sampling time can be shortened considerably. The rapid acquisition and

analysis of flow data are achieved with autocorrelation detection. Fewer transmitted pulses are applied along the scan line compared with PW spectral analysis, and consequently autocorrelation is less sensitive to slow flow and flow in small vessels.

Quadrature Detection

Color Doppler signal processing is initiated with a quadrature detection (QD) circuit, which forms two output signals (in-phase QD and out-of-phase QD) by mixing the reference signal with the detected echo wavetrain. The pulsed technique is necessary to obtain positional information, which necessitates discrete sampling of these QD signals during the observation time. Observation time is time during which Doppler information is acquired along one color scan line (usually about 1 ms).

A succession of echoes from the same reflector is collected by sequential transmitted pulses, processed through the QD circuit, segmented by depth, and placed in a depth-specific hold circuit. In the time following a transmitted pulse the output from each quadrature channel is segmented into different depths by echo ranging. Each transmitted pulse contributes one data point to the composite in-phase and out-of-phase signals at each depth. Multiple transmitted pulses allow the buildup of time-dependent quadrature signals. The time between data points is equal to the pulse repetition period. This scheme allows quadrature signals to be generated from many depth segments during the dwell time for each scan line. The sampling interval along the scan line can be made 0.5 mm or smaller.

Signal Processing

The time-varying output from each quadrature channel is a complex function of amplitude and phase of the echo signals. Both stationary and moving reflectors contribute to the QD waveform. The phase of the received signal from a stationary reflector is constant, whereas the phase of the received signal from a moving reflector fluctuates with time. Consequently, sampling with another pulsed sound wave at a later time introduces a change in the QD signal level at the point in the waveform corresponding to the depth of a moving reflector (Fig. 15-3). Each QD output is partitioned according to depth by sequentially clocked gates. A plot of QD output from successive transmitted pulses, segmented according to depth, indicates that moving reflectors produce signals with varying magnitude. Note that two time measurements are required to obtain the color information. First, the elapsed time following the transmitted pulse assigns depth; each transmitted pulse contributes one data point to the QD signal at every depth segment. Second, intermittent sampling of the QD signal at a particular depth is achieved by a succession of transmitted pulses. Data points are separated by a time interval equal to the pulse repetition period.

Autocorrelation is a comparison of measurements acquired from the same reflector. Processing of the echoes received from multiple depths is done concurrently. The stream of echoes along the entire scan line is examined by delaying the previous echo wavetrain obtained from the immediately preceding excitation pulse by a time equal to the pulse repetition period. This places the successive echo wavetrains on the same relative time scale, and thus reflector location is designated by the time interval following the transmitted pulse. Each echo wavetrain is divided into segments by depth.

At every location the individual echoes from consecutive samplings are multiplied together, and the product is added in the integrator to the values from other samplings (Fig. 15-4). Registers store the computational results while the data are accumulated for one line of sight.

Both channels of the QD circuit provide input to the autocorrelation detector. For each depth two separate registers hold the output from the autocorrelation detector. At the conclusion of sampling along the line of sight, velocity and phase are computed at each depth from the values stored in registers corresponding to that depth. The autocorrelation detector does not depict spectral analysis of the Doppler signal but rather provides the mean frequency of all moving reflectors within each sample volume.

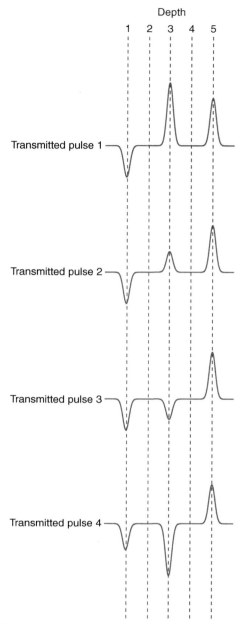

Figure 15-3 Quadrature channel output from four successive pulses along the line of sight. Motion is detected by changes in the signal level at a particular time (depth). The reflectors at depth segments 1 and 5 are stationary, while that at depth segment 3 is moving.

Dwell Time

A minimum of three observations is required to determine the Doppler shift frequency. Generally, each scan line is sampled 4 to 10 times, although it may be sampled as many as 32 times. Packet size or ensemble length describes the number of pulses used to interrogate a single color scan line. Large packet size (long integration time) provides high color definition (more accurate frequency estimates), but a long dwell time lowers the frame rate.

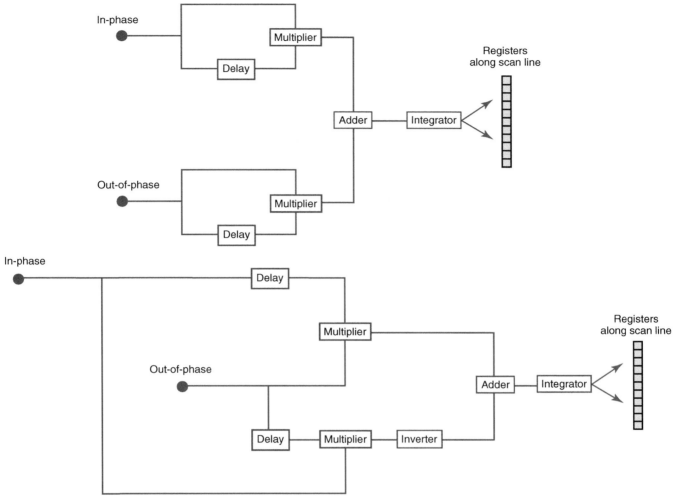

Figure 15-4 Autocorrelation detector. The in-phase and out-of-phase quadrature detection signals from two consecutive transmitted pulses are segmented by depth and then manipulated in a series of multiplication and addition steps. An integrator sums the computational results at each depth from repeated samplings and stores them in registers.

Fixed Echo Canceller

To lower the dynamic range of the input to the autocorrelation detector, strong echoes from stationary structures are often eliminated. Echoes from stationary reflectors remain unchanged in successive echo wavetrains; otherwise varying echoes would be attributed to moving reflectors. Echoes from stationary reflectors are removed by subtracting identical echoes in consecutive transmit pulses through the introduction of a fixed echo canceller.

IMAGE ACQUISITION

A linear array will be used to demonstrate that the gray-scale and flow data are acquired separately and later color is superimposed on gray-scale to form the color flow image. The gray-scale scanning is accomplished by generating sequential dynamically focused beams along the physical extent of the array. Parallel scan lines compose the gray-scale component, which provides sampling perpendicular to the

blood movement (the vessel is assumed to be parallel to the skin surface). This geometry is ideal for imaging but not for assessing flow (for which the interrogation angle would be 90 degrees). To achieve a more favorable Doppler angle, the beam for flow measurements must be steered at an angle to the array (Fig. 15-5).

Separate complete sweeps for gray-scale and then color across the field of view displace stationary tissue and flow in time. At each location the time separation between gray-scale and flow measurements is long. Consequently, to improve the time registration, small groups of steered and unsteered scan lines are alternated in a time-sharing scheme. These scan lines are interwoven in a digital scan converter to compose the final color image (Fig. 15-6).

In an asynchronous autocorrelation system, separate transmitters form either the steered or the unsteered beam. If the beam is steered, the induced signal is directed to the Doppler channel. Otherwise the gray-scale channel is active. The image data are processed and sent to the scan converter. In the Doppler channel a quadrature detector

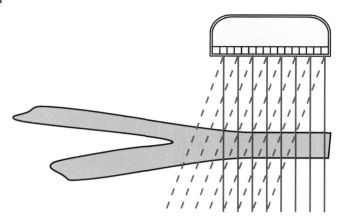

Figure 15-5 Asynchronous linear array with gray-scale lines of sight *(red)* and steered color lines of sight *(blue)*.

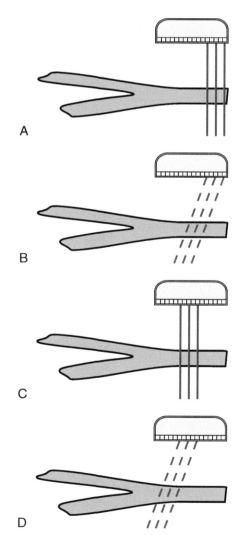

Figure 15-6 Asynchronous linear array with time sharing. A small portion of the field of view (FOV) is sampled with gray-scale scan lines *(red)* **(A)** and then color scan lines *(blue)* **(B)** before the next section of the FOV is probed **(C,D)**.

coupled with autocorrelation quantifies forward and reverse flow signals, which are numerically encoded and placed in the scan converter. The numerical values in the scan converter are translated into gray and color levels before image display on the monitor.

The asynchronous autocorrelation scanner allows the transmitted beam to be optimized for both Doppler and gray-scale because each component is collected independently of the other. The transducer frequency and transmit power may be adjusted for each component. Transmitted pulses can be switched between a gray-scale frequency of 5 MHz and a Doppler frequency of 3 MHz. Although a narrow beam width is desirable for good lateral resolution in the gray-scale mode, it causes spectral broadening in the Doppler mode. Doppler transmitted power is increased to improve detection of weak flow signals.

Most of the acquisition time is devoted for data collection of the color component. Only one pulse per scan line is required for gray-scale, although multiple pulses are necessary to compose a color line. To compensate for the longer acquisition time, low color scan line density, reduced color field of view, a small packet size, or a combination of these is used for color acquisition (Figs. 15-7 and 15-8). Interpolating between color scan lines fills in the gaps (spatial persistence). Doppler and gray-scale spatial resolution are not necessarily matched. Indeed, the axial sampling interval for Doppler is usually greater (as much as several millimeters).

OPERATOR CONTROLS

Commercially available color Doppler instruments have multiple controls that affect the color image. These operator-adjustable parameters contribute markedly to the overall complexity of color Doppler imaging. Fortunately, many of the controls have a function similar to that described for CW and PW Doppler. The terminology used to label the controls has not become standardized, however, and each manufacturer has adopted its own set of descriptors.

Color box or region of interest (ROI) size, position (left-right), and depth are typically controlled by the trackball and a three-way selector switch that sequentially activates each function (Fig. 15-9). To maximize the frame rate, the color box size should be kept reasonably small, setting the optimum width to include the organ of interest and no larger.

In cardiac applications, the color box is not "steered" (angled off-axis to the gray-scale sound beam). This is typically true of any sector-type transducer. The color angle to flow is established by defining the probe position relative to the direction of flow as well as by positioning the cursor box to the left or right on the display. In other applications the color box may be slanted to the left or right to vary the color angle to flow. As the angle of insonation relative to the vessel segment approaches 90 degrees, low-frequency Doppler shifts are generated that may not be depicted in the image. When a steered beam collects the Doppler signal, the angle of insonation can be selected to provide a

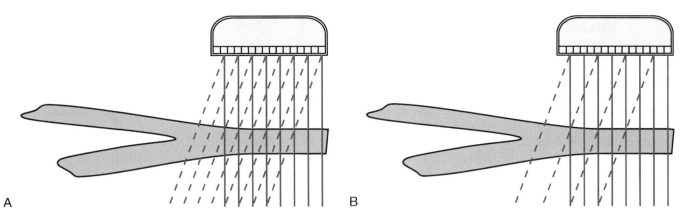

Figure 15-7 Frame rate can be increased by reducing the color line density across the field of view. Color lines of sight are shown as dotted lines. **A,** High density. **B,** Low density.

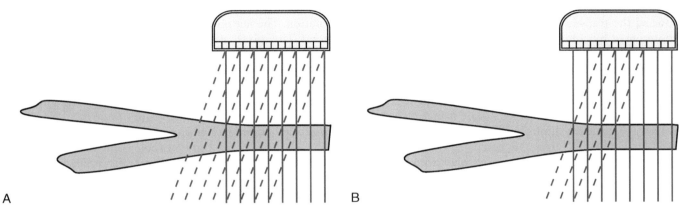

Figure 15-8 Frame rate can be increased by reducing the width of the color field of view (FOV). Color lines of sight are shown as dotted lines. **A,** Wide FOV. **B,** Narrow FOV.

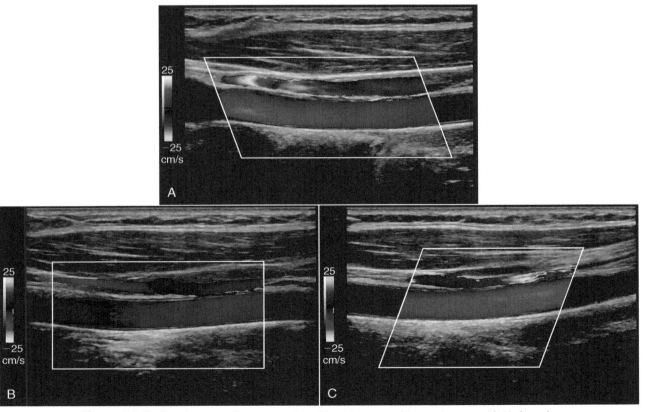

Figure 15-9 The color region of interest (ROI) box defines the portion of the two-dimensional field of view for color display. **A-C,** The color box is shown with three possible sampling directions for the color scan lines.

more favorable geometry between the direction of flow and the ultrasound beam.

The color velocity scale specifies the range of velocities that are presented in the color display. The pulse repetition frequency (PRF) is set by the velocity scale and has a maximum limit established by the depth of scanning. For applications in peripheral vascular imaging, where low-velocity flow is encountered, decreasing the PRF lowers the maximum detectable velocity and improves the velocity resolution. Some manufacturers alter the transducer frequency in response to a shift in velocity scale.

The orientation of the color bar indicates the assignment of colors to the positive and negative flow directions. The color at the top of the bar is assigned to depict flow toward the transducer. Flow in the opposite direction is represented by colors on the bottom half of the bar. The color-map invert control reverses the colors on the color scale bar as well as the colors in the image where flow is present. This inversion may be applied to preferentially show the vessel or cardiac structure as red or blue.

The zero point of the velocity scale is initially set midway so the velocity limits for forward and reverse flow are equal. The color baseline control shifts the center of the velocity scale up or down to display a greater range of velocities in one direction. The total velocity range is unchanged. For example, if the initial velocity range was −50 to 50 cm/s, an adjustment in baseline could establish a new velocity range as −20 to 80 cm/s. Higher velocities in the forward direction can now be displayed without aliasing.

Color gain is the amplification applied to the Doppler signal during processing. High color gain increases the likelihood a pixel is encoded in color and expands the number of pixels encoded with color. Color gain set too low prevents color from adequately "filling" the vessel. If color gain is set too high, the color extends outside the borders of the vessel or heart chamber.

Color reject sets the threshold below which weak flow signals are not included in the color display. The basis for rejection is the signal strength and not the frequency of the Doppler signal. This is a noise-reduction technique. Lowering the threshold increases the amount of color within the image. Color reject is independent of gray-scale gain and time gain compensation.

Echoes from blood are weak compared with echoes from tissue. This property (in the form of signal level) is evaluated using an echo-versus-color threshold to differentiate flow from moving tissue. Strong reflections that exceed the threshold value are assigned a gray level. Weak echoes from tissue are sometimes depicted in color at low-gain settings. Proper gray-scale gain creates an image in which tissue is free of color. Excessive gray-scale gain can suppress color within the vessel and mask the flow.

The number of pulses transmitted along a single color scan line is called the packet size or ensemble length. Large packet size improves the accuracy of the Doppler shift frequency assessment, but with a resultant loss of temporal resolution (decreased frame rate). On some scanners the sonographer can adjust the packet size. The optimal packet size for a given situation is a tradeoff between accurate determination of Doppler shift frequency and temporal resolution.

Frame rate is affected by color line density, the number of color scan lines across the color field of view. Increased color line density improves color lateral resolution, however, acquisition time for a frame is lengthened.

The color gate adjusts the axial length of the Doppler sampling volume along the color scan line. Increasing the color gate enlarges the volume from which color Doppler signals are examined. The ability to separate flow and nonflow is improved but with a sacrifice in spatial resolution. The sampling interval can extend several millimeters. The pixel size encoded with color may not be identical to the gray-scale pixel size.

Some instruments allow adjustment of the color transmit frequency. Low color transmit frequency decreases the Doppler shift frequency, thereby reducing the potential for color aliasing. A low color transmit frequency can also be useful to extend penetration.

Color persistence combines color flow data in successive frames to provide a smoother appearance of blood flow. The time display of a color pixel is extended beyond the time associated with a single frame. This allows the sonographer to better appreciate the extent of a mitral valve regurgitant jet or a high-velocity carotid artery stenosis. Color persistence can obviously be excessive which leads to an inconsistency of color flow information. Also, as averaging is more pronounced, the temporal resolution is degraded. With color persistence turned completely off, the color flow image often has a grainy and very transient appearance.

Doppler shift frequencies below a specific frequency set by the color wall filter are eliminated from the color flow image. These low frequencies tend to represent slow-moving structures, such as vessel walls and heart muscle. In most circumstances, color generated from these structures are considered artifactual. Wall-motion artifacts appear on the display if the color wall filter setting is too low. If the color wall filter is too high, flow information may not be displayed (Fig. 15-10).

The color flow image is not limited to a display of mean velocity, however. Additional information (e.g., the spread of velocities within a sampled region) can also be depicted. The variance is a statistical measure of the velocity distribution within each sampled volume. Regions with plug flow demonstrate little spread, whereas those with laminar flow exhibit more variation. Selection of the variance map in lieu of a color map provides a two-dimensional spatial presentation of flow dissimilarity within each color pixel.

The capture function displays the highest mean velocity detected at each pixel during an elongated acquisition time (one to several seconds). Each small region within the field of view is scanned repeatedly for moving reflectors. On the first pass, if motion is detected at a particular pixel, the color level associated with the mean velocity is

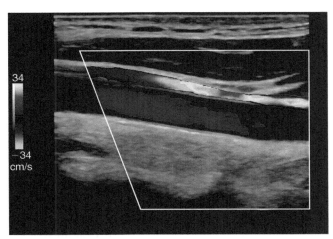

Figure 15-10 Color wall filter. High frequency setting which removes some velocity components near the vessel wall.

displayed on the monitor. This initial color level remains until replaced by a new value. As the data collection continues, measurements may yield a subsequent velocity of greater magnitude at that location. The color level associated with this velocity replaces the existing color level on the monitor. Low-velocity color levels are discarded. Thus, an image is formed of the maximum mean velocity detected at each pixel. For vessels with intermittent flow, the capture function is useful in defining the extent of flow.

COMBINED DOPPLER MODE

In the color flow image a single parameter, usually the mean velocity represented by the variation in color, is spatially registered in two dimensions. A more detailed presentation of the distribution of the velocity profile at a point of interest requires range-gated PW Doppler with FFT analysis. The combined Doppler mode displays the color flow image with Doppler spectral analysis (Fig. 15-11). A specific sampling volume for spectral analysis is identified on the color

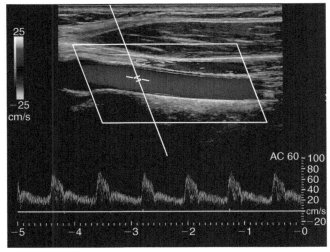

Figure 15-11 Combined Doppler mode. The color Doppler image with the sampled region identified is shown with the Doppler spectral analysis.

flow image. Since the beam must be shared between grayscale, color Doppler, and PW Doppler, the refresh rate of the color flow image is slowed to a new frame every 1 to 5 seconds. Since areas with abnormal flow pattern are rapidly identified, color flow imaging reduces examination time by facilitating placement of the sampling volume for spectral analysis.

POWER DOPPLER

Power Doppler imaging (also called energy mode Doppler imaging) portrays the intensity (amplitude) of the Doppler signal without an indication of the velocity (Fig. 15-12). The signal intensity depends on the number of RBCs within the sampled volume and the attenuation of the intervening tissue. Power Doppler emphasizes the quantity of blood flow. The autocorrelation detector used to estimate flow velocity also yields the total power of the Doppler signal. Consequently, on many scanners, the operator can switch easily from velocity mode to power mode.

Because all phase shifts (moving reflectors) contribute to the amplitude signal, power Doppler imaging is essentially nondirectional and therefore not subject to aliasing. The total power Doppler signal is relatively independent of the insonation angle. However, the color coding does not indicate the velocity or direction of flow; pulsatility and flow reversal cannot be evaluated. This flow information must be obtained from the color flow image.

Vessel wall definition is usually improved with power Doppler imaging. Compare the relative signals arising from a sampling volume near the vessel wall with one partially overlapping the vessel wall. For velocity measurements, the frequency shift will be small because both sampling volumes contain moving RBCs. The color mapping will display the pixels in similar shades. However, for the power Doppler measurements, the total number of RBCs is very different, creating a much lower signal for the sampling volume that includes the vessel wall.

The major advantage of power Doppler imaging is the ability to differentiate between regions with flow and

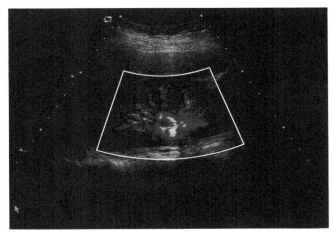

Figure 15-12 Power Doppler image of the kidney.

those with no flow. This is usually described as increased sensitivity to depict small vessels in color, which is derived from expanded dynamic range to extend the color priority to weaker signals. Increased persistence is also employed to image flow in small vessels. Tissue motion (e.g., of the heart) often creates flash artifacts, which limits the applicability of this imaging mode to regions where tissue motion is more subdued.

Power Doppler flow information is used in conjunction with three-dimensional imaging. Regions of flow are color encoded and superimposed on the two-dimensional or three-dimensional gray-scale presentation of anatomy. The vasculature of the organ or structure of interest is portrayed (Fig. 15-13).

The characteristics of Power Doppler imaging are summarized in Table 15-1.

COLOR DOPPLER IMAGE QUALITY

Color Doppler image quality is characterized by four factors: motion discrimination, temporal resolution, spatial resolution, and uniformity. The term *color sensitivity* has also been applied to describe this collection of factors.

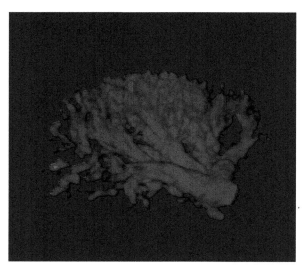

Figure 15-13 Three-dimensional power Doppler image of the kidney. (Courtesy Siemens Medical Solutions USA, Inc., Ultrasound Division, Malvern, PA.)

Table 15-1	Characteristics of Power Doppler Imaging	
Advantages		**Disadvantages**
Visualization of flow in small vessels		Motion artifacts
		No velocity information
Independent of flow direction		No directional information
Independent of velocity		Low temporal resolution
Reduced angle dependence		Qualitative observations
No aliasing		
Good luminal definition		

Color is associated with movement, but it does not necessarily indicate flow. Movement of the transducer, peristaltic motion, and cardiac motion all may contribute spurious color to the image and give an artifactual impression of flow or mask true flow. The ability to distinguish moving blood from moving tissue and at the same time depict subtle flow patterns is the ultimate goal. Low-frequency shifts from slowly moving tissue are selectively removed with a color wall filter. Unfortunately, this technique is not completely effective in eliminating high-amplitude, low-frequency Doppler shifts associated with vessel wall movement. Also, this high-pass filter excludes low-velocity flow components. To better differentiate flowing blood from stationary fluid and moving soft tissue, the amplitude and the phase shift are examined. Weak reflections are associated with blood and other fluids. Gray-scale values are assigned to strong echoes. Motion discrimination evaluates several parameters of the motion (not only velocity and amplitude but also dynamics) to ascertain whether the motion is characteristic of tissue or flowing blood.

Flow hemodynamics varies throughout the cardiac cycle. The ability to detect changing flow patterns depends on the frame rate. Temporal resolution is improved as the frame rate is increased. A high frame rate is achieved by reducing the number of color scan lines, the lateral extent of the color field of view, the dwell time, or a combination of these. For asynchronous autocorrelation scanners, the color region of interest selected by the operator designates that portion of the gray-scale image, which is subjected to Doppler analysis. The width of the color region has a considerable impact on frame rate. The dwell time for a color line is long because multiple pulse repetitions are required for the Doppler analysis (denoted by packet size). *In general, as the color field of view is expanded, more lines of sight are necessary and the frame rate is reduced.* Many scanners, however, automatically adjust packet size and color line density as a function of field width to optimize the frame rate for a particular application.

Spatial resolution characterizes a scanner's ability to depict small structures at the proper location. The axial dimension of the Doppler sampling volume is defined by the sampling time interval (color gate). The out-of-plane dimension (slice thickness) is determined by the beam width along that direction. The beam width and scan line density affect the lateral resolution. As the interrogated volume is reduced in size, weak-amplitude signals that are less likely to be encoded in color are generated. The precision of the mean frequency measurements also deteriorates. Spatial filtering is a technique to diminish random color variations throughout the image. Pixels are encoded in color only if they neighbor other pixels previously encoded in color. Small vessels with weak flow must be visualized with the spatial filter inactivated. Another type of spatial filtering (sharp or smooth processing) manipulates the presentation of the boundary between color and gray-scale pixels.

Uniformity implies that vessels with identical properties are depicted in a similar manner regardless of their respective locations within the field of view; that is, vessel size and color pattern should not be altered by a change in position. Color voxel size and color scan line density should be consistent throughout the field of view. Dynamic focusing improves spatial registration.

ARTIFACTS

Because color flow imaging is a spatial presentation of the Doppler shift frequencies in two dimensions, artifacts associated with B-mode imaging and PW Doppler are also possible. These potential artifacts include shadowing, reverberation, mirror image, misregistration from secondary lobes, depth ambiguity, and aliasing. In addition, artifacts such as color bleed, color flash, and color noise are unique to color flow imaging.

Attenuation

Enhanced attenuation by overlying structures may cause no color to be displayed within the vessel although flow is present. In Fig. 15-14, shadowing by a calcified plaque masks flow through the vessel.

High Pulse Repetition Frequency

Under conditions of high pulse repetition frequency (PRF), high gain, and low transmitter frequency, flow may be incorrectly depicted in a more superficial location. This depth ambiguity occurs because echoes that originate beyond the displayed scan range are associated with the most recent transmitted pulse and not the transmitted pulse that formed the echoes. Flow can be portrayed in a region where no flow actually exists. Because attenuation reduces the echo amplitudes from deep-lying reflectors, color reject often excludes these signals from color encoding.

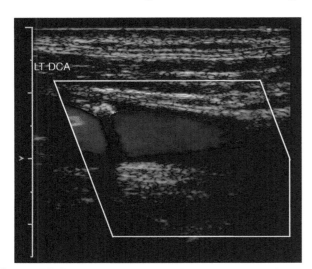

Figure 15-14 Shadowing by a calcified plaque obscures flow in the common carotid artery.

Color Aliasing

Because moving reflectors are sampled intermittently along the color scan line, color aliasing occurs if the flow exceeds the velocity range set by the operator. A high-frequency shift above the Nyquist limit, but less than twice the Nyquist limit, is detected as a low-frequency shift with opposite phase. The reversal in phase is interpreted as flow in the opposite direction, and thus a color change is induced. Often, aliasing is readily identified as an inappropriate color progression in which a pale shade of red or blue is surrounded by a light shade of the contrasting color, or, in the case of the rainbow color map, colors representing maximum flow in opposite directions are contiguous (Fig. 15-15). At a very high velocity (i.e., greater than twice the Nyquist limit) flow is depicted incorrectly, with a low-velocity color level but in the proper direction.

Aliasing may be eliminated by expanding the velocity scale, changing the baseline, increasing the Doppler angle, decreasing the frequency of the transmitted pulse, or shortening the depth by moving the transducer (Fig. 15-16).

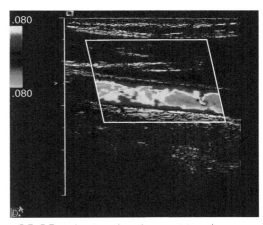

Figure 15-15 Color Doppler aliasing. Note the improper color progression—red to yellow to green to blue. If reverse flow were present, red and blue would be separated by a black region.

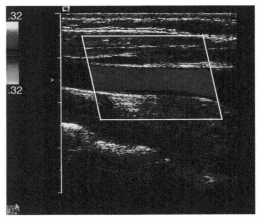

Figure 15-16 Increasing the velocity scale range removes the aliasing artifact in Figure 15-15.

Multiple-Angle Artifact

A phased array transducer interrogates a linear segment of a vessel oriented parallel to the skin surface with a variable angle of insonation (Fig. 15-17). The Doppler angle is greatest in the center of the field of view and decreases toward the periphery. Progressing across the field of view, a vessel with constant flow is depicted first by color in the reverse direction, then with no color, and finally by color in the forward direction (Fig. 15-18).

Comparatively, a linear array with a constant angle of insonation demonstrates uniform color throughout the field of view. Power Doppler imaging, because of its independence with respect to insonation angle, is less susceptible to this artifact (Fig. 15-19).

Nonuniform angle of insonation can also occur when a tortuous vessel is imaged with a linear array transducer.

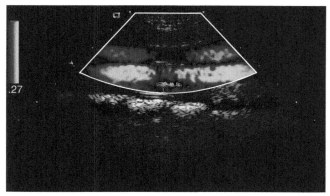

Figure 15-19 Power Doppler image of two vessels acquired with a vector transducer.

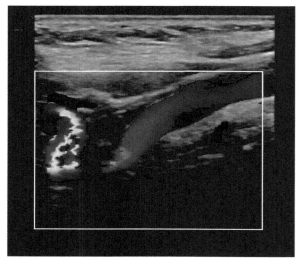

Figure 15-20 A tortuous vessel with unidirectional flow is depicted in changing colors, which suggests a reversal of flow.

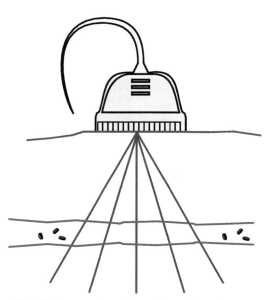

Figure 15-17 A steered beam from a linear phased array interrogates the vessel at different insonation angles.

An apparent velocity deviation at the bend of the vessel is attributed to a change in Doppler angle (Fig. 15-20).

Flow reversal must be distinguished from aliasing and multiple-angle artifact. The color filter removes low-frequency Doppler signals, thereby setting a velocity threshold below which color is not assigned to the image. Flow reversal is characterized as a black region separating areas with forward and reverse flow depicted in contrasting low-velocity colors (Fig. 15-21).

Mirror Image Artifact

A mirror image of the color flow is produced when the vessel lies proximal to a highly reflective interface, which results in an additional color encoding of the vessel at the wrong location. Spectral analyses of the real and virtual images are identical. For example, the lung acts as a strong reflector to form a mirror image of the subclavian artery (Fig. 15-22). Reducing the power, decreasing the color gain, changing the angle of insonation, or a combination of these eliminates this artifact.

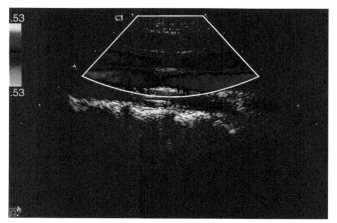

Figure 15-18 Color Doppler image of two vessels acquired with a vector transducer.

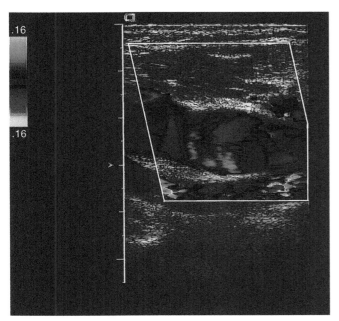

Figure 15-21 Flow reversal. Regions of dark red and dark blue are separated by black.

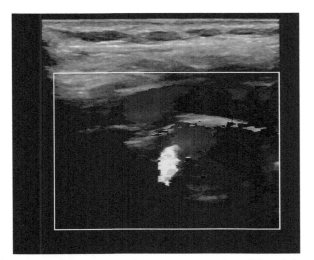

Figure 15-22 Color Doppler mirror image artifact of the subclavian artery.

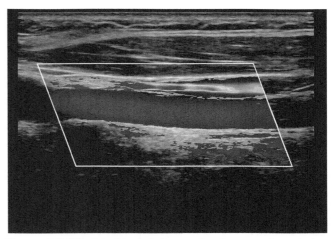

Figure 15-23 Color bleed. Color extends to the regions beyond where flow is present.

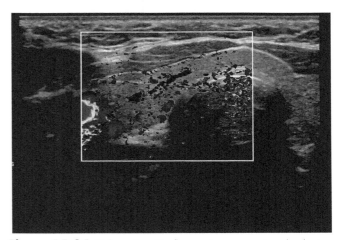

Figure 15-24 Color noise. Nonflow regions are assigned color in a mosaic pattern.

Color Bleed

Color bleed is the extension of color beyond the region of flow to the adjacent tissue (Fig. 15-23). This artifact is eliminated by decreasing the transmit power or color gain or both.

Color Noise

Induced signal strength is often used as a factor to suppress color. Strong echoes are assigned a gray-scale value, but weak echoes are permitted a color assignment if other criteria are met. If color gain is set too high or the color reject is set too low, random variations in echo measurements are interpreted as movement and cause hypoechoic regions to fill with color (Fig. 15-24). Fluid collections or thrombosed vessels may be color encoded by color noise. Color noise can be differentiated from flow by spectral analysis.

Misregistration of Color

The flash artifact is a sudden burst of color that encompasses a wide region within the frame. The improper assignment of color is caused by movement of the transducer or tissue (Fig. 15-25). Cardiac motion, general pulsatility of the arteries, and respiratory movements are all responsible for a change in interface position, which is color encoded. The flash artifact is suppressed by increasing the color wall filter, decreasing the persistence, and reducing the width of the color field of view. Increasing the color wall filter removes low-velocity components associated with these motions. On a more limited basis, tissue movements are conveyed to nonvascular structures with low echogenicity, which are color encoded. Motion discriminators

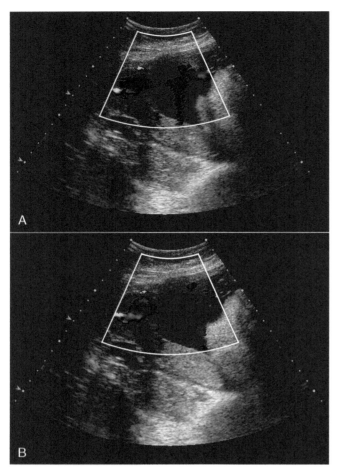

Figure 15-25 Flash artifact. **A,** Color is improperly assigned to non-flow regions caused by movement, which is eliminated by the repeat scan **(B)**.

are less effective when applied to weak signals. Doppler spectral analysis is necessary to distinguish tissue movement from flow.

Color Bruit

A bruit is a low- to high-pitched squirting sound caused by severe stenosis of the vessel (usually between 60% and 95% stenosis). The sound occurs during systole and can be auscultated with a stethoscope. The strong vibrations are radiated into the surrounding tissues, which are encoded in color. These color disturbances around the vessel are centered at the stenotic source of the bruit. The color bruit in the color flow image provides a valuable diagnostic tool for the location of the stenotic area and for identification of the involved vessel. Decreasing the velocity scale enhances the color disturbance caused by the bruit.

APPLICATIONS

The presence of flow, direction of flow, characteristics of flow, and existence of focal differences in velocity within the vessel are all assessed by color Doppler imaging. For cardiac applications, temporal resolution is essential. To achieve high frame rates, the color box width, scanning depth, and color scan line density are minimized. Often, when a larger color box is selected, color scan line density is adjusted automatically to maintain a high frame rate. Slow flow in peripheral vessels is analyzed by a low pulse repetition frequency, long dwell time, and low wall filter setting. The Doppler transmit frequency influences the limit for the lowest velocity that can be detected. High frequency reduces the low-velocity limit. Under the same conditions the low-velocity limit is 15 cm/s and 6 cm/s for 3 MHz and 7.5 MHz, respectively. Deep slow flow in the abdomen requires a low frequency to penetrate tissue and a narrow color box to counteract the effect of a long dwell time and low PRF on the frame rate.

The major advantage of color Doppler imaging is that the pattern of flow throughout the vessel within the color box is visualized instantaneously as the hemodynamics change during the cardiac cycle (Fig. 15-26). Vessels too small to be discerned with real-time gray-scale imaging are located with color Doppler imaging. Improved ease of vessel identification allows for examination of large vascular territories. In addition, vascular and nonvascular structures are more readily differentiated. Determination of the presence or absence of flow in peripheral vessels is also enhanced.

Color coding is based on the average rather than the peak Doppler shift frequency. Measurement of peak velocity from the color Doppler image is not appropriate. Velocity estimates do not include the correction for Doppler angle. Short pulses optimized for gray-scale imaging are interspersed with longer pulses that provide Doppler information. The pulsing sequence and extensive computations limit the frame rate.

The color encoding is not a sensitive indicator of velocity variation. Color assignment is based on the direction of flow but can be reversed. The direction of flow in the

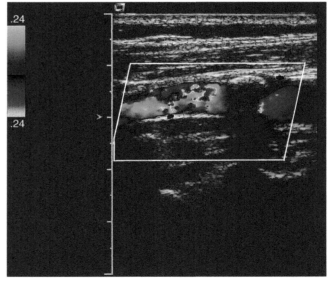

Figure 15-26 Turbulence distal to the stenosis is readily identified.

vessel of interest should be established by the orientation of the vessel with respect to the transducer or by reference to another vessel of known origin.

The presence of gas also produces color artifacts because the velocity of sound in air is not the same as it is in tissue. The highly focused beam is readily attenuated by a calcified plaque. Shadowing obscures the lumen of the artery and gives the impression of an absence of flow. Vessel tortuosity, poor scanning technique, and weak Doppler signal may also lead to the failure to visualize flow in an image.

SUMMARY

Color flow imaging combines gray-scale with two-dimensional spatial mapping of flow velocity in real time. Motion is depicted throughout the field of view by color encoding the flow information. In color flow imaging, the mean velocity at each sampling site is depicted in color as prescribed by the color velocity scale. In power Doppler imaging, the signal strength of moving reflectors at each sampling site is encoded by color. Global flow patterns within the color field of view are portrayed. The characteristics of color Doppler imaging are summarized in Table 15-2.

Autocorrelation is based on frequency differences in the detected echoes and compares successive echo wavetrains to compute the mean velocity. The distribution of velocity components is not available from autocorrelation and must be obtained by another method, such as fast Fourier transform spectral analysis.

Table 15-2	**Characteristics of Color Doppler Imaging**

Advantages	Disadvantages
Spatial display of blood flow	Aliasing
Global overview of flow	Motion artifacts
Real-time frame rates (10 frames per second)	Limited frame rate
	Mean velocity displayed
More sensitive than B-mode to show flow in vessels	Accuracy of velocity limited by sampling time
Guides placement of pulsed-wave sampling volume	Low-density scan lines or limited field of view
	Qualitative observations

Motion discrimination, temporal resolution, spatial resolution, and uniformity all contribute to overall image quality. Numerous controls are available to manipulate the collection and processing of the color flow data.

Potential artifacts associated with color flow imaging include shadowing, reverberation, mirror image, misregistration, depth ambiguity, and aliasing. *Color bleed, color flash,* and *color noise* describe the incorrect assignment of color to tissue.

Vessel tortuosity, poor scanning technique, and weak Doppler signal may lead to the failure to visualize flow in an image.

M-Mode Scanning

16

Chapter Objectives

To understand the principle of M-mode scanning
To describe the informational content of the M-mode trace

Key Terms

Color M-mode imaging   M-mode scanner

MOTION DETECTION

The first motion-detection device used in diagnostic ultrasound was the M-mode (or motion-mode) scanner. The two-dimensional display of reflector depth as a function of time emphasizes the movement of interfaces, including velocity, amplitude, and pattern of motion. Also called time-motion (TM) or position-motion (PM) mode, it is often used to interrogate heart valves in cardiac ultrasonography.

EFFECT OF MOTION

A nonstationary reflector moving toward or away from the transducer exhibits a changing horizontal position on the A-mode display corresponding to the depth of the interface. Accurate depiction of the motion depends on the pulse repetition frequency. Because most A-mode scanners are pulsed at least 1000 times per second, the motion appears continuous. However, recording and analysis of the A-mode signal for the study of motion is not feasible.

B-mode scanning allows visual portrayal of moving structures, but the sampling rate must be fast compared with the motion to prevent blurring. Temporal resolution describes the ability to image the motion dynamics with fidelity. The limitation imposed on the frame rate by the field of view and scan line density have been discussed previously. In spite of many advantages, B-mode scanning does not readily allow quantitative analysis of the motion. For that application M-mode scanning excels.

M-MODE FORMAT

The spatial locations of reflectors are combined with the time of observation to form a two-dimensional recording called an M-mode trace. The transmitted beam is repeatedly directed along a single line of sight with a pulse repetition frequency of less than 500 Hz (Fig. 16-1). Echo-ranging measurements following each transmitted pulse compute the depths of the various reflectors encountered along the propagation path. For each reflector a line drawn from the previous axial position to the current axial position shows the movement between sampling. A time sweep of the connected data points for each interface proceeds across the screen at a constant rate. Tick marks

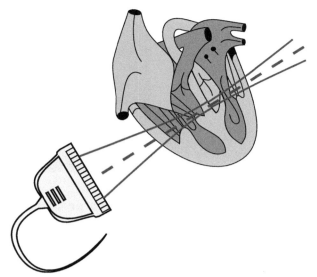

Figure 16-1 M-mode sampling is along a single line of sight.

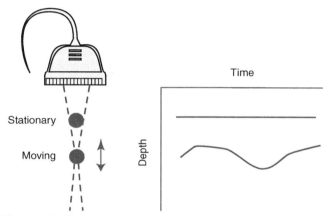

Figure 16-2 Principle of M-mode scanning. The depth of each interface encountered along the line of sight is monitored by repeated measurements during the observation time. M-mode display of showing stationary and moving interfaces within the pulsed sound beam.

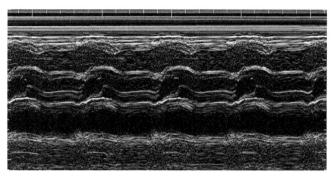

Figure 16-3 M-mode trace of an aortic valve.

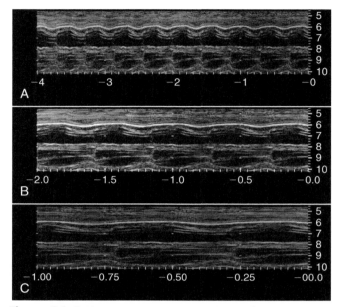

Figure 16-4 Variation in sweep rates. **A,** 4 seconds per sweep. **B,** 2 seconds per sweep. **C,** 1 second per sweep. The pattern is changed (expanded along the time direction) as the trace time is reduced.

show the timing interval. The sweep rate can be varied to improve temporal resolution or to extend the plot over a longer time interval. Stationary interfaces produce straight lines on the display, whereas moving interfaces are associated with fluctuating waveforms (Fig. 16-2). An M-mode trace can be acquired by using dedicated units with a circular pencil-type fixed-focus single-element transducer or with a multielement transducer. Sampling for a new line of sight is accomplished by moving the single-element transducer or steering the beam.

Echo intensity varies greatly depending on the properties of the interface. The strength of the detected echo is represented in the display by shades of gray, color brightness, or different hues of color. With gray-scale encoding the brightness of the dot increases as signal level is increased. Color encoding is useful to enhance subtle signal differences. *The M-mode trace contains four types of information: reflector depth, signal level of each reflector, relative positions of the reflectors along the line of sight,* *and change in axial position of each reflector with time.* Motion in the lateral direction or scan plane in the B-mode image is not known because sampling is limited to one line of sight.

The M-mode trace in Figure 16-3 illustrate strong specular reflection from the ventricular wall and the low-amplitude tissue scatterers. The sweep rate can change the pattern of the M-mode trace depending on the speed of the moving interface (Fig. 16-4).

M-MODE WITH B-MODE IMAGING

The screen is divided into two sections to show a B-mode image and the M-mode trace. A line cursor is placed on the gray-scale image to designate the sampling direction for the M-mode acquisition (Fig. 16-5). Updates of the B-mode image are suspended (or less frequent) while the M-mode trace is collected. The visualized anatomy in the gray-scale image facilitates sampling of the desired structures and provides correlation between the two scanning modes.

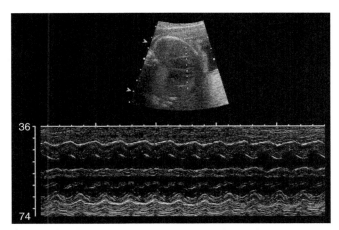

Figure 16-5 M-mode with two-dimensional B-mode imaging. Four-chamber view of the fetal heart. The line of sight for the M-mode trace is denoted on the B-mode image.

COLOR M-MODE

Color M-mode imaging combines the M-mode trace with color Doppler imaging. A line cursor on the color Doppler image denotes the M-mode sampling direction with respect to flow. Scan data along one line of sight are evaluated for both interface motion and blood flow. The flow data and M-mode trace are displayed in conjunction with the corresponding segment of the cardiac cycle given by the electrocardiogram.

OPERATOR CONTROLS

In many ways the informational content of the single line of sight M-mode acquisition is similar to B-mode imaging. The operator controls are also similar in function. These include gray-scale map, gain, dynamic range, filter, sweep rate, freeze, and magnification.

The gray-scale map or color map is selected as a display option. Signal strength is translated into brightness level or color depending on the selected map. Gain, independent of the B-mode receiver gain, amplifies the induced signals from along the sampling direction. Log compression changes the dynamic range and usually is applied to suppress low signals and noise. Filtering is a processing technique to sharpen or smooth borders of moving structures. Sweep rate adjusts the scale along the time axis of the M-mode trace. High sweep rate improves the temporal resolution and low sweep rate extends the time interval of a single trace.

The freeze function suspends M-mode data collection and captures the last few seconds of the M-mode trace for prolonged viewing or recording. By reducing the length of the line cursor to limit sampling to a particular range of depths, the spatial component of the M-mode trace improves the axial resolution. The effect is that structures in close proximity can now be more easily separated in the M-mode trace.

VELOCITY MEASUREMENT

M-mode is a two-dimensional graphic presentation that provides a plot of distance (i.e., the depth of the interfaces relative to the face of the transducer along one line of sight) versus time. The M-mode trace is descriptive of the speed of the reflector, the distance traveled by the reflector, and the direction and type of motion of the reflector. The velocity of the interface is obtained by the slope of the trace (Fig. 16-6). A line drawn tangent to the trace at the point of interest yields the instantaneous velocity (change in position with time). M-mode scanning gives an excellent evaluation of the object's size and amplitude of motion in the axial direction.

ADVANTAGES AND DISADVANTAGES

The M-mode scan is interpreted by pattern recognition, but it does not replicate the usual structural anatomy as depicted in real-time imaging. Although the axial and temporal resolution are excellent, motion in the lateral direction (perpendicular to the beam axis) is not portrayed because of the limited field of view (sampling is along one line of sight only).

Another limitation of M-mode scanning is the assumption of geometric shape when measurements along one dimension are extrapolated to calculate area and volume. Only real-time B-mode imaging can portray lateral motion and depict reflector shape.

Because of its simplicity, high axial resolution, and superior temporal resolution, M-mode scanning provides motion dynamics not easily obtained by other scanning modes.

SUMMARY

M-mode scanning evaluates the motion of an interface. Reflector depth and position relative to other structures, signal level, and changes in position with time (velocity and amplitude of the motion) are depicted by the M-mode trace. A single line of sight is repeatedly sampled.

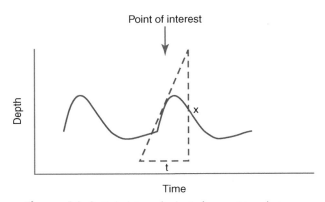

Figure 16-6 Calculation of velocity from an M-mode trace.

The detected echoes from each transmitted pulse are registered with respect to distance from the transducer, and multiple transmitted pulses provide the temporal changes in each reflector's position. The high pulse repetition frequency allows very rapid motion to be characterized faithfully. However, motion is evaluated only along the sampling direction. When combined with B-mode imaging or color Doppler imaging, the M-mode sampling direction can be specified with respect to the visualized structures.

Clinical Safety

17

Chapter Objectives

To identify the three interactions by which ultrasound may cause damage

To understand the indication of risk quantified by the thermal index and the mechanical index

To apply the principle of "as low as reasonably achievable" (ALARA) during sonography

Key Terms

Cavitation

Derating factor

Epidemiologic studies

Mechanical index (MI)

Output display standard (ODS)

Radiation force

Stable cavitation

Thermal index (TI)

Threshold

Transient cavitation

POTENTIAL RISK

The widespread acceptance of ultrasound is attributed in large part to one especially attractive feature—ultrasound is not a type of ionizing radiation. Furthermore, no *acute* harmful effects have been reported after diagnostic ultrasound examinations. Obstetrics seems particularly well suited for ultrasonography, which include amniocentesis, fetal heart monitoring, estimation of fetal age, determination of fetal position, diagnosis of multiple pregnancy, and placental localization. Nevertheless, when large populations are exposed to any agent, it is appropriate to investigate any potential long-term effects, which may not be evident on an individual case-by-case basis.

RISK ASSESSMENT

A risk (i.e., potential harmful effect) versus benefit (i.e., diagnostic information derived) analysis is necessary to assess medical efficacy. Quantification of risk from ultrasound examination is not currently available and will never be precisely known. The potential harmful effects to the exposed human population must be inferred from various investigational findings.

Because of the observed bioeffects, most research has been conducted at higher intensity levels and with longer exposure times than those used clinically. *The validity of results from these studies is limited when extrapolated to predict potential effects from exposure to diagnostic ultrasound.* The problem posed is not unique to ultrasound. If we wanted to know the hazard of the thermal effects resulting from taking a warm bath, the effect to 100°C could readily be measured using relatively few subjects. However, we would encounter some difficulty in constructing a model that permitted the extrapolation of resulting data to temperatures slightly above 37°C. To perform the study at 40°C, for example, would require an epidemiologic comparison of possibly a million subjects in which the control and test populations were matched perfectly. For the study of any effect, as the probability of that effect approaches zero, the number of individuals necessary to quantify this probability approaches infinity. In most situations we attempt to avoid large risks and accept risks that may be nonzero but that are too small to measure accurately.

Intensity levels below a certain value may be incapable of inducing an effect if a threshold exists. If the biological response has a threshold, effects reported for high intensity levels are not present at levels lower than the threshold. If the biological response has no threshold, however, any exposure to the physical agent carries some risk; the question then becomes whether effects observed at high intensity can accurately predict the risk at low intensity based on theoretical models.

Unfortunately, much of the early work published in the scientific literature is seriously flawed. The conditions of exposure were not specified, particularly with respect to defining the ultrasound field intensity. The early animal experiments did importantly demonstrate that acute functional or gross structural alterations could occur at very high intensity levels. Some research results involving reflex responses for rodents suggest that ultrasound exposure in utero may affect prenatal growth and development. Recently, more study has been directed toward elucidating potential effects at intensity levels produced by diagnostic devices.

MECHANISMS OF BIOLOGICAL DAMAGE

Three mechanisms by which ultrasound interacts with matter have been identified: acoustic radiation force, thermal, and cavitation. Cavitation and radiation force are often classified together as nonthermal interactions.

Mechanical Interactions

The first mechanism by which damage can be induced, radiation force, is sometimes called direct and generally includes all but thermal and cavitational effects. The ultrasound wave propagates through the medium by interactions between neighboring particles. The particles undergo considerable changes in velocity and acceleration. An object with a density different from that of the surrounding medium experiences a force in the ultrasound field because acoustic pressure is applied over its surface. This causes translational or rotational motion of the object. The rotational motion may give rise to acoustic streaming (i.e., circulatory flow of the fluid), and spinning of intracellular particles may be induced. At high intensities, high-velocity gradients are formed near solid boundaries. The resulting microstreaming (i.e., rapid movement of fluid in a localized area) can fragment the macromolecules in these regions.

Thermal Interactions

The second mechanism by which damage can be induced is thermal. As the ultrasound beam propagates through the medium, absorption of sonic energy is converted into heat. The increased temperature has the potential to cause irreversible tissue damage. The rate of temperature rise depends on the temporal average intensity, the absorption coefficient of the medium, the cross-sectional area of the beam, the duration of exposure, and the heat-transport processes (thermal conductivity and blood flow). Within the frequency range of 1 to 20 MHz, the absorption coefficient increases with frequency. Thermal effects dominate the low-megahertz frequencies and tend to mask other (nonthermal) effects.

Cavitation

The third mechanism by which damage can be induced is cavitation. As the ultrasound wave propagates through the medium, regions of compression and rarefaction are created. Thus localized regions are subjected to increases and decreases in pressure in an alternating fashion, and these cause gas bubbles to form and grow and to exhibit dynamic behavior. This phenomenon is known as cavitation, and it can be either stable or transient.

Stable Cavitation

In stable cavitation, microbubbles already present in the medium expand and contract during each cycle in response to the applied pressure oscillations. The bubbles may also grow as dissolved gas leaves the solution during the negative-pressure phase. Each bubble oscillates about the expanding radius for many cycles without collapsing completely. At a characteristic frequency (which is a function of the size of the bubble), the vibration amplitude of neighboring liquid particles is maximized.

The action of the gas bubble in the liquid is analogous to a child's swinging on a swing. An external force (push) applied to the child at the proper point in the oscillatory path increases the height of the swing. If the force is repeated over and over at the proper frequency, the motion of the swing is amplified. If the child is pushed opposite the direction of movement, the height of the swing decreases. The interplay between the rate of pushing and the physical characteristic of the swing (e.g., length of rope between the pivot point and the seat) is essential for maximum effect. Similarly, in cavitation, the interaction between the size of the gas bubble (i.e., the swing) and the frequency becomes critically important.

A free air bubble in water undergoes resonance at 1 MHz when its radius is 3.5 microns. At higher frequencies, the size of the bubble required for resonance decreases. Bubbles somewhat smaller than resonance size tend to grow, whereas those significantly larger than resonance size do not sustain stable cavitation. Oscillations of a gas bubble may produce high shearing forces in the nearby surrounding areas. Stable cavitation may also give rise to microstreaming. The radial oscillatory motion of the bubble is not always spherically symmetrical. An adjoining solid boundary may distort the motion of the bubble and cause eddies near the air-liquid interface. High-velocity gradients are created in the localized region of the oscillatory boundary layer. Biomolecules or membranes subjected to such gradients can fragment or rupture.

Transient Cavitation

Transient cavitation is a more violent form of microbubble dynamics in which short-lived bubbles undergo large size changes over a few acoustic cycles before completely collapsing. During the rarefaction phase, bubbles may be formed by dissolved gases leaving the solution or bubbles of submicron dimensions may already exist in the medium. High viscosity and surface tension inhibit bubble growth. A rarefaction phase of long duration enhances growth in bubble size.

During the compression phase, changing pressure causes the bubbles to collapse and produce highly localized shock waves. In addition, very high temperatures (up to 10,000°K) and pressures (10^8 pascals or higher) are created within the bubbles, resulting in the decomposition of water to free radicals. These pressures and temperature changes may also drive chemical reactions.

The general consensus is that transient cavitation is a threshold effect. The intensity levels necessary for cavitation to develop in tissue are a matter of debate. The pressure threshold for transient cavitation in water is 0.3 MPa at 1 MHz if gas bodies of optimal size are present. *The threshold of the peak negative pressure increases with frequency, exhibiting an $f^{0.5}$ dependence.* Transient cavitation has been demonstrated in mammalian systems at pressure levels generated by diagnostic imaging equipment. Lung hemorrhage attributed to cavitation has been observed at a pressure threshold of 1 to 2 MPa for a frequency range 0.5 to 5 MHz.

MUTAGENIC POTENTIAL

The conflicting results obtained from mutagenicity studies of mammalian cells in culture remain unresolved. If ultrasound is a mutagen, its mutagenic action is relatively weak compared with that of x-rays. Furthermore, high intensity levels sufficient to produce cavitation are required. The site of cavitation must be close to the DNA so the free radicals produced can migrate to the DNA.

TERATOGENIC EFFECTS

Thermal-induced damage is a threshold phenomenon; that is, fetal abnormalities are not observed unless the temperature elevation exceeds a particular value for a minimum time duration. For example, a temperature increase of 2.5°C must be present for 2 hours to cause fetal abnormalities. At higher temperatures, the time necessary to induce damage is shortened dramatically (e.g., 1 minute at 43°C and 5 minutes at 41°C).

EPIDEMIOLOGIC STUDIES

Although experimentation on animals has provided some insight into and reassurance regarding the potential effects from ultrasound exposure at diagnostic levels, the application of these data to human populations is limited. The ultimate assessment of biological effects induced in human populations exposed to ultrasound lies with epidemiologic studies. Observational investigations of human populations attempt to answer the question whether individuals exposed to a particular agent have a higher risk of developing impaired health than nonexposed individuals do. If the additional risk to an exposed population is small, large sample sizes are required to distinguish the agent-induced effects from disorders that occur spontaneously. The possibility of a long latent period (i.e., the delay between exposure and observable effect) must be considered. To assess risk factors accurately, it is often necessary to examine these populations over a period of many years. Collecting data for a large population over a long time is an extremely expensive undertaking and subject to many difficulties.

A major complication in epidemiologic studies is the influence of other risk factors. The agent of interest is most likely not the sole determinant of an adverse effect; furthermore, the risk of a potential effect is not the same for all members of the population. Modification of the incidence of an adverse effect by other factors is called confounding.

Rarely does a single study become the definitive work regarding identification of an adverse effect and the level of risk from exposure to a particular agent. The overall assessment must be based on multiple studies conducted under diverse conditions involving different populations. Epidemiologic studies are often flawed, either in experimental design or by incompleteness of the data. To establish an agent as potentially harmful, a pattern must develop whereby the results from different studies associate the same biological effect(s) with prior exposure to the agent, produce a dose-dependent rate of occurrence, and demonstrate a similar time sequence with respect to onset of the adverse effect.

Low birth weight, fetal chromosome abnormalities, structural fetal anomalies, altered neurologic development, cancer, and hearing disorders have been investigated as possible adverse effects from fetal exposure to ultrasound. No association between in utero ultrasound exposure and fetal chromosome abnormalities, congenital malformations, cancer, and hearing disorders has been demonstrated. Several studies, including three randomized clinical trials, have found no association between low birth weight and in utero exposure. The finding of reduced birth weight in two retrospective studies has little clinical importance. Suggestions of delayed speech and abnormal reflexes from in utero exposure in isolated surveys are not generally supported by multiple studies that show negative findings.

Results of the epidemiologic studies have been generally negative, which indicates that damage, if any, is subtle, delayed, or infrequent. The number of subjects in a study reporting negative results places an upper limit on the incidence rate of an adverse effect, but it does not exclude the induction of the effect by ultrasound. The association of ultrasound exposure with a particular outcome does not absolutely establish ultrasound as the causative agent. The association may be the result of shared underlying factors. The overall assessment is that no firm epidemiologic evidence exists to conclude that a causal relationship exists between diagnostic ultrasound and adverse effects.

RISKS VERSUS BENEFITS

Although harmful effects of ultrasound have not been demonstrated after exposure at diagnostic levels, the data are not sufficient to permit unquestioned acceptance of its safety. The prudent course of action must be to apply objective criteria in the selection of patients for an ultrasound examination and to minimize exposure. Exposure in this sense consists of the intensity (or peak pressure) and the exposure time.

A diagnostic ultrasound examination should be conducted only when medically indicated. *Medically indicated* implies that some benefit can be expected from the information obtained. Furthermore, an intensity consistent with the objectives of the examination should be used. A low intensity that reduces the ultrasound exposure but does not provide the desired diagnostic information exposes the patient unnecessarily. Although the exposure is low, no benefit is gained. The same principles apply to an examination so limited in time as to compromise the validity of the study.

THERMAL CONSIDERATIONS

For life processes to be maintained, the body temperature must stay within a narrow range. Although a variation of 1°C is tolerable (and indeed common), thermally mediated fetal abnormalities can result from temperature elevation. Avoiding a local rise in temperature above 1°C should ensure that no biological effects are induced.

Acoustic energy is converted to heat as the ultrasound beam passes through tissue. The heat production rate in a small volume is determined by the absorption coefficient of the tissue and the local time-averaged intensity of the ultrasound beam. The rate of absorption for most tissues increases linearly with frequency. Variations in the heat production rate occur because of different tissue types and nonuniformity of the ultrasound field.

For example, the initial temperature rise caused by an ultrasound beam (3.5 MHz, 1000 mW/cm² temporal-averaged intensity) incident on soft tissue is compared with one incident on bone. The heat capacity of a substance is the amount of energy required to raise the temperature 1°C. Dividing the heat production rate by the heat capacity yields the initial temperature rise. The initial temperature rise is approximately 50 times higher in bone.

The initial rate of temperature rise cannot be maintained. Heat removal by conduction and perfusion quickly slows it. Focused beams create small, localized regions of heating. The removal of heat from small volumes is very rapid. Continuous insonation ultimately produces a steady-state condition in which the maximum temperature does not change. Results of experiments quantifying the heating of rat skull bone exposed to a focused ultrasound beam form the basis for thermal models involving the insonation of bone.

TEMPERATURE PROFILES

Temperature profiles along the axis of a focused beam through a homogeneous medium can be calculated for a given set of conditions: transducer diameter, frequency, intensity, absorption coefficient of tissue, and degree of perfusion (Fig. 17-1). From the temperature profiles for a wide range of parameters, a conservative estimate of the acoustic power output necessary to maintain the maximum temperature rise to less than 1°C at any point along the ultrasonic path is determined. As the total absorbed energy encompasses a larger volume, the effectiveness of heating tissue becomes less; therefore an increased diameter of the transducer raises the acoustic power limit. The energy of the sound beam is more readily converted to heat as the frequency is increased, which reduces the acoustic power limit.

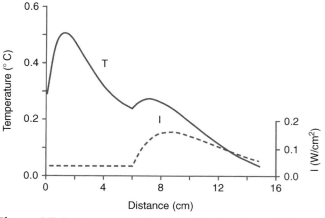

Figure 17-1 Temperature and intensity profiles along the axis of a focused beam. Exposure conditions include frequency 3 MHz, transducer diameter 2 cm, radius of curvature 10 cm, absorption coefficient 1.3 dB/cm, power 0.1 W. (Adapted from American Institute of Ultrasound in Medicine: *J Ultrasound Med.* 7:S1-S38, 1988.)

OUTPUT DISPLAY STANDARD

In 1992 the American Institute of Ultrasound in Medicine (AIUM) and the National Electrical Manufacturers Association (NEMA) adopted the voluntary standard for display of acoustic output information (Output Display Standard [ODS]). Two acoustic output parameters, called the thermal index (TI) and the mechanical index (MI), are defined as indicators of the potential for biological effects. The thermal index, in essence, gives the maximum temperature rise in tissue that can be predicted as a result of the diagnostic examination, and the MI describes the likelihood of cavitation.

Determining acoustic intensity distributions along various tissue paths for diverse equipment and operating modes in use today is an overwhelming task. Thermal and mechanical indices are generated from simplified models using conservative worst-case situations. The indices provide upper limits for the assessment of risk. The agreement among manufacturers to standardize acoustic output information allows sonographers to apply the same safety principles to all diagnostic ultrasound equipment regardless of manufacturer.

A homogeneous tissue model is assumed for soft tissue. Tissue in this model has low fat content and does not contain calcifications or large gas-filled spaces. Thermal conduction is the same as in water. The attenuation coefficient is uniform and equal to a value of 0.3 dB/cm-MHz. The probability of scatter is low, which allows the absorption rate to be represented by the attenuation coefficient.

Acoustic output is generally denoted by the power at the radiating source or by an intensity descriptor that characterizes the ultrasonic field. Peak negative pressure is also used as an output parameter. Intensity (or pressure) is measured at multiple points throughout the ultrasound field in a water medium. To quantify the tissue exposure to ultrasound, the free-field intensity or pressure must be converted to an in situ (localized) value.

When soft tissue replaces water along the ultrasonic pathway, a decrease in the intensity is expected because soft tissue has a much higher rate of attenuation. The fractional reduction in intensity caused by attenuation is calculated using the derating factor.

THERMAL INDEX

Temperature elevation depends on power, transducer aperture, tissue types, beam dimensions, and scanning mode. *Scanned mode* or *autoscanning* refers to the steering of successive ultrasound pulses through the field of view. In scanned modes where no bone is present, the highest temperature rise occurs near the surface where the beam enters the patient. In the nonscanned modes (pulsed-wave Doppler and M-mode), emission of ultrasound pulses occurs along a single line of sight, which does not change until the transducer is moved to a new position. In this circumstance, if bone is not present, the highest temperature rise is between the surface and the focal zone.

Three thermal indices corresponding to soft tissue (TIS), bone (TIB), and cranial bone (TIC) have been developed depending on whether bone is encountered along the path, and if it is, whether bone is located near the transducer or in the interior of the body. TIS applies when the ultrasound beam passes through soft tissue only and bone is not present (examinations of the abdomen and fetus during the first trimester). If bone is encountered near the transducer, then TIC is used (examinations of pediatric and adult head). TIB applies if the ultrasound beam, after passing through soft tissue, impinges on bone near the focal zone (examinations of the fetus during the second and third trimesters). Six thermal models have been developed to mimic possible clinical situations (Table 17-1).

The thermal index is defined as the ratio of the in situ acoustic power ($W_{0.3}$) to the acoustic power (reference value) required to raise tissue temperature by 1°C (W_{deg}). In situ acoustic power is calculated from the measured power in water corrected for attenuation by the derating factor. The subscript 0.3 indicates the attenuation rate is assumed to be 0.3 dB/cm-MHz. The equation defining the thermal index is the 13th essential equation of sonography:

$$17\text{-}1 \qquad TI = \frac{W_{0.3}}{W_{deg}}$$

The reference power depends on the model and is calculated using parameters defined by the model. The reference power necessary to cause a 1°C temperature elevation in bone is considerably less, since acoustic energy absorption by bone is higher than by soft tissue.

Along a poorly attenuating path, as when fluid is present, the derated peak rarefactional power is lower than the in situ value, and an underestimate of the thermal index occurs. For those situations in which a long sound path is encountered before reaching the point of interest (obese patients, large muscular patients, and deep-lying structures), the TI may overestimate the temperature rise for that region. In the circumstance of nonlinear propagation, the thermal index may underestimate temperature rise in tissue at high power levels.

Table 17-1	Thermal Models		
Number	Composition	Mode	Specification
1	Soft tissue	Nonscanned	Large aperture
2	Soft tissue	Nonscanned	Small aperture
3	Soft tissue	Scanned	Evaluated at surface
4	Soft tissue and bone	Scanned	Soft tissue at surface
5	Soft tissue and bone	Nonscanned	Bone at focus
6	Soft tissue and bone	Nonscanned or scanned	Bone at surface

For poorly perfused tissue in contact with the transducer, the temperature rise may be higher than that predicted by the thermal index. TIS is calculated at the transducer surface and overestimates the temperature rise in tissue at the focus. The dwell time from scanning is often less than the time required to reach steady state; in that circumstance, the thermal index overestimates the temperature rise in tissue.

MECHANICAL INDEX

The pulsed ultrasound wave, consisting of multiple cycles, causes large fluctuations in pressure as it moves through the medium. Cavitation is more likely to occur at high pressures and low frequencies. Scientific research has indicated that cavitation-induced effects may be possible at peak pressures and frequencies within the operational range of diagnostic equipment. Specifically, lung and intestinal hemorrhages in mice have been reported at diagnostic output levels. The cavitation threshold under optimal conditions with pulsed ultrasound is predicted by the ratio of the peak negative pressure in situ to the square root of the frequency.

Measurement of peak rarefactional pressure is performed in water for the transducer under well-defined operating conditions. The location of measurement is specified at the point along the beam axis where the derated intensity in the pulse is a maximum. The measured values of the pulse intensity as a function of depth along the beam axis are corrected for attenuation using the homogeneous tissue model. At the point of maximum derated intensity, the peak rarefactional pressure is measured in water and then corrected for attenuation for the tissue path. The derated peak rarefactional pressure in megapascals ($p_{r.3}$) is used to calculate the mechanical index (MI). The equation defining the mechanical index is the 14th essential equation of sonography:

$$17\text{-}2 \qquad MI = \frac{Cp_{r.3}}{\sqrt{f}}$$

where f is the frequency in MHz and C is a unit constant equal to $(1\ MHz)^{0.5}/(1\ MPa)$ to express the mechanical index as a dimensionless quantity. For water, cavitation is not produced if the mechanical index is less than 0.7 over the frequency range 1 to 10 MHz.

The position in tissue at which the mechanical index is calculated may shift as output power is changed. ODS indicates the numerical value of the index, but the site of highest value is not communicated to the operator. The spatial distribution of pressure amplitudes is unknown. Along a poorly attenuating path, as when fluid is present, the derated peak rarefactional pressure is lower than the in situ value, and an underestimate of the mechanical index occurs. For those situations in which a long sound path is encountered before reaching the point of interest, the mechanical index may overestimate the pressure for that region. In the circumstance of nonlinear propagation,

mechanical index may underestimate the pressure in tissue at high power level.

In 1976 the U.S. Food and Drug Administration (FDA) established the maximum I(SPPA) (pulse-averaged intensity at spatial peak, averaged over the duration of the pulse) limit as 190 W/cm^2, which is a historic standard based on the acoustic output of devices on the market at that time. An alternative standard sets the limit as an mechanical index value of 1.9. Manufacturers, at their option, are permitted to meet either of these criteria for the introduction of new equipment. A mechanical index of 1.9 corresponds to a peak negative pressure of 3.3 MPa at a frequency of 3 MHz. The pulse-averaged intensity at a mechanical index of 1.9 is 360 W/cm^2, which is an effective increase in acoustic power level permitted by the FDA guidelines.

DISPLAY OF OUTPUT INDICES

The following display guidelines apply to all thermal and mechanical indices. Ultrasound equipment, which has the potential to produce an index value above 1, must be able to display that index. If the index value falls below 0.4, it is unnecessary to display it. The display increments are no greater than 0.2 for index values less than 1 and no greater than 1 for index values greater than 1.

TIS and TIB may be displayed simultaneously or independently. If the equipment is intended for adult cephalic applications exclusively, only the display of TIC is necessary. When operated in B-mode, scanners are not capable of producing a temperature rise above 1°C; thus the MI will be displayed during this mode of operation. Display of mechanical index and thermal index should be possible, although not necessarily simultaneously, for a transducer that operates in a mode other than real-time B-mode. For multiple modality ultrasound equipment, the mechanical index is displayed during real-time B-mode imaging and the thermal index during pulsed-wave Doppler, M-mode, and Doppler imaging provided that the display criteria mentioned earlier are met.

OUTPUT INDICES AS RISK INDICATORS

The determination of thermal index is a conservative estimate based on a worst-case scenario. Although the calculated temperature elevation is subject to many uncertainties, it provides an upper limit of the actual temperature rise from typical clinical examinations. Insonation of long duration is necessary to achieve the steady-state temperature rise predicted by the thermal index.

Cavitation is generally believed to be a threshold phenomenon. The presence of gas cavities escalates the potential for cavitation. Gaseous spaces in the aerated lung, undissolved gas in the gastrointestinal tract, and gaseous contrast agents are the principal areas of concern. Lung hemorrhage has been observed for peak negative pressure ranging from 0.6 to 2.2 MPa in the frequency range of 1 to

4 MHz (MI values vary from 0.6 to 1.4). The cavitation threshold for the fetal lung is much higher because this tissue does not contain undissolved gas.

By tracking peak rarefactional pressure and frequency, the mechanical index provides an estimate of the potential for mechanical biological effects. Even if cavitation does occur at isolated sites, however, the affected area is extremely small and a small number of cells may be killed. The only situation in which the loss of a few cells would be of concern is when the subject is a fetus.

The acoustic output indices serve as risk indicators. If the index value is below the threshold level for bioeffects (considered to be 0.5), a further decrease in acoustic output would not improve safety and could compromise the quality of the diagnostic examination. At an index value less than 0.5, the possibility of adverse effects associated with tissue heating and cavitation is low. If the index value is greater than 0.5, the physician must evaluate the risks associated with a particular ultrasound procedure against the diagnostic information to be gained. TIBs for commercially available systems range from 0.1 to 10 for fetal scanning. At the highest thermal index values, scanning for more than a few seconds may cause harm.

An additional protective measure is to limit the exposure time when the thermal index exceeds 1. Experiments on the effects of temperature elevation on fetal development have shown no abnormalities if the time and temperature elevation were less than 10 minutes and 3°C. The maximum safe exposure time in minutes is calculated as

$$17\text{-}3 \qquad t = 10 \times 0.25^{(TI-3)}$$

However, if the patient is febrile, the exposure time limit is reduced by incrementing the term -3 in the exponent by $+1$ for each degree centigrade the body temperature exceeds 37°C. For example, if the patient's body temperature is 38°C, the maximum safe exposure time is reduced to 2.5 minutes for a TI of 3.

Practical guidelines using the thermal and output indices have been published by Nelson and colleagues.[3] The prenatal examination should be conducted with a TI less than 0.5 if possible. If the TI exceeds 2.5, the time should be limited to less than 1 minute; if the TI is 0.5 to 1, the time can be extended to 30 minutes. A mechanical index of less than 0.4 is recommended. For the postnatal examination, a TI less than 2 may be used for scanning times on an extended basis. If the TI exceeds 6, the time should be limited to less than 1 minute; if the TI is 2 to 6, the time can be extended to 30 minutes. A mechanical index of less than 0.4 is recommended, but in the absence of gas bodies, MI as high as 1.9 can be used if needed.

NONLINEAR PROPAGATION

The calculation of ODS indices requires estimates of the in situ values for pressure, intensity, and power. The acoustic field parameter is measured in water, then a derating factor is applied to obtain the value in tissue. For low-power waveforms, this method works reasonably well. However, if measurements are performed under high-power conditions, the derated pressure (or intensity) underestimates the actual pressure (or intensity) in tissue.

As power levels are increased, nonlinear propagation distorts the wave shape and creates harmonic frequencies. The relationship between the source intensity and pressure at the focal point is no longer linear. The presence of harmonics accelerates the attenuation loss. (The high-frequency components are removed more rapidly.) The consequence of this nonlinear behavior is that the negative peak pressure derated from water underestimates the value in tissue by a factor of 2 or more.

The generation of harmonics increases the rate of local absorption and thus the heat production per unit volume. As power is raised further, local absorption becomes greater, until at very high power levels the intensity at the point of interest is nearly constant. The heating at the point of interest is now independent of source power.

Fortunately the effect of nonlinear propagation on the steady-state temperature rise in soft tissue is small. The highest temperatures occur in the near field, but the predicted increase is less than 20% (insignificant compared with the other uncertainties in the calculation of TI). The centrally peaked heating pattern is modulated by heat diffusion to the surrounding area. In the application of thermal index to the homogeneous tissue model, the temperature rise depends on the total energy converted into heat. Even though the axial heating rate is greater during nonlinear propagation, the heat transfer across the entire beam at the focal distance compared with linear propagation is less. Therefore, the effect of nonlinear propagation can be ignored if intensity is specified by the source intensity and not by the measured nonlinear propagation intensity in water.

AMERICAN INSTITUTE OF ULTRASOUND IN MEDICINE

The Bioeffects Committee of the AIUM was established to examine current knowledge concerning bioeffects and to assess the risks of clinical diagnostic ultrasound. This committee regularly publishes critiques of research reports and issues statements regarding the safety of diagnostic ultrasound. Its conclusions are acknowledged as the governing safety guidelines throughout the ultrasound community.

In August 1976 the Bioeffects Committee reviewed all the data pertaining to biological effects attributable to ultrasound irradiation of mammalian tissue. Its evaluation of the scientific literature was summarized in a statement that was subsequently revised in November 2008:

Information from experiments utilizing laboratory mammals has contributed significantly to our understanding of ultrasonically induced biological effects and the mechanisms that are most likely responsible. The following statement summarizes observations relative to specific diagnostic ultrasound parameters and indices.

In the low-megahertz frequency range there have been no independently confirmed adverse biological effects in mammalian tissues exposed in vivo under experimental ultrasound conditions, as follows.

1. Thermal Mechanisms

   a. No effects have been observed for an unfocused beam having free-field spatial-peak temporal averaged (SPTA) intensities* below 100 mW/cm^2, or a focused† beam having intensities below 1 W/cm^2 or thermal index values less than 2.

   b. For fetal exposures, no effects have been reported for a temperature increase above the normal physiologic temperature ΔT, when $\Delta T < 4.5 - (\log t/0.6)$, where t is exposure time ranging from 1 to 250 minutes, including off time for pulsed exposure.[2]

   c. For postnatal exposures producing temperature increases of 6°C or less, no effects have been reported when $\Delta T < 6 - (\log t/0.6)$, including off time for pulsed exposure. For example, for temperature increases of 6.0°C and 2.0°C, the corresponding limits for exposure durations t are 1 to 250 minutes.[4]

   d. For postnatal exposures producing temperature increases of 6°C or more, no effects have been reported when $\Delta T < 6 - (\log t/0.3)$, including off time for pulsed exposure. For example, for temperature increases of 9.6°C, the corresponding limit for exposure duration is 5 seconds (=0.083 minutes).[4]

2. Nonthermal Mechanisms

   a. In tissues that contain well-defined gas bodies (e.g., lung), no effects have been observed for in situ peak rarefactional pressures below approximately 0.4 MPa or mechanical index values less than approximately 0.4.

   b. In tissues that do not contain well-defined gas bodies, no effects have been reported for peak rarefactional pressures below approximately 4.0 MPa or mechanical index values less than approximately 4.0.[1]

The low-megahertz frequency range is considered to be 0.5 to 10 MHz. Continuous-wave and pulsed-wave ultrasound as well as focused and unfocused beams are included. The intensity is designated SPTA as measured under free-field conditions. With the availability of later information, the committee's statement has been modified to incorporate specifications that are more suitable for the clinical environment with the inclusion of acoustic output indices. Generally, bioeffects data have been obtained under the conditions of high-power, broad-beam, and continuous-wave irradiation. A focused beam is less damaging than an unfocused beam of equal I(SPTA). Most bioeffects are attributable to the thermal mechanism, and the temperature rise is a critical function of beam width. A small beam (less than 4 mm in diameter) transfers heat more rapidly from the irradiated volume than a large beam does, and the corresponding increase in temperature is only 1/10 to 1/100 that for a wide beam. The I(SPTA) estimate of 1 W/cm^2 for a focused beam is conservative, since this level is 10 times the level for an unfocused beam.

Thermal damage is dependent on the temperature elevation and the duration of exposure, which is addressed by the mathematic relationship between thermal index and exposure time. The threshold for nonthermal damage is considered a peak pressure of 0.4 MPa or a mechanical index of 0.4.

A summary of bioeffects and clinical applications demonstrating the prudent use of ultrasound is published by the AIUM as *Medical Ultrasound Safety,* second edition, 2009. This document is must reading for every sonographer.

CLINICAL EFFICACY IN OBSTETRICS

Because ultrasound yields excellent anatomic visualization and is generally considered to be without harmful effects, it has become widely used in the practice of obstetrics. In the United States at least 70% to 80% of the 4 million children born each year were examined in utero with ultrasound. Although ultrasound is assumed to contribute to the improved management and outcome of pregnancy, its clinical efficacy has not been demonstrated. In a randomized clinical trial, the Routine Antenatal Diagnostic Imaging with Ultrasound (RADIUS) study tested the hypothesis that routine screening reduces perinatal morbidity and mortality. The results did not improve outcome compared with selective ultrasound examination when clinically indicated. This does not mean that no benefit is gained—merely that for low-risk populations, routine screening with ultrasound has not reduced perinatal mortality and morbidity beyond that achieved by selective examination based on clinical judgment. Nevertheless, routine screening with ultrasound for every pregnant patient is conducted in some European countries.

As a guide for practitioners, the National Institutes of Health reviewed the available scientific information and concluded that ultrasound has clinical benefit for certain applications. Currently the routine screening of every pregnancy is not recommended by the National Institutes of Health. Ultrasonography during pregnancy should be performed for a specific medical indication and should be discouraged for the sole purpose of viewing the fetus by the mother or determining its sex (these are potential secondary benefits of a medically indicated examination). Additionally, feedback—in the form of viewing the monitor screen with explanation of the images—may improve maternal perception of the fetus and maternal-infant bonding. The maternal attitude can influence fetal outcome by causing prenatal behavioral changes (e.g., cessation of smoking). Educational and commercial demonstrations of ultrasound imaging during pregnancy without medical benefit are inappropriate.

---

*Free-field SPTA for continuous wave and pulsed exposures.

†Quarter-power (−6 dB) beam width smaller than four wavelengths or 4 mm, whichever is less at the exposure frequency.

OPHTHALMIC CONSIDERATIONS

The cornea, lens, and vitreous body of the eye do not have a direct blood supply, and heat removal by perfusion is slow. The lens is a collagenous structure that readily absorbs ultrasound energy. Thus the lens is susceptible to high levels of heating. Therapeutic levels of ultrasound have been demonstrated to induce cataracts. Clinical studies with diagnostic exposure levels have yet to be conducted to determine bioeffects. The FDA recognizes the potential for damage to the eye by establishing lower output limits for ophthalmic applications. The I(SPTA) is 50 mW/cm^2 and the mechanical index is 0.23 instead of 720 mW/cm^2 and 1.9 for all other applications.

RESPONSIBILITY OF USERS

Diagnostic ultrasound has well-established medical applications with known benefits and recognized efficacy. The statement on clinical safety by the AIUM recommends prudent use of ultrasound in the clinical environment. The term *prudent use* was not defined initially. In a subsequent statement in May 1999, nonmedical use of ultrasound for psychosocial and entertainment purposes is discouraged. Viewing the fetus without medical indication is inappropriate.

Objective criteria should be applied in the selection of patients for an ultrasound examination. Furthermore, qualified health professionals should conduct the examination at minimum intensity levels and exposure times to obtain the desired diagnostic information (medical benefit). The principle of "as low as reasonably achievable" (ALARA) is applied to evaluate whether the conditions of use are appropriate to conduct the examination with the lowest reasonable exposure to the patient. The sonographer must practice ALARA using the displayed output indices provided at the time of examination. Exposure of the patient may be minimized by adjusting acquisition parameters while maintaining the desired informational content.

ODS indices provide an indication of the change in risk as operator controls are adjusted. The final benefit/risk assessment should be performed by a user who is knowledgeable in ultrasound dosimetry and biological effects and who takes into account the index values and the particular details of the patient being examined. Users should be helped and encouraged by development of educational materials designed specifically for evaluating benefits and risks of diagnostic ultrasound procedures. Laboratory guidelines for making these decisions and training in these decisions should be documented.

For each application, default settings for the diagnostic ultrasound system should be implemented, or reviewed, and documented by the user. The output indices should be assigned values based on the best available information on bioeffects and also on knowledge of the lowest values at which the system employed will yield the required diagnostic information. For example, operation when mechanical index is less than 0.5 and thermal index is less than 1 poses negligible risk under most conditions. For some situations, the desired diagnostic information can be obtained with settings of the indices in these ranges, while for others, higher outputs should be used when justified by consideration of risk and benefit to the patient. The user may find it helpful to employ a feature of the equipment that provides a reminder signal when a user-selected value of a relevant index is exceeded.*

EDUCATION AND TRAINING

In a perceptive editorial, Ziskin[5] advocates educating physicians and sonographers as the major safeguard for patients. Well-designed instrumentation to limit exposure of the patient is an alternative measure. However, equipment safeguards can be bypassed by the operator. Knowledgeable users conduct the examination at the minimum intensity levels necessary to obtain the desired diagnostic information. In addition, the examination time is usually reduced. More important, misdiagnoses because of lack of education, inexperience, and poor examination technique are more likely to cause harm than is the potential damage from ultrasound itself.

The diagnostic efficacy of ultrasound is strongly operator-dependent. Unfortunately only about half of obstetric and gynecologic sonographers are certified. The training and education requirements for physicians are not standardized. The ability of physicians to perform and interpret ultrasound examinations varies considerably. Minimum standards of education and training for clinical users of ultrasound (both physician and sonographer) must be established by certification organizations, by regulatory agencies, or by medical specialty societies.

SUMMARY

Three mechanisms for the interaction of ultrasound with matter have been identified: radiation force, thermal, and cavitation. Pressure across the surface may cause the object to twist or rotate in the ultrasonic field by the induced radiation force. Absorption of sound causes heating of tissue (thermal effects). Cavitation describes the dynamic behavior of microbubbles subjected to pressure fluctuations. These physical processes may give rise to the secondary actions of microstreaming and altered chemical reaction rates.

Early studies using high-intensity levels and long exposure times reported numerous biological effects—including protein denaturation, changes in membrane permeability, membrane rupture, chromosomal breakage, nerve block,

---

*Modified from National Council on Radiation Protection and Measurements: *Exposure Criteria for Medical Diagnostic Ultrasound; II. Criteria Based on All Known Mechanisms*, NCRP Report No. 140, Bethesda, Md, December 2002, NCRP.

cataracts, brain lesions, and fetal developmental anomalies. Much of this work lacks the necessary dosimetric details.

Although animal studies provide a good indication of potential damage and can aid in the establishment of reasonable levels of safety, they possess certain limitations when extrapolated to humans. Species sensitivity variation has been demonstrated, and there is no assurance that humans will respond in the same manner as certain species of animals. The amount of attenuation and the relative target size are also factors that must be considered. Nevertheless, dose-effect observations in animals are critically important in determining the mechanisms of interaction and assessing the risk in humans.

At current diagnostic intensity levels and scan times, no biological effects of ultrasound have been observed in humans. However, no high-quality epidemiologic studies have been conducted since the introduction of increased power levels by the output display standard.

The AIUM has reviewed available data and established intensity guidelines. A safe level of 100 mW/cm^2 I(SPTA) is often mentioned in the literature. The adoption of 1 W/cm^2 I(SPTA) as a safe level for focused beams by the AIUM has also become widely accepted.

Ultrasound is not a form of ionizing radiation. This attractive feature has resulted in its extensive use for the evaluation of pregnancy, fetal age, and fetal condition. Nevertheless, sufficient data do not exist to state categorically that ultrasound is absolutely safe. The continued use of diagnostic ultrasound examinations in obstetrics and other areas is justified because the potential risk appears to be minimal and the benefit high. This does not imply that ultrasound should be employed indiscriminately. The selection of patients should be a result of well-defined conscious processes, and steps should be taken to minimize exposure during the examination (the practice of ALARA). Thermal and mechanical acoustic output indices offer a uniform approach to controlling ultrasonic exposure of patients and providing assurance of safety. The wide acceptance of the Output Display Standard shifts the responsibility to reduce patient exposure from the manufacturer to the operator of the ultrasound device. Standards for education and training to perform sonography must be instituted by medical speciality societies, and those standards must then be widely accepted by regulatory agencies. Two essential equations of sonography (thermal index and mechanical index) were introduced.

References

1 Church CC, Carstensen EL, Nyborg WL, et al: The risk of exposure to diagnostic ultrasound in postnatal subjects: nonthermal mechanisms, *J Ultrasound Med* 27:565–592, 2008.
2 Miller MW, Nyborg WL, Dewey WC, Edwards MJ, Abramowicz JS, Brayman AA: Hyperthermic teratogenicity, thermal dose and diagnostic ultrasound during pregnancy: implications of new standards on tissue heating, *Int J Hyperthermia* 18:361–384, 2002.
3 Nelson TR, Fowlkes JB, Abramowicz JS, et al: Ultrasound biosafety considerations for the practicing sonographer and sonologist, *J Ultrasound Med* 28:139–150, 2009.
4 O'Brien WD Jr, Deng CX, Harris GR, et al: The risk of exposure to diagnostic ultrasound in postnatal subjects: thermal effects, *J Ultrasound Med* 27:517–535, 2008.
5 Ziskin: The prudent use of diagnostic ultrasound, *J Ultrasound Med* 6:415–416, 1987.

Performance Testing

18

Chapter Objectives

To describe the performance testing of B-mode scanners using tissue-mimicking phantoms

To state the recommended quality control tests for B-mode scanners

To identify the Society of Motion Picture and Television Engineers (SMPTE) test pattern and explain its use

Key Terms

Axial resolution
Dead zone
Focal zone
Horizontal distance accuracy

Lateral resolution
Maximum depth of visualization
Sensitivity

Tissue-mimicking (TM) phantoms
Uniformity
Vertical distance accuracy

PURPOSE

Axial resolution, lateral resolution, and sensitivity affect the overall quality of the B-mode image. The purpose of this chapter is to discuss the ways in which these parameters and others can be measured to evaluate scanner performance. Testing by independent laboratories allows confirmation that the manufacturer's specifications are factual and provides guidance for purchase decisions. Acceptance testing is the initial evaluation of equipment after installation to assess performance and to establish baselines for quality control tests. Such tests are conducted at regular intervals to ensure continued operation at an acceptable level.

PHANTOM MATERIALS

A wide variety of test objects and phantoms have been developed to monitor the performance characteristics of B-mode scanners. A test object usually consists of material in which the acoustic velocity is the same as that in tissue (1540 m/s); but other properties with respect to ultrasound propagation vary from those of tissue. The test object of the American Institute of Ultrasound in Medicine (AIUM) uses a uniform liquid medium with poor scattering characteristics. The incorporation of tissue-mimicking (TM) material into ultrasound phantoms has essentially eliminated the need for test objects.

Tissue-mimicking (TM) phantoms have properties similar to those of tissue with respect to acoustic velocity, scattering, and attenuation throughout the diagnostic frequency range (2 to 15 MHz). The acoustic velocity in TM material is typically within 1% of the average velocity in soft tissue (1540 m/s). The attenuation rate is specified as either 0.5 dB/cm-MHz or 0.7 dB/cm-MHz. A linear response of attenuation with frequency (mathematically stated as f^1) is recommended by AIUM. Backscatter by TM material is similar to that produced by liver parenchyma. With the development of tissue harmonic imaging, nonlinear propagation has become an important consideration, but phantoms are not generally specified with respect to the nonlinearity parameter.

The TM phantom is composed of water-based polymer impregnated with small-diameter particles (graphite or polysaccharide and glass). The concentration of particles controls the attenuation rate and the backscatter levels. Small, strong reflectors (e.g., nylon rods 0.1 mm in diameter) are placed within the gel matrix in well-defined geometric patterns. This small rod size is necessary to avoid reverberation artifacts at frequencies above 5 MHz. Normally, two sets of nylon rods (one along the vertical direction and the other along the horizontal direction) are spaced at precise intervals. These rods assess distance accuracy in the respective directions. Different nylon rod groups are also used to evaluate axial resolution, lateral resolution, and dead zone. Hypoechoic and hyperechoic cylindrical or spherical objects are often distributed throughout the TM material. The amount of scattering from an object is controlled by varying the concentration of scattering material. Reducing the concentration of scattering material by a factor of 2 results in a −3 dB backscatter level. Increasing the concentration of scattering material by a factor of 2 has the opposite effect (backscatter level increases by 3 dB).

To preserve its acoustic properties, the tissue-mimicking phantom should be maintained at a temperature between 32°F and 150°F in a dark place, preferably in an airtight container to inhibit dehydration. Improved design of water-based phantoms now incorporates a polymer laminate covering the acoustic window to act as a vapor barrier. Proper storage prolongs the useful life of the TM phantom, in some cases to 4 to 8 years. Loss of water content is monitored by periodically weighing the phantom. Manufacturers have programs to replace or regenerate the phantom when water content becomes too low.

Urethane rubber-based phantoms have also been developed to mimic the attenuation and scattering of tissue. However, the acoustic velocity in this material is about 1460 m/s. Urethane is more stable and has a longer life than the water-based TM material, but care must be taken in performing distance measurements using rubber-based phantoms. Generally, the object placement in the axial direction is less than the stated value, so that an echo-ranging distance measurement using the calibrated velocity of 1540 m/s yields the stated separation of objects. Inaccurate focusing of the ultrasound beam caused by timing-delay errors limits the assessment of axial resolution, lateral resolution, and cyst fill-in.

GENERAL-PURPOSE PHANTOMS

Most clinical facilities are limited by cost considerations so that only a single phantom is available for testing. The most commonly used phantoms have multiple applications and are designed for general purpose testing. *General-purpose phantoms commonly test for dead zone, axial resolution, lateral resolution, penetration, image uniformity, distance accuracy, focal zone, and cyst characteristics (size, shape, and fill-in).* The phantom properties of velocity, scattering, and attenuation should emulate soft tissue throughout the diagnostic frequency range. Therefore a TM phantom is the best choice for testing scanners under conditions that simulate the clinical environment.

Phantoms are also useful in the training of student sonographers in the proper operation of various controls including time-gain compensation (TGC), receiver gain, power, transmit focal zones, and write zoom.

Two commonly used general-purpose TM phantoms are manufactured by CIRS Inc., Norfolk, Virginia (Model 40 and new version Model 040GSE) and Gammex-RMI, Middleton, Wisconsin (Model 403 series). Figures 18-1 and 18-2 illustrate the structures contained within these phantoms. The specifications for these phantoms are listed in Tables 18-1 and 18-2. Both manufacturers have models that contain gray-scale targets. The Model 40 phantom is divided vertically in half so that one side has an attenuation rate of 0.5 dB/cm-MHz and the other has an attenuation rate of 0.7 dB/cm-MHz. The Model 403 is uniform in its attenuation, either 0.5 dB/cm-MHz or 0.7 dB/cm-MHz, which is selected at purchase. Since

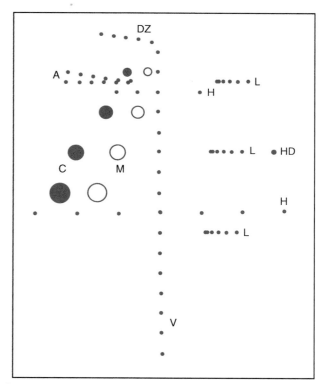

Figure 18-1 Diagram of the Model 40 tissue-mimicking phantom. Vertical rod group (V), horizontal rod groups (H), dead-zone rod group (DZ), axial resolution rod group (A), lateral resolution rod groups (L), simulated cysts (C), simulated solid mass (M), and high-density (HD) attenuator are indicated.

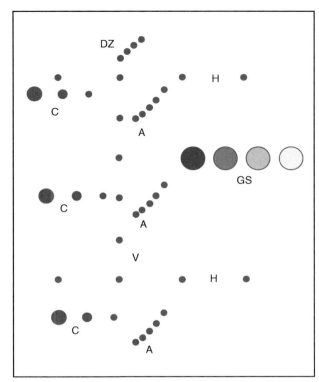

Figure 18-2 Diagram of the Model 403GS tissue-mimicking phantom. Vertical rod group (V), horizontal rod groups (H), dead-zone rod group (DZ), axial resolution rod groups (A), simulated cysts (C), and gray-scale targets (GS) are indicated.

Table 18-1	Specifications of the CIRS Model 40 TM Phantom	
Objects	**Description**	**Specification**
Near-field group	Number of rods	5
	Depth range	1–5 mm
	Vertical spacing	1 mm
Vertical group	Number of rods	15
	Depth range	1–16 cm
	Vertical spacing	10 mm
Horizontal groups	Number of groups	2
	Depth of each group	3 cm and 9 cm
	Number of rods	4 and 7
	Horizontal spacing	10 mm and 20 mm
Axial resolution group	Depth	2.5 cm
	Number of rods	12
	Axial separation between rods	5, 4, 3, 2, 1, 0.5 mm
Lateral resolution group	Number of groups	3
	Depth of each group	2.5 cm, 6 cm, 10 cm
	Number of rods	6
	Horizontal spacing	5, 4, 3, 2, 1 mm
Simulated cysts	Number of cysts	4
	Attenuation coefficient	0.07 dB/ cm/MHz
	Diameter	2 mm, 4 mm, 6 mm, 8 mm
	Depth	2 cm, 4 cm, 6 cm, 8 cm
High-contrast masses	Number of masses	4
	Attenuation coefficient	1.23 dB/ cm/MHz
	Diameter	2 mm, 4 mm, 6 mm, 8 mm
	Depth	2 cm, 4 cm, 6 cm, 8 cm
High-density target	Material	Acrylic
	Diameter	1/16-in
	Depth	6 cm

penetration at high frequency has improved dramatically in the past few years, the higher value of 0.7 dB/cm-MHz is recommended for penetration measurements using a phantom with a uniform attenuation rate. Extended field-of-view sonograms of these phantoms are presented in Figures 18-3 and 18-4.

Phantoms in which the tissue-mimicking material is replaced with urethane rubber are reasonable alternatives for routine monitoring of scanner performance. Figures 18-5 and 18-6 illustrate the design for two phantoms. The specifications for these phantoms are listed in Tables 18-3 and 18-4. Note the relatively low acoustic velocity in urethane compared with soft tissue. Three sides of the phantom provide an acoustic window, which allows structures to be interrogated at different depths depending on the side of access. Extended field-of-view scans of these phantom are presented in Figures 18-7 and 18-8.

If the attenuation frequency dependence is greater than f^1, then the attenuation would be greater in the phantom than in tissue at high frequency, and penetration depth measurement would be in error. The nonlinear attenuation response at high frequencies is a disadvantage of the urethane material. However, for routine quality control testing where consistency is the primary consideration, the stability, ruggedness, ease of transport, and absence of a requirement for a vapor barrier are positive factors. All the materials conform to the recommendation that changes in velocity due to temperature change be less

than 3 m/s-°C. The effect of temperature on backscatter is negligible. Nevertheless, testing with phantoms should be conducted at room temperature.

SPECIALIZED PHANTOMS

Special-purpose TM phantoms have been designed for specific applications (e.g., contrast resolution, slice thickness, elasiticity, beam shape determination, accommodation of endoscopic probes, and various types of speciality imaging including breast, thyroid, prostate, heart, and fetus). Contrast-resolution phantoms assess object size resolvability for varying levels of contrast. Some phantoms have limited scan depth (a few centimeters) to test small-parts transducers only. A common configuration for endosonography transducers enables the probe to be inserted into a cavity surrounded by TM material.

Table 18-2	Specifications of the Gammex-RMI Model 403GS TM Phantom	
Objects	**Description**	**Specification**
Dead-zone group	Number of rods	4
	Depth range	1–10 mm
	Vertical spacing	3 mm
Vertical group	Number of rods	9
	Depth range	1–16 cm
	Vertical spacing	10 mm and 20 mm
Horizontal groups	Number of groups	2
	Depth of each group	2 cm and 12 cm
	Number of rods	4
	Horizontal spacing	30 mm
Axial resolution groups	Number of groups	3
	Depth	3 cm, 8 cm, 14 cm
	Number of rods per group	5
	Axial separation between rods	2, 1, 0.5, 0.25 mm
Simulated cysts	Number of cyst groups	3
	Attenuation coefficient	0.05 dB/cm/MHz
	Diameter	2 mm, 4 mm, 6 mm
	Depth	3 cm, 8 cm, 12 cm
Gray-scale targets	Diameter	10 mm
	Depth	6 cm
	Backscatter	12 dB, 6 dB, –6 dB, anechoic

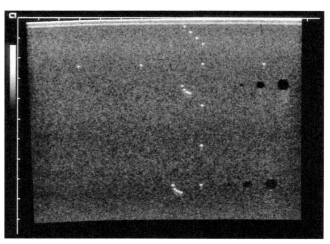

Figure 18-4 Extended field-of-view sonogram of the Model 403 tissue-mimicking phantom. The width of the field of view was 12 cm and the scan depth was 10 cm. The center frequency was 6 MHz.

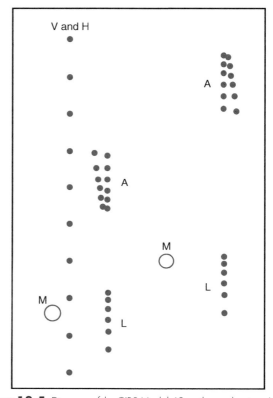

Figure 18-5 Diagram of the CIRS Model 42 urethane phantom. Vertical and horizontal rod group (V and H), axial resolution rod groups (A), lateral resolution rod groups (L), and simulated anechoic masses (M) are indicated.

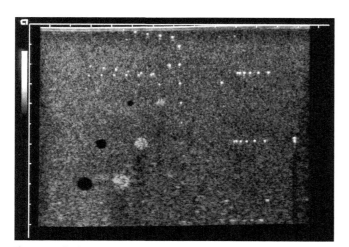

Figure 18-3 Extended field-of-view sonogram of the Model 40 tissue-mimicking phantom. The width of the field of view was 12 cm and the scan depth was 10 cm. The center frequency was 6 MHz.

PERFORMANCE TESTING

Numerous methods using assorted phantoms have been developed to evaluate different aspects of B-mode scanner performance. Tests for dead zone, axial resolution, lateral resolution, penetration, uniformity, vertical distance accuracy, horizontal distance accuracy, focal zone, and cyst characteristics (size, shape, and fill-in) are described. Measurements of power, intensity, bandwidth, and echo-response patterns require expensive electronic test equipment and are usually the purview of the manufacturer and independent research laboratories.

A well-designed phantom allows the use of clinically appropriate operator settings during testing. Dynamic range, gray-scale map, power, gain, and TGC should be recorded for each combination of transducer and

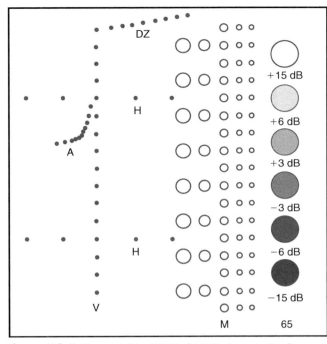

Figure 18-6 Diagram of the ATS Model 539 phantom. Dead zone rod group (DZ), vertical and horizontal rod group (V and H), axial and lateral resolution rod group (A), simulated anechoic masses (M), and gray-scale targets (GS) are indicated.

Table 18-3	Specifications of the CIRS Model 42 Urethane Phantom	
Objects	**Description**	**Specification**
Vertical group	Number of rods	10
	Depth range	1–19 cm
	Vertical spacing	10 mm and 20 mm
Horizontal group	Number of groups	1
	Depth	3 cm and 10 cm
	Number of rods	10
	Horizontal spacing	18.6 mm
Axial resolution group	Number of groups	2
	Depth	2, 5, 8, 11 cm
	Number of rods	12
	Axial separation between rods	5, 4, 3, 2, 1, 0.5 mm
Lateral resolution group	Number of groups	2
	Depth of each group	2 cm, 5 cm, 8 cm, 11 cm
	Number of rods	6
	Horizontal spacing	5, 4, 3, 2, 1 mm
Anechoic masses	Number of stepped masses	2
	Attenuation coefficient	0.2 dB/cm/MHz
	Diameter	2, 4, 6, 8 mm
	Depth	2, 5, 8, 11, 13, 16 cm

Table 18-4	Specifications of the ATS Model 539 Urethane Phantom	
Objects	**Description**	**Specification**
Dead-zone group	Number of rods	9
	Depth range	2–10 mm
	Vertical spacing	1 mm
Vertical group	Number of rods	17
	Depth range	1–18 cm
	Vertical spacing	10 mm
Horizontal group	Number of groups	2
	Depth	5 cm at surface 1 and 5 cm at surface 3
	Number of rods	5 per group
	Horizontal spacing	20 mm
Combined axial and lateral resolution group	Number of groups	1
	Depth	7, 11, 4, 16 cm (multiple scan surfaces)
	Number of rods	11
	Axial separation between rods	5, 4, 3, 2, 1 mm
Anechoic masses	Number of stepped mass groups	5
	Number per group	17 or 8
	Diameter	2, 3, 4, 6, 8 mm
	Depth	1 to 17 cm
Gray-scale targets	Number of groups	1
	Number of targets	6
	Spacing	20 mm
	Diameter	15 mm
	Contrast	−15, −6, −3, +3, +6, +15 dB

performance test. Scan range and focal zone settings are adjusted as needed. TM phantoms are well suited for assessing the focusing at various depths in systems that have variable transmit focal zones.

Dead Zone

The dead zone corresponds to the region adjoining the transducer in which no useful information is collected, in part because of the pulse length (transducer ringing) and reverberations from the transducer-phantom (or patient) interface. The dead zone occurs because the transducer cannot send and receive at the same time. Generally, as frequency is increased, the depth of the dead zone is decreased. However, acoustic output influences the depth of the dead zone.

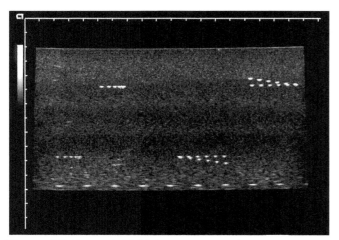

Figure 18-7 Extended field-of-view sonogram of the CIRS Model 42 urethane phantom. The scanning surface was oriented parallel to the vertical/horizontal rod group. The width of the field of view was 18 cm and the scan depth was 10 cm. The center frequency was 6 MHz.

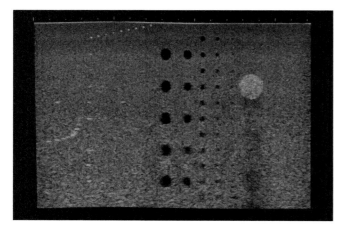

Figure 18-8 Extended field-of-view sonogram of the ATS Model 539 phantom. The scanning surface was oriented parallel to the horizontal rod groups. The width of the field of view was 16 cm and the scan depth was 11 cm. The center frequency was 6 MHz.

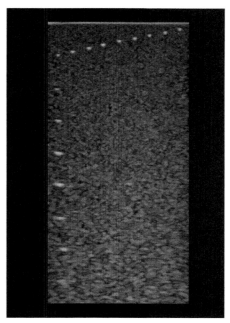

Figure 18-9 Dead-zone measurement with a Model 539 phantom. The distance from the face of the transducer to the beginning of the tissue-texture pattern is less than 2 mm. Linear array transducer operating at 6 MHz.

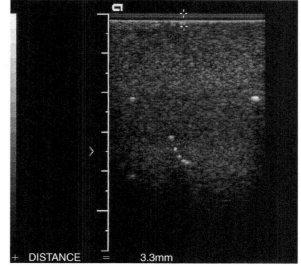

Figure 18-10 Dead-zone measurement with a Model 403 phantom for a transducer manufactured in 1993. The distance from the face of the transducer to the beginning of the tissue-texture pattern is 3.3 mm (cursors). Linear array transducer operating at 7 MHz.

The transducer with coupling gel is placed in contact with the scanning surface of the phantom. Extra gel may be required when a mechanical sector transducer is tested. The instrument settings (e.g., gain, TGC, power) are adjusted to the established baseline values (commonly a default application for the transducer) and the rods in the dead-zone target group near the surface are scanned. For the Model 403 phantom, the rods are spaced 3 mm apart vertically and offset horizontally. For the Model 539 phantom, the rods are spaced 1 mm apart vertically and offset horizontally.

The dead zone is the distance from the front face of the transducer to the first identifiable echo. The tissue scatter from parenchyma is not present in the dead zone. Beyond the dead zone, the tissue texture pattern, similar to liver parenchyma, is observed. The depth of the rod that can be visualized closest to the surface or the depth at which "normal tissue texture" is first seen indicates the axial

extent of the dead zone (Figs. 18-9 and 18-10). Electronic calipers are used to measure the depth of the dead zone.

A shift in the depth of the dead zone reflects a change in the transducer, pulsing system, or both. Specifically, an elongated pulse caused by a cracked crystal, a loose backing or facing material, a broken lens, or a longer excitation pulse deepens the dead zone.

In recent years improvements in transducer design have reduced the extent of the dead zone compared with past performance. Guidelines for dead-zone depth with respect

Table 18-5	Performance Criteria for Dead-Zone Measurements
Frequency (MHz)	**Depth of Dead Zone (mm)**
<3	<7 mm
3–7	<5 mm
≥7	<3 mm

to frequency are listed in Table 18-5. If the depth of the dead zone exceeds the guideline value, an attempt should be made to correct the problem.

Axial Resolution

Axial resolution describes the ability of an ultrasound system to resolve two closely spaced objects along the axis of the beam. It also indicates the smallest object that can be faithfully represented with respect to the axial direction. The axial resolution is dictated by spatial pulse length, which depends on power, transmit frequency, and ringing. Reduced ringing and higher frequency improves the axial resolution. If the integrity of the transducer is altered (cracked crystal, loose facing material, or loose backing material), a change in the pulse length and hence a degradation in resolution will result.

Axial resolution is evaluated by scanning closely-spaced rods oriented vertically. To prevent shadowing from the rods above, they are situated at a 15-degree angle or offset in the horizontal direction. The smallest distance between any two rods in the group that can be differentiated yields the axial resolution. In order to conclude that overlap does not occur in the axial direction, an imaginary horizontal line of is drawn between adjacent rods. Line placement is at the maximum axial extent of one rod toward the overlying rod. To be recorded as a true separation both rods cannot touch the line (Fig. 18-11). Most phantoms allow testing of axial resolution at several depths (e.g., both TM phantoms contain axial resolution rod groups at three depths: 3 , 8, and 14 cm or 3, 6.5, and 10.5 cm).

The instrument settings (e.g., gain, TGC, power, transmit focal zone) are adjusted to the established baseline

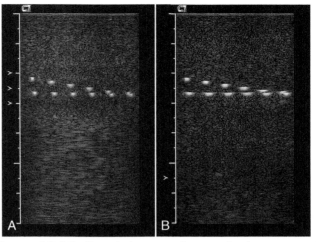

Figure 18-12 Effect of placement of transmit focal zone on axial resolution for a linear array transducer using the Model 40 phantom. The center frequency is 4 MHz. **A,** Transmit focal zone at a depth of 2 to 3 cm corresponding to the location of the axial resolution rod group. **B,** Transmit focal zone at a depth of 6.5 cm. Axial resolution group is located outside the focal zone.

values (a default application for the transducer). The axial resolution is determined by measuring the smallest distance between any two rods that can be visualized as separate entities (i.e., a gap between rods). The spacing of the rods for the Model 403 phantom is 2, 1, 0.5, and 0.25 mm; for the Model 40 phantom, it is 4, 3, 2, 1, 0.5 and 0.25 mm. Figure 18-12 shows scans obtained with a linear array transducer that has a resolution of 1 mm. Note that the lateral extent of the rods does not effect the measurement. Figure 18-13 illustrates the axial resolution at various depths for a transducer with multiple transmit focal zones and dynamic receive focusing. For this transducer, the axial resolution is relatively uniform at all measured depths. Switching to a high-frequency transducer improves axial resolution (Fig. 18-14).

The axial resolution should be within the manufacturer's specifications. Typical values range from 0.5 to 2 mm. The consistency from week to week should not vary by more than 1 rod gap for the same instrument settings.

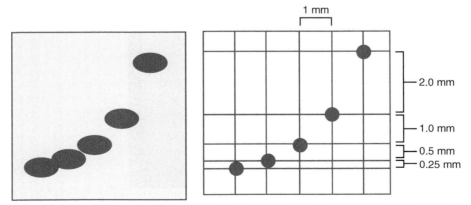

Figure 18-11 Assessment of axial resolution. To be resolved, the spatial representation of adjacent rods must not overlap in the vertical direction. In this example for the illustrated sonogram on the left the axial resolution is 1 mm.

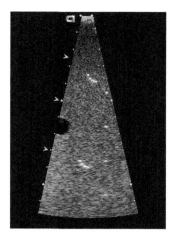

Figure 18-13 Axial resolution for a phased array transducer with multiple focal zones using the Model 403 phantom. The center frequency is 4 MHz. Write zoom was applied to narrow the width of the field of view to emphasize the resolution rod groups. Good axial resolution is maintained throughout the scan range of 11 cm.

Lateral Resolution

Lateral resolution is the ability to distinguish two objects adjacent to each other within the scan plane in the direction perpendicular to the beam axis. Decreasing the beam width by focusing improves the lateral resolution. A single object smaller than the ultrasound beam produces scattered echoes when it is intercepted by the beam; thus the object appears to be the same size as the width of the beam. A small beam width with high scan line density enables small objects to become distinguishable. Lateral resolution is altered by loss of transducer elements or problems with the beam former.

The lateral resolution, which depends on beam width, is evaluated by scanning closely spaced rods oriented horizontally. The lateral resolution is expressed as the smallest distance between any two resolvable rods at a particular depth. In the Model 40 phantom, a lateral resolution group is located at depths of 3, 6.5, and 10.5 cm. This placement allows assessment of the lateral resolution for different focal zones and transmission frequencies. For transducers with fixed focus, lateral resolution can be determined within or very near the focal zone by selecting the appropriate rod group. If variable transmit focusing is available, the focal zone can be selected to correspond with a particular lateral resolution group (Figs. 18-15 and 18-16). Switching to a higher-frequency transducer generally improves the lateral resolution. For those phantoms that do not contain lateral resolution rod groups, lateral resolution can be assessed by scanning the vertical rod

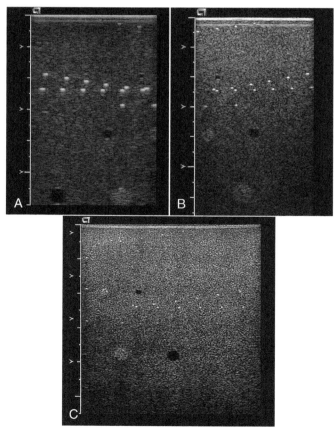

Figure 18-14 Axial resolution measured by a Model 40 phantom is improved by increasing the frequency. **A,** The axial resolution is 1 mm for a frequency of 4 MHz. **B,** The axial resolution is 0.5 mm for a frequency of 6 MHz. **C,** The axial resolution is less than 0.5 mm for a frequency of 14 MHz.

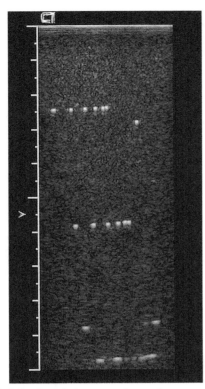

Figure 18-15 Effect of placement of a single transmit focal zone on lateral resolution for a linear array transducer. The lateral resolution within the single focal zone at a depth of 6 cm is 1 mm. The lateral resolution deteriorates markedly when the focal zone is displaced from the region of interest. At a depth of 10 cm, the lateral resolution rod group is blurred. The center frequency is 4 MHz.

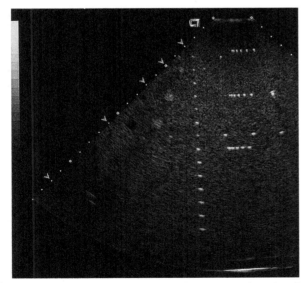

Figure 18-16 Effect of multiple transmit focal zones on lateral resolution for a phased array transducer. The lateral resolution is improved throughout the field of view by applying multiple transmit focal zones. The center frequency is 4 MHz.

group. The horizontal extent of the image of the rod varies with beam width.

A linear transducer acquired the image in Figure 18-15. The lateral resolution is 1 mm at a depth of 6 cm. Typical

Table 18-6	Performance Criteria for Lateral Resolution Measurements	
Depth (cm)	Frequency (MHz)	Lateral Resolution (mm)
>10	<3.5	<4
<10	3.5–5	<3
<10	≥5	<1.5

values range from 0.5 to 3 mm for the B-mode scanners, depending on the degree of focusing, frequency, and the depth of measurement. Guidelines for lateral resolution measurements are listed in Table 18-6. Lateral resolution should not vary by more than 1 mm.

Vertical Distance Measurement

To facilitate the measurement of distance, area, and volume, most ultrasound systems are equipped with distance indicators, calipers, or both. Timing marks are usually superimposed on the image, which must be properly calibrated by the manufacturer to provide accurate values. Vertical distance is measured along the axis of the beam. The location of a reflector with respect to the face of the transducer can be determined if the velocity of ultrasound in the medium and the time of flight of the ultrasonic pulse are known. In practice, the acoustic velocity is assumed to be constant (1540 m/s). The elapsed time between the transmitted pulse and the returning echo is measured, which permits the calculation of the distance to the interface.

The transducer is positioned over the vertical set of rods in the phantom, and scan data are acquired. The instrument settings (e.g., frequency, power, and transmit focal zone) are adjusted to the established baseline values (a default application for the transducer) except that gain and TCG are adjusted to produce an image with moderate brightness. Pressing down on the phantom with the transducer while acquiring the image may displace the rods and cause an error in the distance measurement. Scanning should be performed by applying as little pressure as possible to the acoustic window membrane. Vertical distance accuracy is checked by comparing distance indicators (markers or calipers) in the vertical direction with the known separation between rods in the phantom. The image is analyzed by measuring the distance between rods located at the extremes of the field of view (Fig. 18-17). This measurement is most likely to identify vertical distance miscalibration, because errors are compounded with longer distances. Some sector scanners have distance markers on the outside edge of the sector image with no other indicators available. In this case, handheld calipers in conjunction with the calibration scale must be used for distance measurements on the hard-copy image. Alternatively, images can be transferred to PACS for distance measurements.

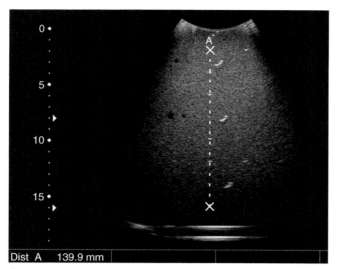

Figure 18-17 Check of vertical distance accuracy. Measurement when the separation includes several rods in a Model 403 phantom over the scanning range. For a known distance of 140 mm, the measured separation is 140 mm. Curvilinear array transducer operating at 4 MHz.

The vertical distance indicators should be accurate to within 2% or 2 mm, whichever is less restrictive. Scanner velocity miscalibration, degradation of phantom TM material, or excessive pressure on the acoustic window of the phantom can cause an error in distance measurement.

Horizontal Distance Measurement

Horizontal distance is measured perpendicularly to the central beam axis within the scan plane. The ultrasound image is a composite of many scan lines, each representing the depth information gathered along the axis of the beam. The two-dimensional image, however, depicts spatial relationships perpendicular to the beam axis. The autoscanning mechanism determines placement of each scan line, which in turn governs the horizontal mapping of the detected signals. Often, information regarding the size of an object in the horizontal direction is desirable. This spatial representation depends on the number of scan lines, resolution of the scan converter (pixel size), resolution of the display, and beam width (lateral resolution). Changes in beam formation by a defective transducer and mechanical motor wear can degrade horizontal distance accuracy.

A scan of the horizontal rods in the phantom is performed, and the internal calipers are used to measure the separation of rod echo positions in a manner similar to the vertical measurement procedure (Figure 18-18). The horizontal distance indicators should be accurate to within 3% or 3 mm, whichever is less restrictive. If the phantom material does not have an acoustic velocity of 1540 m/s, then horizontal distance measurements with sector formats may not agree with stated separation distance (Figure 18-19). Often, horizontal and vertical distance measurements are obtained from the same image (Figure 18-20).

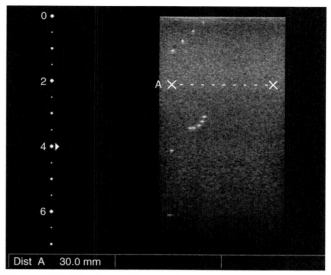

Figure 18-18 Check of horizontal distance accuracy. Measurement when the separation includes horizontal rods in a Model 40 phantom at a scan depth of 2 cm. For a known distance of 30 mm, the measured separation is 30 mm. Linear array transducer operating at 14 MHz.

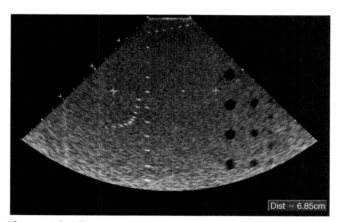

Figure 18-19 Horizontal distance measurement may not accurate if the acoustic velocity is not 1540 m/s in the phantom. For a known distance of 60 mm, the measured separation is 68 mm. Vector transducer operating at 4 MHz.

Focal Zone

The maximum intensity and narrowest beam width occur at the focal point of the transducer. The focal zone is the region surrounding the focal point in which the intensity is within 3 dB of the maximum intensity. This is also the region of the best lateral resolution. The beam pattern (i.e., the beam width at various depths) is obtained by scanning equally spaced vertical rods. Each rod appears as a line on the display in which the length of the line signifies the width of the beam at the depth of the rod. The beam pattern generated by scanning a set of rods positioned at various depths permits visualization of the ultrasonic field (Fig. 18-21).

Ultrasound can be focused either electronically (multiple-element arrays) or internally with lenses or curved crystals

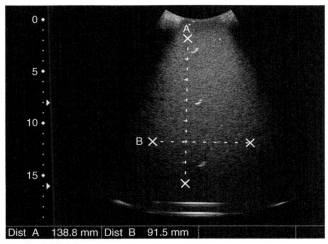

Figure 18-20 Horizontal and vertical distance measurements on the same image. For a known vertical distance of 140 mm, the measured separation is 139 mm. For a known horizontal distance of 90 mm, the measured separation is 91.5 mm. Curvilinear array transducer operating at 4 MHz.

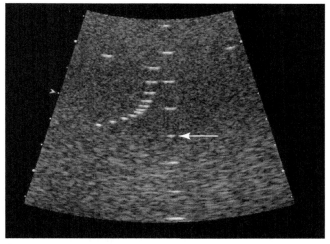

Figure 18-22 Write zoom of the vertical rod group using a single focal zone. The vertical rods within the focal zone are depicted with a narrower width than the rods located above or below this region. The observed focal zone is slightly offset from the indicated focal zone at 7 cm. Curvilinear array operating at 4 MHz.

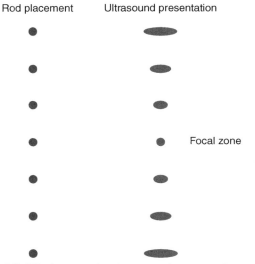

Figure 18-21 The vertical rod group within a TM phantom when scanned yields an image of the rods with variable width. The minimum width of the imaged rod indicates the focal zone.

Figure 18-23 Sonogram of the vertical rod group within a TM phantom using seven focal zones throughout the scan range from 1 to 14 cm. This narrows the in-plane beam width in the region of each focal zone. Note the lateral extent of the vertical rods throughout the entire scan range. Linear array operating at 5 MHz.

(mechanical sector) to reduce the beam width and improve lateral resolution at a certain depth. In scanning a patient, it is important that the focal zone coincide with the depth of interest. Therefore the location of the focal zone must be verified. The depth of the depicted focal zone should agree with the manufacturer's specifications and should not change with time. Variable and dynamically focused transducers are checked by selecting different focal zones throughout the scan range. The location of the focal zone can be affected by the properties of the medium (acoustic velocity offset from the calibrated value), which is outside the control of the sonographer.

A scan of the vertical rods in the phantom is performed. Rods inside the focal zone form a shorter line than the rods above or below the focal zone (Fig. 18-22). For a variable focused transducer, scans with several different focal zone settings should be performed. Figure 18-23 is a scan obtained with a linear array in which five focal zones were selected. In-plane beam width is relatively uniform throughout the scan range.

Sensitivity

Sensitivity refers to the ability of the B-mode scanner to detect weak echoes from small scatterers located at specified depths in an attenuating medium. Weak signals approaching noise levels may not be detected in the presence of noise. The inability to perceive weak echoes restricts the tissue volume that is probed. In addition, the internal detail of organs from nonspecular reflections is degraded with a loss in sensitivity. Factors that influence the signal-to-noise ratio include frequency, power, degree of focusing, attenuation by the medium, distance to the reflector, composition of the interface, and geometry of the reflector. Typically, sensitivity is related to maximum penetration of the ultrasound beam under specified conditions.

The transducer is coupled to the phantom, in which a uniform section of the TM material wider than the field of view is scanned. Nylon rod depth markers may be included within the field of view. Most scanners have application presets optimized for specific examinations that set scan range, frame rate, scan line density, transmit focal zone, persistence, and dynamic range. Often, some of these scanning parameters cannot be adjusted individually by the operator. Instrument settings are adjusted to maximum output, high gain, deepest focal zone, wide dynamic range (>50 dB), reject off or minimum, and time-gain compensation set at full gain where signal falloff occurs. Note the slider positions so that depth dependent gain can be reproduced in future measurements. The maximum depth, at which parenchyma scatterers are visualized without the dominance of noise, is measured (Figs. 18-24 and 18-25). Reduced sensitivity decreases the maximum depth at which this pattern can be observed. A general-purpose TM phantom relatively free of embedded objects throughout the field of view is highly desirable for this test.

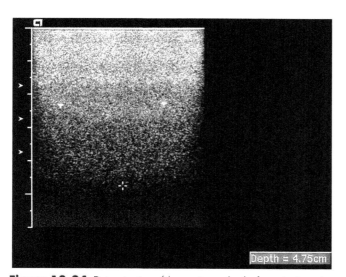

Figure 18-24 Determination of the maximum depth of penetration using a tissue-mimicking phantom. The fading of parenchymal scatterers indicates that the maximum depth of penetration is 4.8 cm for this linear array transducer operated at a frequency of 14 MHz.

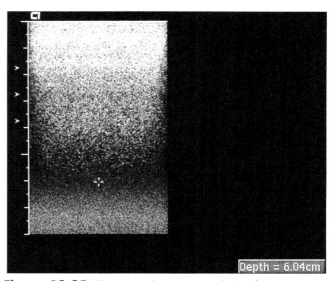

Figure 18-25 Change in the maximum depth of penetration as frequency is reduced. The fading of parenchymal scatterers in a tissue-mimicking phantom indicates that the maximum depth of penetration is 6 cm for the same linear array transducer as in Figure 18-24. The center frequency was lowered to 8 MHz.

The depth of penetration for a particular transducer should not shift by more than 1 cm for identical settings. Variations of output intensity and loss of transducer channels reduce sensitivity, which decreases the maximum depth of visualization.

Uniformity

Uniformity refers to the ability of the imaging system to display structures of equal reflectivity with the same brightness on the monitor. *Ideally a scan of a uniform object should produce an image with a consistent speckle pattern and uniform brightness throughout the field of view.* This is not achieved in practice because of imprecise attenuation compensation and altered beam intensity due to focusing. Nevertheless, the brightness level at a specific depth should appear unvarying. Image nonuniformities can conceal subtle variations in tissue texture. Because TGC modifies the amplitude of the received signal, the echoes originating at the same depth must be compared across the field of view. Autoscan malfunction with a loss of information along scan lines is identified by uniformity testing.

The scanning procedure is the same as the procedure described for maximum depth of visualization. However, images should be obtained with single and multiple focal zones. Mechanical sector and curvilinear transducers may not produce a uniform pattern at the edges of the field of view; this is caused by poor coupling with the phantom surface. To evaluate the entire length of the curvilinear surface, the transducer must be rotated back and forth to establish good contact with the phantom.

This is a qualitative measurement, which is not assigned any numerical control limits. The tissue texture pattern of

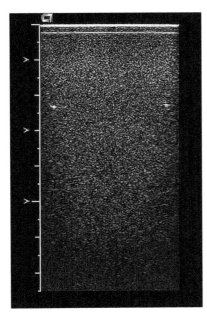

Figure 18-26 Uniformity testing using the Model 403 phantom. At each depth the brightness is relatively constant across the field of view. Linear array transducer operating at 6 MHz.

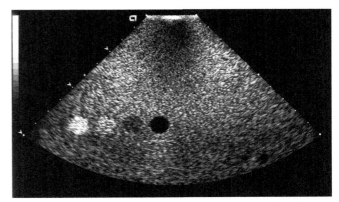

Figure 18-28 Example of poor uniformity in the central field of view at shallow depths for a vector transducer.

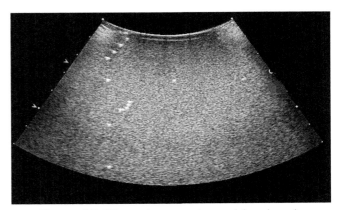

Figure 18-29 Curvilinear transducer with loss channels.

the phantom should be uniform in intensity at a particular depth (Fig. 18-26). Sonograms in Figures 18-27 and 18-28 demonstrate poor uniformity. Occasionally defective scan lines are readily apparent from the clinical or phantom images (Fig. 18-29). More often, the loss of information from defective crystal elements is more subtle because beam

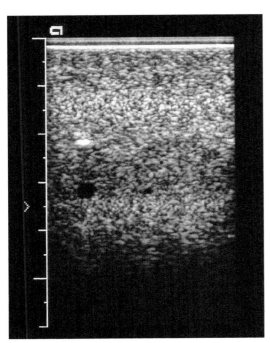

Figure 18-27 Example of poor uniformity for a linear array transducer. A single-transmit focal zone was set at 3.5 cm. A low-intensity band is present across the image near a depth of 3 cm. This suggests that time gain compensation was not properly applied, but the banding is not constant across the width of the field of view.

former combines signals from multiple channels. Lost channels cause reduced signal levels for multiple scan lines but is difficult to recognize as the cause of poor image quality since scan-line dropout is not present (Fig. 18-30).

TM phantoms are sometimes defective and exhibit a nonuniform response throughout the scattering material (Fig. 18-31). The phantom was readily identified as the source of the signal variation by scanning the phantom with multiple transducers from different B-mode scanners. All images demonstrated the same appearance with bright dots distributed throughout the tissue-mimicking material. Upon receipt of a new phantom, the phantom should be scanned immediately to confirm that manufacturing defects are not present. TM phantoms degrade with time and may develop air pockets between the scanning surface and the tissue-mimicking gel, producing reverberation artifacts (Figure 18-32).

Simulated Cysts and Masses

Cysts are fluid-filled structures that are hypoechoic and usually weakly attenuating. They also have slower velocities than the surrounding tissue. Solid masses are normally more attenuating and produce more internal echoes than soft tissue does. The velocity of ultrasound

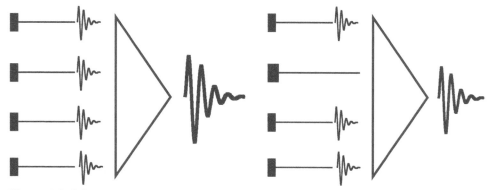

Figure 18-30 Loss of a single channel in the receive beam former results in reduced signal level. Left, proper operation. Right, channel malfuction.

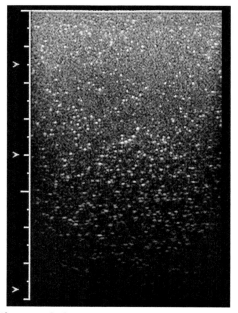

Figure 18-31 Defective tissue-mimicking phantom.

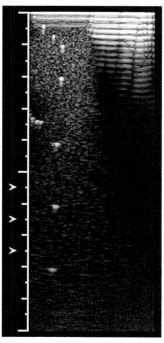

Figure 18-32 Degradation of tissue-mimicking phantom in which an air pocket is formed between the scanning surface and the gel producing reverberation artifacts.

is also usually faster in these structures than in normal tissues. Often, cylinders, cones, or spheres of varying size are incorporated within the TM matrix. These structures are weak scatterers appearing anechoic or strong scatterers appearing hyperechoic compared with the phantom background.

The image of the simulated cyst has a distinctive pattern that should represent its size, shape, and consistency. A nonuniform echo pattern across the cyst is referred to as cyst fill-in. Changes in output, beam width, and gain can affect cyst fill-in. Because the reflector surface is curved, fill-in occurs more readily outside the focal zone, where the beam width is greater. When a cyst is scanned with low scan line density, the smooth, round border is misrepresented as an irregular border.

The simulated cysts are evaluated for size, fill-in, accuracy of shape, and enhancement distal to the simulated cyst. Some ultrasound units are limited in their depth of penetration and may not be able to image deep-lying

structures. Often, bright spots occur at the tops and bottoms of the anechoic objects (Figure 18-33). These are normal specular reflections from the simulated cyst-tissue interface.

The size of each displayed simulated cyst is measured in both vertical and horizontal directions by means of electronic calipers. The shape of each simulated cyst and the brightness throughout the structure are noted (Fig. 18-34). The measured size of each simulated cyst should be within 1 mm of the actual size. The geometric shape should be circular, but often linear array transducers and systems with limited numbers of scan lines tend to square the edges of the simulated cysts. The cysts should be of uniform brightness (hypoechoic) with normal scan settings. Refraction defocusing artifact may be observed at the edge of the simulated cyst.

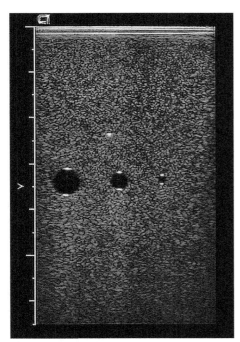

Figure 18-33 The sonogram of simulated cysts often shows bright areas at the boundary caused by specular reflections from the cyst–tissue interface.

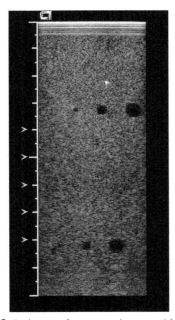

Figure 18-34 Evaluation of cyst size, shape, and fill-in using a tissue-mimicking phantom. Three simulated cysts at a depth of 3 cm and two simulated cysts at a depth of 8 cm are seen. Fill-in is observed for the simulated cysts located at the deeper depth (displaced from the mechanical focal depth).

The scanner should be able to differentiate between solid masses and normal tissue structures. Solid structures are evaluated for size, accuracy of shape, and shadowing distal to the simulated mass. The shape of the structures should be round with uniform brightness (Fig. 18-35). The size of each simulated mass should be measured in

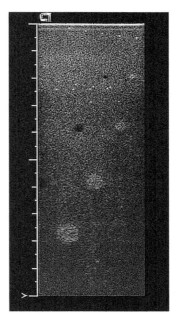

Figure 18-35 Evaluation of mass size and shape plus shadowing behind the mass using the Model 40 phantom. Four high-contrast masses with respective diameters of 2 mm, 4 mm, 6 mm, and 8 mm are seen.

both the vertical and horizontal directions using electronic calipers. The measured size of each simulated mass should be within 1 mm of the actual size. Shadowing behind the simulated solid mass may occur. Refraction defocusing artifact may be seen at the edges of the simulated mass.

Gray Scale

Contrast resolution characterizes a scanner's ability to distinguish structures with similar reflection and attenuation properties. For the purpose of evaluating contrast resolution, some TM phantoms have a set of gray-scale targets in the form of solid cylinders with different scattering properties. Commonly, backscatter levels of the targets are denoted in increments of 3 dB. Each target produces a characteristic signal level, which is translated into a corresponding brightness level on the monitor.

The transducer is positioned over the gray scale targets and scan data are acquired using write zoom (Fig. 18-36). The instrument settings (e.g., frequency, power, and transmit focal zone) are set to the established baseline values except that gain is adjusted so that the signal level in the

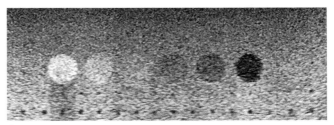

Figure 18-36 Sonogram of gray-scale targets in the Model 539 phantom.

anechoic target is low (approximately 1) as measured by the region-of-interest tool. For each gray-scale target, a region of interest is placed completely inside the respective image and the signal level is recorded. The signal level corresponding to the background material is also measured. Control limit is ± 10% of the baseline average pixel value for each target within 6 dB of background.

IMAGE DISPLAY

Manufacturers have incorporated various video test patterns in B-mode scanners to evaluate the image quality exhibited by monitors and hard-copy cameras. These test patterns usually include a set of gray-scale bars with varying brightness levels and a grid of equally spaced parallel horizontal and vertical lines. The gray scale from black to white represents the entire dynamic range of potential signal levels. The grid makes possible an assessment of geometric distortion across the screen.

The brightness and contrast controls on the monitor are adjusted at the initial setup to achieve the proper gray-scale presentation. The settings must be checked periodically to confirm that all gray levels are seen. The fidelity of image display is assessed by displaying the gray-scale test pattern. Each bar in the test pattern should be distinguished as a separate shade of gray. The gray levels must range from black to white, with midscale bars depicted in gray tones. If tearing or blurring of letters in the text occurs, the brightness adjustment is too high. Once brightness and contrast controls have been adjusted to achieve the proper gray-scale presentation, the knobs can be taped in place (or at least labeled) to inhibit modifying the settings.

The most practical test pattern for the evaluation of monitors is one developed by the Society of Motion Picture and Television Engineers (SMPTE) (Fig. 18-37).

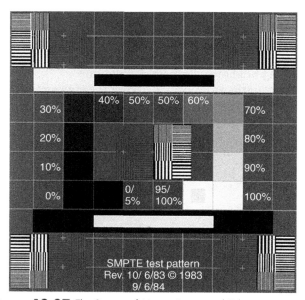

Figure 18-37 The Society of Motion Picture and Television Engineers (SMPTE) test pattern.

Note that the background is a uniform gray at 50% signal level. Low- and high-contrast bar patterns are placed at the center and at each corner. The size of the bars varies, but the smallest bar is limited by the pixel size of the digital system (i.e., the width of the smallest bar is one pixel). The low-contrast bars are modulated in contrast from 1% to 5%. The high-contrast bars have maximum contrast of 100%. Boxes with varying brightness levels are arranged in stepwise fashion throughout the central portion of the test pattern. The entire dynamic range of potential signal levels is represented in 11 steps from 0% to 100%, with 10% increments. An incremental patch with 5% contrast is inset in the 0% and 100% boxes. For example, a 95% patch is positioned within the 100% box. Failure to visualize all 11 gray-level steps or the 5% contrast boxes signifies that the brightness and contrast of the monitor are not properly set.

Unfortunately, ultrasound-equipment manufacturers have not universally adopted the standardized SMPTE test pattern. The ready accessibility of the SMPTE pattern as a display option facilitates quality control of display monitors, hard-copy cameras, and PACS. In addition, more uniform image recording by equipment from different manufacturers would then be possible.

IMAGE RECORDING

The potential end product of an ultrasonic scan is a high-quality photographic reproduction of the display—a hard-copy visual representation of the interactions of ultrasound with tissue. *The image recorded on film must be a faithful reproduction of the image viewed on the display monitor.* The fidelity of any recording with respect to resolution, distortion, and contrast is checked by comparing the displayed test pattern with the final hard-copy image. *Proper adjustment of the display monitor does not ensure similar gray-scale presentation by the processed film.* The image-recording device is not affected by brightness or contrast controls on the display monitor. The translation of input signals to optical density by the hard-copy camera are regulated independently via internal controls for contrast, brightness, exposure time, and gray-scale map.

The photographic film should duplicate the structural detail of the B-mode image. Additionally, the display monitor and processed film must have the potential to exhibit gray levels extending from black to white with multiple intermediate shades. Hard-copy image quality depends on the matched response between display monitor and image-recording device as well as on proper film processing. The photographic system may distort the image on the display when the image is recorded on film. The integrity of the hard-copy process is evaluated by comparing direct measurements of rod separation on film with those determined from the display. Hard-copy images derived from testing also provide documentation of scanner performance, whether proper or improper.

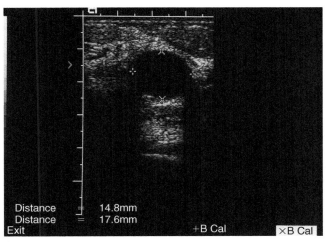

Figure 18-38 Sonogram of a breast containing a cyst. Cursors mark the dimensions of the cyst. A properly adjusted multiformat camera recorded the hard-copy image.

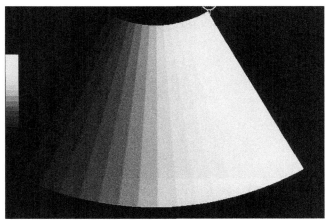

Figure 18-40 Gray-scale test pattern with an improperly adjusted multiformat camera. The bars in the low-optical density range are not resolved.

Figure 18-38 shows a sonogram of a breast containing a cyst. The sonogram was recorded with a properly operating hard-copy camera. Distance measurements in the horizontal and vertical directions obtained by the internal calipers agree with measurements by handheld calipers. Furthermore, the graduated distance scales in both directions are equal; that is, the separation between any two points in the hard-copy image should be the same whether the horizontal or vertical calibration scale is used.

A full sheet of gray-scale test pattern images is recorded in the format and size normally used clinically (i.e., a 6:1 format requires the pattern to be printed six times). Dark borders between printed images prevents glare and improves contrast resolution. The maximum optical density for film viewed on a conventional light box is usually set at 3.2 to 3.5. The clear area must have an optical density less than 0.1 above base-plus-fog. All bars in the test pattern should be distinguishable (Fig. 18-39). A gray-scale test

pattern recorded with an improperly adjusted hard-copy camera is shown in Figure 18-40.

Hard-copy recording of the image, including the demographic information displayed on the monitor, requires data transfer to the image-recording device. To prevent geometric distortion, the aspect ratio of the monitor screen (ratio of width to height) must be maintained on the recording medium. The hard-copy image is often minified to accommodate various film formats (e.g., 15:1 on 14- by 17-in. film or 6:1 on 8- by 10-in. film). The aspect ratio of the recorded image is the same regardless of film format. The typical aspect ratio for ultrasound scanners is 4:3. A change in this ratio is accompanied by unequal magnification (or minification) in the horizontal and vertical directions.

Unequal magnification causes distortion. Circular shapes on the display monitor are elongated in the direction of higher magnification and appear elliptical on the hard-copy. For example, a fetal head that is round on the display monitor would be recorded as an oval. In addition, a distance measurement along any diagonal path through the hard-copy image would yield an incorrect result. Figure 18-41 illustrates the effect of unequal magnification in the recording of a sonogram of the kidney. The size and shape of the kidney are distorted by being protracted in the horizontal direction. The calibration scale indicates that the distance between cursors is 145 mm instead of 108 mm as measured by the internal calipers. If distortion is introduced by the image-recording device, the internal calipers are unaffected by this malfunction and, consequently, the measured value for distance as designated by the cursors is correct.

The most likely circumstance for an improperly adjusted image-recording device is an incorrect initial setup (1) during installation of the scanner or (2) during replacement of the hard-copy recording device. To ensure that the image-recording device is functioning properly, acceptance testing following these events is essential.

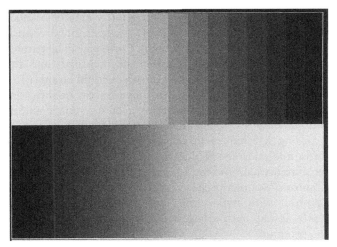

Figure 18-39 Gray-scale test pattern with a properly adjusted multiformat camera. All 16 bars are resolved.

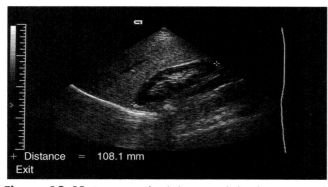

+ Distance = 108.1 mm
Exit

Figure 18-41 Sonogram of a kidney recorded with an improperly adjusted laser camera. Whereas internal calipers measure the craniocaudal dimension as 108 mm, the calibration scale indicates incorrectly that the distance (between cursors) is 145 mm.

IMAGE CAPTURE (PACS)

Many facilities have discontinued film as a image recording option and instead electronically transfer images to PACS. Standards for PACS technology have been developed by the American College of Radiology and the National Electrical Manufacturers Association. The collection of standards is called Digital Imaging and Communication in Medicine (DICOM). DICOM established standardized file formats for patient data and images as well as criteria for the transfer, storage, and display of this information.

Ultrasound scan data are communicated to the network digital interface, which transfers the image and demographics directly to the network from the scanner. Most ultrasound scanners can be purchased with DICOM output for this direct communication link to a PACS. The fidelity of the transferred data with respect to contrast and distortion is evaluated by sending the SMPTE test pattern from the scanner to PACS. In some scanners the test pattern must be incorporated into a patient study prior to transfer. All 11 gray level steps and the dark and light contrast boxes should be visualized. Distance accuracy in two directions is evaluated with the workstation distance measurement tool.

Gray-scale targets with varying reflectivity (usually, in 3-dB increments) are incorporated in many phantoms and can be used to quantify gray-level response. An image of the phantom is sent from the scanner to PACS. The workstation region-of-interest tool is placed over each gray-scale target to measure signal level. The respective values depend on image processing but are reproducible within 10% over time if all acquisition parameters are consistent. The change in signal level with dB scattering content exhibits a nonlinear response, which also depends on image processing.

QUALITY CONTROL

An effective quality control (QC) program is required to obtain consistent high-quality images and ensure proper scanner performance. It must be simple to implement

and easy to maintain. One that is overambitious in terms of complexity or frequency of testing will often cease to be performed at all. At the same time, to be meaningful, the tests must be comprehensive and capable of detecting common system problems.

QC tests provide objective assessment of instrument stability and performance. They have proved to be beneficial in diagnostic imaging facilities when conducted regularly. One of the most important advantages is the documentation of gradual degradation of system performance when compared with clinical impressions of image quality. Long-term performance is evaluated by periodically testing ultrasound equipment under well-defined conditions (e.g., specified instrument settings using appropriate phantoms).

The sonographer who routinely uses the equipment for patient examinations should perform the QC procedures. A more sensitive check on machine malfunction and technical error can thus be made. Administrative support to allot time for access to the unit, analysis of image data, and documentation of results is essential.

A wide variety of general-purpose TM phantoms have been developed to monitor the performance characteristics of ultrasound scanners. Model 403 and Model 40 are recommended for routine QC testing. Phantom design with regions of TM material only that are relatively free of objects improves testing for sensitivity and image uniformity. Manufacturers are receptive to requests to modify multiple-purpose phantoms so that all structures except that vertical and horizontal rods are eliminated from the gel matrix.

Rubber-based urethane phantoms have also been developed for QC applications. The low velocity and frequency dependence of the attenuation coefficient limit the application to monitoring consistency but not accuracy of scanner performance. The physical separation of the vertical rods is 18.6 mm, so that the measured axial distance is the stated 20 mm (corrected for the difference in acoustic velocity between urethane and tissue). When the rods are oriented perpendicularly to the direction of propagation, the measured distance should correspond to actual separation of 18.6 mm.

While extensive testing is appropriate when the scanner is installed, the purpose of QC is to use tests that are sensitive indicators of overall scanner performance. The parameters to be tested, the results to be recorded, and the performance limits for each parameter should be specified. The following tests are recommended for the quality control program: penetration, distance accuracy, image uniformity, fidelity of image display, and fidelity of image recording. Mechanical inspection of the transducers, power cords, and console should also be included. Low contrast detectability has not been demonstrated as yet to be a useful monitor of scanner performance. Since a specially designed phantom with hypoechoic spherical objects at various depths is required, this test is not recommended for the QC program.

The transducer acoustic surface, housing, and cable should be inspected for cracks and other damage each day of use. If liquids enter the housing, damage to the transducer will result. This also poses an electrical hazard to the operator. The connector should be examined for bent or loose prongs. The power cord should be inspected periodically for wear. Indicator lights and scan parameter displays on the console should function properly.

The most frequently used transducers should be monitored on a semiannual basis, and all other transducers should be tested at least yearly. Mobile scanners are more susceptible to failure and should be tested more frequently, at least quarterly. Image-recording devices should be tested at least on a quarterly basis for gray-scale contrast and at least semiannually for distortion. A scan of the TM phantom should be obtained after the unit is repaired (preferably before the service representative leaves) to confirm proper operation.

An important aspect of any QC program is documentation. QC test procedures are of little value without an effective means of recording the results for future reference. The primary concern is long-term operating performance of an imaging system, which this information provides. It is essential that all instrument settings (e.g., TGC and power) be specified for all future testing. To facilitate comparisons of results, they should be easily reproducible. When values exceeding the control limits are obtained, further testing, the results of that testing, any corrective action (including service reports), and the results of that action should be documented.

Documentation provides potential solutions to problems that recur at a later date. Permanent records also aid in identifying problem areas in the system. Documentation of baseline values and abnormal values on a hard-copy format is extremely helpful. Film storage is bulky and time consuming, however; therefore appropriate test results can be recorded on special forms (Fig. 18-42). Hard-copy images of results outside of the control limits are useful for proving malfunctions to service personnel, particularly for intermittent problems that disappear when the service representative arrives.

EVALUATION OF CLINICAL IMAGE QUALITY

An impression of degraded image quality is difficult to assess by viewing clinical sonograms only. Testing with TM phantoms often identifies improper scanner operation. A general complaint of poor image quality from one

Diagnostic Imaging Department
Canton, Ohio

Scanner	
Manufacturer	
Model	
ID	

Transducer	
Model	
Frequency	
S/N	

Date	Image uniformity (ok)	Penetration (cm)	Distance accuracy		Image recording		Initials
			Depth	Lateral	Distortion	Gray levels	

Figure 18-42 Sample quality control form.

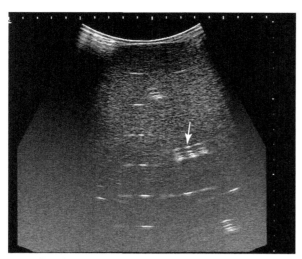

Figure 18-43 Sonogram of a tissue-mimicking phantom with a defective curvilinear array transducer. The axial resolution rod set at a depth of 8 cm is recorded at three different locations in the image (arrow).

real-time unit was rectified by a scan of the phantom, which demonstrated that a curvilinear array transducer was defective (Fig. 18-43). The one-to-one correspondence between scanned subject and the image was corrupted. Whereas anatomic structures in sonograms were blurred and indistinct, the multiple replications of a single rod set in the image of the TM phantom was immediately apparent.

SPECIALIZED TESTING

Elasticity

Elasticity targets with varying stiffness relative to the background material are incorporated in many phantoms to provide image contrast when scanned in elastography mode. These targets range in mechanical properties, diameter, and depth but generally appear isoechoic in the B-mode image.

Slice Thickness

Most multiple-element transducers are focused in the elevation direction by placing a lens in front of the crystal elements. This mechanical focusing fixes the focal length to one specific depth. The focal length is appropriate for the type of transducer and the operational frequency. For example, a small-parts transducer operating at 5 MHz has a minimum slice thickness at a depth from 1.5 to 3.5 cm, while the minimum slice thickness for a general-purpose transducer operating at the same frequency occurs at a deeper depth of 3 to 6 cm.

Mechanical focusing is evaluated qualitatively by scanning anechoic cylindrical objects in a general-purpose phantom with the scan plane oriented parallel to the length of the cylinders. The scan head is rotated 90 degrees from the typical orientation. Cyst fill-in is present where the slice thickness extends beyond the boundary of the cylindrical object. For narrow slice thickness, cyst fill-in is less pronounced and corresponds to the depth of mechanical focus. Assessment is limited by the placement depths of the anechoic objects in the phantom.

Quantitative assessment over a continuous range of scan depths is achieved by using an inclined-plane phantom. The phantom is composed of two sections forming a flat interface oriented at 45 degrees. Both materials are uniform in their attenuation. One material containing backscattering particles forms an inclined plane; the other material containing no backscattering particles is in contact with the surface of the inclined plane. The transducer is positioned so that the scanning plane at a constant depth intercepts the inclined plane with the 45-degree angle. The scattering plane interrogated by the beam appears as a horizontal band in the image. The axial height of the band is equal to the slice thickness. To view the scattering plane at different depths, the transducer is moved along the length of the inclined plane. As slice thickness becomes narrower near the mechanical focal point, the horizontal band is reduced in size.

Contrast-and-Detail Phantoms

Special phantoms with "cysts" and "masses" (solids) embedded in TM material permit testing of the contrast and detail of the imaging system under simulated clinical conditions. A contrast-and-detail phantom with multiple conical targets having varying contrast (echoes vary by 20 dB) tests the system's ability to reproduce contrast and detail in quantitative terms. This evaluation is very helpful in comparing transducers on the same system and in comparing different systems for total performance.

A major criticism of sensitivity test conducted with a general-purpose phantom is that the determination of the maximum depth of visualization is subjective. An alternative method to measure the maximum depth of visualization is to scan a specialized phantom containing multiple randomly distributed, small-diameter (1-5 mm), hypoechoic spherical objects (Fig. 18-44). The judgment of penetration becomes easier, since the depth at which the structures are no longer observed is measured. Objects rather than noise denote the limit of detectability. This method is dependent on the beam width and thus the focusing characteristics of the transducer and tends to underestimate the maximum depth of penetration compared

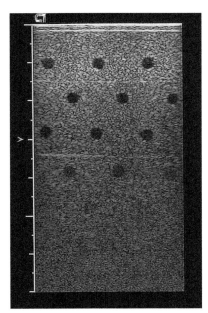

Figure 18-44 *Maximum depth of penetration is 4.5 cm at a frequency of 5 MHz using a Model 44 tissue-mimicking phantom with low scatter, spherical objects.*

with that measured by signal loss from parenchymal scatterers. Since monitoring the consistency of performance is the primary goal of quality control, this type of phantom is a reasonable substitute for testing penetration. However, further expense would be incurred for the purchase of an additional phantom.

SUMMARY

The end product of an ultrasound scan is its image. The quality of the image depends largely on a properly functioning unit. Performance of B-mode scanners is evaluated using phantoms to measure vertical distance accuracy, horizontal distance accuracy, axial resolution, lateral resolution, sensitivity, uniformity, and dead zone. Within well-defined limits, these parameters reflect properly functioning equipment.

The display monitor, hard-copy camera, and film processing all contribute to the image-recording process. To optimize photographic system performance, the recommendations of manufacturers of the image-recording device, film, and processing chemicals should be followed. The image-recording device should exhibit a full range of gray-scale contrast and an accurate portrayal of size, shape, and relative positions of structures in the displayed image. Matching the response of the display monitor and the hard-copy camera is necessary to ensure that what is seen on the monitor is recorded on film.

The performance of B-mode scanners is monitored via a QC program. The essential checks include vertical distance accuracy, horizontal distance accuracy, sensitivity, uniformity, fidelity of image display, and fidelity of image capture. The QC program must be structured so that the testing is performed on a consistent basis. Documentation of routine tests provide the means to compare performance levels over long periods. Service records should be included as part of this record-keeping process.

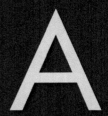
Essential Equations of Sonography

1. Acoustic velocity

$$c = f\lambda$$

2. Intensity reflection coefficient

$$\alpha_R = \left(\frac{Z_2 - Z_1}{Z_2 + Z_1}\right)^2$$

3. Snell's law

$$\frac{c_i}{c_t} = \frac{\sin\theta_i}{\sin\theta_t}$$

4. Echo ranging

$$z = \frac{ct}{2}$$

5. Instantaneous intensity

$$I = \frac{p^2}{\rho c}$$

6. Decibel

$$\text{Level(dB)} = 10\log\left(\frac{I}{I_{ref}}\right)$$

7. Intensity loss

$$\text{intensity loss(dB)} = \mu f z$$

8. Maximum pulse repetition frequency

$$PRF_{max} = \frac{c}{2R}$$

9. Q-value

$$Q = \frac{f_c}{\Delta f}$$

10. B-mode maximum frame rate

$$FR_{max} = \frac{c}{2Rn}$$

11. Doppler shift frequency

$$f_D = \frac{2vf}{c}\cos\theta$$

12. Pulse-wave Doppler velocity limit

$$V_{max} = \frac{c^2}{8fR\cos\theta}$$

13. Thermal index

$$TI = \frac{W}{W_{ref}}$$

14. Mechanical index

$$MI = \frac{p_r}{\sqrt{f}}$$

Physical Descriptors and Symbols

Parameter	Symbol
Acoustic impedance	Z
Acoustic pressure	p
Acoustic velocity	c
Angle	μ
Attenuation coefficient	θ
Bandwidth	Δf
Density	ρ
Doppler shift frequency	f_D
Elapsed time to echo	t
Frame rate	FR
Frequency	f
Intensity	I
Mechanical coefficient	Q
Peak negative pressure	p_r
Power (in situ)	W
Power (reference)	W_{ref}
Pulse repetition frequency	PRF
Reflection coefficient	α_R
Reflector depth	z
Reflector velocity	v
Scan lines	n
Scan range	R
Time to echo	t
Wavelength	λ

Essential Principles of Diagnostic Sonography

- During linear propagation, molecular density exhibits sinusoidal behavior along the transmission path (plot of molecular density as a function of distance at an instant in time is a sine wave).
- For longitudinal waves, the molecular (particle) motion is along the same direction as sound propagation (sound waves in liquids and tissue).
- Acoustic velocity is determined by the properties of the medium (density and bulk modulus).
- Acoustic velocity is independent of frequency.
- The average acoustic velocity in soft tissue is 1540 m/s or 1.54 mm/μs.
- Dividing 1.54 by the frequency expressed in megahertz yields the wavelength in millimeters for soft tissue.
- In any medium an increase in frequency reduces the wavelength.
- At low intensity (no harmonic formation) the wave parameters of frequency, wavelength, and acoustic velocity are unchanged as intensity is varied.
- Reflection at a specular interface causes a fraction of the incident sound energy to be redirected into the medium from which it came.
- Differences in acoustic impedance at an interface affect the fraction of the incident intensity that is reflected.
- Frequency is unchanged when a wave is transmitted across a boundary.
- Scattering causes the sound energy to radiate in all directions after the sound beam strikes a small interface with physical dimensions less than a wavelength.
- Refraction is the change in direction of a sound beam as it enters a medium, which is predicted by Snell's law.
- Angular displacement by refraction is based on the ratio of the velocity of sound in the respective media and obeys Snell's law.
- Interference is the superposition (algebraic summation) of waves, which depends on amplitude, frequency, and phase of the respective waves.
- Absorption is the process whereby sound energy is converted into heat.
- The attenuation rate of soft tissue varies linearly with frequency.

- In echo ranging, the delay time for the echo depends on depth and equals 13 μs/cm if a constant velocity of 1540 m/s is assumed.
- Intensity is the rate of energy flow through a cross-sectional area.
- The hydrophone is a device that measures the time-varying pressure in the ultrasonic field.
- *Free field* describes conditions in which pressure (intensity) measurements are performed in water without reflectors or other disturbances to the ultrasonic field.
- Temporal variation of the pulsed-wave intensity is classified by temporal peak, pulse average, and temporal average.
  - Temporal peak intensity is the maximum intensity when accessed on the basis of time.
  - Pulse average intensity is the time-varying intensity averaged over the duration of a single pulse.
  - Temporal average intensity is time-varying intensity averaged over the pulse repetition period.
- Spatial variation of the pulsed wave intensity is classified by spatial peak and spatial average.
  - The maximum intensity of all temporal intensity values within the ultrasonic field is the spatial peak.
  - Averaging of the temporal intensity over the cross-sectional area of the beam is the spatial average.
- Duty cycle is the fraction of time the transducer is actively generating ultrasound energy.
- Power is the energy radiated per unit time, usually expressed in milliwatts (mW) or watts (W) or joules per second (J/s).
- Relative change in intensity is expressed in decibels (dB).
- Intensity loss along the propagation path is proportional to the attenuation coefficient in dB/cm-MHz, the frequency, and the distance traveled in the medium.
- Decibel losses along path segments are additive to yield the decibel loss for the entire path.
- The 3-dB rule states each 3 dB change corresponds to a factor of 2. For example, if intensity loss is 9 dB, the reduction in intensity is a factor of 8 (factor 2 multiplied three times).

- The average attenuation rate in soft tissue is estimated as 0.7 dB/cm at 1 MHz. For clinical safety, the attenuation rate is assumed to be much lower (0.3 dB/cm at 1 MHz) to provide a conservative estimate of intensity in tissue.
- Detected echo intensity can be 100 dB or more lower than the transmitted intensity.
- The piezoelectric effect is a phenomenon exhibited by crystalline materials in which an electrostatic voltage is produced across the crystal when the crystal is deformed in shape.
- Design criteria for the transducer used in imaging include an ultrasound wave of the proper frequency in the megahertz range, directional control, limited spatial extent (beam width and pulse length), and capability for pulsed-wave operation.
- Crystal thickness is equal to half the natural resonance wavelength.
- Matching layer improves energy transfer from crystal to patient, which shortens pulse duration and increases pulse intensity.
- For pulsed-wave ultrasound, the backing material has an acoustic impedance similar to that of the crystal to reduce ringing and produce a pulse of short duration.
- The time interval between transmitted pulses should be no shorter than for the time for the transmitted pulse to travel to the depth of interest and the echo generated at that depth to return.
- The center frequency or operating frequency is the dominant component in the frequency distribution.
- Bandwidth indicates the range of frequencies present in the transmitted pulse.
- As pulse duration is decreased, the bandwidth becomes greater.
- Higher operating frequency, lower Q-value, increased damping, and shorter pulse duration reduce the spatial pulse length and improve axial resolution.
- Axial resolution is essentially constant throughout the scan range (independent of depth).
- Larger diameter of the crystal and higher operating frequency increase the near-field depth.
- Compared with the nonfocused beam, focusing causes the ultrasound energy to be concentrated in a smaller volume within the focal region for improved spatial localization and stronger echo formation.
- High transmit power causes a proportionate rise in echo intensity and improves the detection of weak reflectors.
- Dynamic range, often expressed in decibels, indicates the range of signal levels that can be preserved as distinct values.
- Noise is variation in signal level, which is not correlated with echo intensity.
- A-mode is a two-dimensional presentation of signal strength versus time (scan depth) on the monitor.
- Static B-mode image is a two-dimensional spatial presentation of detected echoes (tomographic slice).
- Spatial mapping of the echo-induced signals in the real-time image is a combination of echo ranging and directional beam scanning.
- The scan converter retains the echo-induced signals from each scan line and then translates this information into the two-dimensional image format for readout.
- Reducing the number of scan lines, the scan range, or both increases the maximum frame rate.
- A mechanical sector transducer has one or more piezoelectric crystals mounted on a mechanical arm that is moved to different locations during frame acquisition.
- Selected elements in the linear and curvilinear arrays are activated during transmission to control sampling direction.
- In the phased array, elements are activated in a timed sequence during transmission to control sampling direction.
- For multiple-element arrays, electronic transmit focusing enables the focal length to be prescribed for each transmitted pulse.
- Aperture focusing is a form of electronic transmit focusing in which the number of crystals fired in a group depends on the depth of focus.
- Apodization varies the excitation voltage to each element to control that element's contribution to the overall transmit-beam pattern.
- Mechanical focusing in the elevation direction for linear, curvilinear, phased, and vector arrays is fixed.
- Dynamic receive focusing uses beam formation to improve lateral resolution and signal-to-noise ratio.
- The 1.5D transducer permits dynamic focusing in the elevation direction (it replaces fixed mechanical focusing).
- Multiple small rectangular piezoelectric crystals configured in a two-dimensional matrix across the transducer face enable electronic steering in all directions throughout a volume without moving the transducer.
- Grating lobes are secondary lobes caused by the regular periodic spacing of elements in the linear and phased array.
- In spatial compounding, frames acquired with different steered beam angles are combined to reduce speckle, clutter, and noise while improving the border definition of specular reflectors.
- Extended field-of-view imaging expands the field of view by forming a panoramic image composed of multiple frames as the transducer is moved across the patient.
- Binary encoding and frequency modulation (chirp) in coded excitation improve signal-to-noise ratio and/or increase the depth of penetration.

- In zone sonography, the acquisition time for a frame is greatly reduced by sampling a large region with a broad transmit beam (e.g., 20 pulse/receive cycles across the field of view).
- The contributions from clutter, grating lobes, and side lobes at the fundamental frequency are suppressed in tissue harmonic imaging.
- Elastography measures the displacement of tissue (strain) following the application of a compression force (stress).
- 3D ultrasound depicts the spatial relationships within a scanned tissue volume as a set of tomographic slices, a surface-rendered image, or a volume-rendered image.
- In 4D ultrasound, the fourth dimension of time is combined with volumetric sampling to depict the dynamic behavior of structures.
- Time gain compensation is the exponential amplification of signals as a function of elapsed time following the transmitted pulse to compensate for attenuation along the beam path.
- Receiver gain, the primary control for image brightness, increases the amplitude of all signals (and consequently noise) by the same factor.
- Reject control, adjustable by sonographer, eliminates low signals and noise below a threshold value from the image.
- Operator control of compression (also called dynamic range and logarithmic compression) adjusts the displayed dynamic range and often increases image contrast by removing low or high signals.
- Write zoom is a magnification technique to distribute the pixels in the image matrix over a smaller field of view to improve resolution.
- Panning allows the operator to move the displayed field of view to a new anatomic location during scanning without repositioning the transducer.
- Persistence or frame averaging adds successive frames to reduce noise.
- Gray-scale mapping establishes the relationship between pixel value and brightness displayed on the monitor.
- Speckle is a composite interference pattern from numerous scattering events.
- Clutter is spurious signals arising from echoes induced by ultrasound transmission unrelated to the main beam (e.g., multipath scattering).
- Contrast resolution is the ability to discern reflectors that have different acoustic properties; it depends on the magnitude of the signal difference as well as the size of the object.
- Geometric distortion is the inaccurate presentation of spatial relationships.
- An artifact is a structure in the image that does not correlate directly with actual tissue.
- Partial volume effect occurs when simultaneous sampling of tissues with different acoustic properties yields an intermediate result.

- Regions distal to a low-attenuating structure are depicted with stronger signals compared with adjacent similar tissues, which were interrogated by beam paths that did not include the low-attenuating structure.
- Regions distal to a high-attenuating structure are depicted with weaker signals compared with adjacent similar tissues, which were interrogated by beam paths that did not include the high-attenuating structure.
- Reverberation artifacts often occur between an interface with a high acoustic impedance mismatch (soft tissue-gas, fat-muscle, or fluid-gas) and the transducer.
- Multiple internal reflections within a small but highly reflective object create multiple echoes, which are recorded in the image as a series of short bands distal to the object.
- Mirror image artifact is formed when an object is located proximal to a highly reflective surface at which strong reflection occurs.
- Refraction along the beam path causes an object to be misregistered in the image (the assigned location differs from the true position of the object).
- A highly reflective object along the path of a secondary lobe produces an echo that is incorrectly assigned a location along the direction of the main beam.
- At high pulse repetition frequencies and short scan range, structures distal to the displayed field of view may be misregistered near the transducer.
- If the acoustic velocity along the propagation path to a reflector deviates from the assumed 1540 m/s, the depicted spatial location of that reflector is displaced from its true position.
- The Doppler effect describes the change in the frequency of sound observed if there is relative motion between the source of the sound and the receiver of the sound.
- The Doppler shift frequency depends on the relative velocity between source and receiver, the transmitted frequency, the acoustic velocity of the medium, and the Doppler angle as given by the Doppler shift equation.
- For a constant reflector velocity, the detected Doppler shift frequency decreases as the Doppler angle is increased.
- If the Doppler angle is 90 degrees, the Doppler shift frequency is zero.
- For a stationary transducer, the Doppler shift equation predicts that an increase in reflector velocity will cause a higher Doppler shift frequency.
- Uncertainty in the measurement of Doppler angle, particularly at large angles, introduces error in the velocity computation.
- The optimal transmitted frequency for Doppler is usually lower than that for B-mode imaging.
- Measurement of the Doppler shift frequency is based on wave interference, in which the echo-induced radio-frequency signal is combined with the reference signal to yield a complex waveform that varies with the beat frequency.

- Reflectors moving with a range of velocities produce multiple beat frequencies, which form a complex Doppler signal.
- The wall filter removes low-frequency Doppler shift frequencies associated with large, slow-moving reflectors (e.g., vessel walls) that can produce intense signals.
- Small differences in flow velocity can be detected with continuous wave (CW) Doppler.
- Echo ranging to ascertain depth of the moving reflectors is not possible with CW Doppler.
- In pulsed wave (PW) Doppler, the echo-ranging principle is applied to provide depth information regarding the origin of the Doppler signal.
- The sample-and-hold circuit in PW Doppler is a buffer that assembles point-by-point measurements acquired at the rate of the pulse repetition frequency to form the complex Doppler signal.
- Aliasing is the misrepresentation of the Doppler shift frequency as a lower frequency than the true value.
- The Doppler shift frequency must be sampled at a minimum of two times per cycle to detect movement without aliasing (Nyquist criterion). If the pulse repetition frequency is 16 kHz, the highest Doppler shift frequency that can be accurately presented is 8 kHz.
- Duplex Doppler scanners combine real-time B-mode imaging with CW or PW Doppler detection.
- Spectral analysis is the determination of the individual Doppler shift frequencies that compose the complex Doppler signal.
- Spectral analysis, when repeatedly rapidly in time, characterizes the flow in vessels.
- Fast Fourier transform (FFT) is a mathematical algorithm that converts the complex Doppler signal into a series of single-frequency sine wave components.
- The power spectrum shows the amplitude (or magnitude) of the individual Doppler shift frequency components plotted as a function of frequency or velocity via the Doppler shift equation.
- A graphic plot of the power spectrum as a function of time is called the Doppler spectral waveform.
- Aliasing in the Doppler spectral waveform is characterized by wraparound, whereby the high-velocity components above the Nyquist limit appear at lower velocity and in the reversed flow direction.
- Techniques to eliminate aliasing include higher pulse repetition frequency, baseline adjustment, increased angle of insonation, decreased depth to sample volume, and lower transmitted frequency.
- A time-varying trace of the highest Doppler shift frequency converted to velocity is the maximum velocity waveform, the most commonly displayed descriptor of Doppler spectral analysis.
- Doppler imaging combines, in real time, two-dimensional flow information depicted in color with gray-scale B-mode imaging.
- By displaying the two-dimensional spatial distribution of velocities and the temporal changes in the velocity patterns, Doppler imaging enables global visualization of flow.
- Color flow imaging detects the mean velocity at each sampling site where motion is present, which is then color-encoded by hue.
- Power Doppler imaging displays the amplitude of the Doppler signal at each sampling site where motion is detected, which is then color-encoded by hue.
- Color flow imaging depicts flow toward and flow away from the transducer simultaneously.
- Packet size or ensemble length is the number of transmit pulses that interrogate a color scan line.
- The rapid acquisition and analysis of color-flow data is accomplished with autocorrelation detection.
- An asynchronous scanner acquires B-mode and flow data separately, which are later superimposed to form the color Doppler image.
- Color aliasing is readily identified by adjoining regions shown with contrasting colors, representing maximum flow in opposite directions.
- Color flash is a sudden burst of color that encompasses a wide region within the frame, which is caused by transducer or tissue movement.
- Color bleed is the extension of color beyond the region of flow to the adjacent tissue.
- Color noise is the color fill-in of hypoechoic regions caused by random variations in Doppler signal measurements.
- M-mode scanning depicts the depth of the reflectors as a function of time in a two-dimensional graphic display.
- The information content of the M-mode trace contains reflector depth, signal level for each reflector, relative positions of the reflectors at each sampling time, and change in the axial position of each reflector with time.
- Visualized anatomy in the B-mode image facilitates the placement of the line cursor so that the desired structures are depicted in the M-mode trace.
- Ultrasound is not a form of ionizing radiation.
- No *acute* harmful effects have been reported following diagnostic medical sonography.
- *Radiation force* describes damage induced by mechanical motion.
- Absorption of sound causes heating of tissue (thermal effects).
- The dynamic behavior of microbubbles subjected to pressure fluctuations is called cavitation.
- Fetal abnormalities in mammals are not observed unless the temperature elevation exceeds a particular value for a minimal time duration (threshold effect).
- Epidemiologic studies have considered whether ultrasound exposure in utero at diagnostic intensity levels is harmful to the unborn child.

- Results from epidemiologic studies have been generally negative, which means that biological damage, if any, is subtle, delayed, or infrequent.
- Two acoustic output parameters, thermal index and mechanical index, have been adopted as indicators of potential adverse biological effects.
- The thermal index (TI) calculates the maximum temperature rise (in degrees centigrade) in tissue caused by energy absorption.
- The mechanical index describes the possibility of cavitation, which is more likely to occur at high acoustic pressure and low frequency.
- Cavitation has been demonstrated at peak pressures and frequencies within the operational range of diagnostic medical ultrasound.
- Thermal index is the ratio of the in situ acoustic power to the reference acoustic power required to raise tissue temperature by $1\,^{\circ}\text{C}$.
- Mechanical index is a dimensionless quantity and directly proportional to the derated peak negative pressure and inversely proportional to the square root of the frequency.

- The "as low as reasonably achievable" (ALARA) principle (lowest power and exposure time consistent with the objectives of the examination) should be practiced for diagnostic medical sonography.
- The AIUM's statement on mammalian in vivo biological effects concludes that no adverse thermal effects in mammalian tissues exposed in vivo have been independently confirmed for I(SPTA) below $100\,\text{mW/cm}^2$ (unfocused) and $1\,\text{W/cm}^2$ (focused).
- Tissue-mimicking material in phantoms has properties similar to those of tissue with respect to velocity, scattering, and attenuation.
- General-purpose tissue-mimicking phantoms commonly test for dead zone, axial resolution, lateral resolution, penetration, image uniformity, distance accuracy, and focal zone.
- Tests for penetration, vertical and horizontal distance accuracy, image uniformity, fidelity of image display, and fidelity of image recording are considered the most sensitive indicators of B-mode performance.
- The SMPTE test pattern is most appropriate means to evaluate the display monitor and hard-copy recording device.

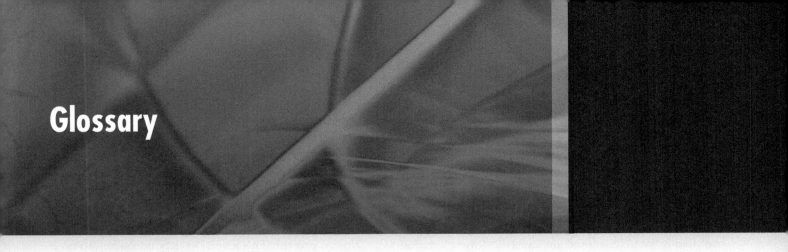

Glossary

3D ultrasound: An imaging mode in which spatial relationships of structures within a scanned volume are represented in three dimensions. The display of tomographic data is by a surface-rendered image, volume-rendered image, or multiple format planes.

4D ultrasound: An imaging mode in which three-dimensional echo data of the sampled volume are displayed in real time.

A-mode: Type of scanning mode in which the amplitude of the signal is plotted against the depth of the interface. The signal strength of the detected echo is represented by the height of the vertical deflection of the trace.

absorption: The process whereby ultrasound energy is dissipated to a medium by conversion to other energy forms, primarily heat. Intensity loss from absorption exhibits an exponential decrease and is the major factor in the total attenuation of the beam.

acoustic impedance: A measure of the resistance of a medium to the transmission of sound. Acoustic impedance is expressed as the product of acoustic velocity and the density of the medium.

acoustic velocity: The speed at which sound propagates through a medium. The average velocity of sound in soft tissue is 1540 meters per second (m/s).

aliasing: An artifact in pulsed-wave Doppler in which Doppler shift frequency is incorrectly interpreted as a lower frequency. Aliasing is caused by the intermittent sampling of moving reflectors.

amplitude: Normally refers to the particle displacement, particle velocity, or acoustic pressure of a sound wave. Amplitude also indicates the strength of the detected echo or the voltage induced in a crystal by a pressure wave.

analog-to-digital converter (ADC): A device that translates continuously variable signals (analog) into discrete values (digital). The digital form can then be manipulated and stored by computers.

annular phased array: Type of transducer in which the crystal arrangement consists of a central disk surrounded by concentric rings. Electronic focusing narrows the beam width for both in-plane and out-of-plane directions. Sampling along different lines of sight is achieved by the mechanical movement of the crystal array.

apodization: A technique applied during transmission and reception to reduce secondary lobes and enhance beam formation. During transmission, the excitation voltage is varied for each crystal element across the aperture of a multiple-element array. During reception the applied gain is varied for each crystal element in the array.

artifact: A structure in the image that does not provide a true representation of the scanned object. Artifacts are created by the inherent nature of sound interactions (e.g., reflection, refraction, and attenuation) or by equipment malfunction or by improper operation of the equipment.

asynchronous scanner: In Doppler imaging, flow data and gray-scale scan data are acquired independently (separate and distinct transmission for each).

attenuation: The decrease in intensity via scattering and absorption as a sound beam travels through a medium.

autocorrelation: A signal processing technique in Doppler imaging whereby a series of echoes from the same reflector (red blood cell group) are compared to assess motion. This is a very fast data collection method by which the mean frequency and amplitude of the Doppler signal are measured.

axial resolution: The ability to resolve, as separate entities, objects located near each other along the axis of propagation. Axial resolution depends primarily on spatial pulse length.

backing material: The material placed behind the crystal in the transducer to control the ringing of the crystal. In B-mode imaging, the acoustic impedance of the backing material is nearly the same as that for the crystal to dampen ringing.

banding: B-mode image artifact characterized by uneven brightness levels along the depth direction.

bandwidth: A parameter that describes the spread of frequency components in a wave (e.g., transmitted pulse).

baseline: In pulsed-wave spectral Doppler scanning, a control that shifts the center point of the velocity scale to vary the range of velocities displayed in the forward and reverse directions.

beam formation (reception): Echo-induced signals from multiple crystal elements are delayed in time and then summed to maximize the net signal associated with the reflector.

beam formation (transmission): Timed sequence of excitation pulses applied to crystal elements across the aperture to enable focusing of the ultrasound beam, steering of the ultrasound beam, or both.

beam width: The lateral extent of the beam perpendicular to beam propagation. Beam width (in-plane and elevation) varies along the beam axis.

beat frequency: A phenomenon caused by wave interference in which waves of different frequencies, when added together, produce rhythmic cycles or beats. In pulsed-wave spectral Doppler scanning, the transmitted waveform and the received signals are combined to yield the beat frequency (Doppler shift frequency), which indicates the presence of motion.

bilinear interpolation: A scan conversion method to assign echo amplitude to a pixel, which is not interrogated by a scan line. The interpolation is performed in axial and angular directions.

bulk modulus: A physical parameter that quantifies the fractional change in volume when a pressure is applied to material.

cavitation: Dynamic behavior of microbubbles in the medium exposed to an ultrasonic beam. Two types of cavitation are possible: stable and transient.

center frequency: The dominant frequency in the transmitted pulse (highest magnitude in a graph of frequency components).

channel: A communication pathway between a crystal element and the transmitter or summing circuit in the beam former. The total number of channels limits the number of crystal elements that participate in beam formation.

cine loop: Multiple frames of a real-time acquisition stored in computer memory for playback.

clutter: Spurious echo signals originating outside the main beam caused by side lobes, grating lobes, and scattering.

coded excitation: Frequency modulation or binary encoding of the transmitted pulse to improve signal-to-noise ratio. On reception, the echo wavetrain must be manipulated mathematically (deconvoluted) to identify individual reflectors.

color baseline control: In color Doppler imaging, a control that shifts the center point of the velocity scale to vary the range of velocities displayed in the forward and reverse directions.

color box: Designation of the color field of view within the two-dimensional field of view in color Doppler imaging.

color flow imaging: A real-time imaging modality in which flow information encoded in color is superimposed on a gray-scale image depicting stationary structures.

color gain: Doppler imaging control that adjusts the amplification of the Doppler signal.

color gate: Doppler imaging control that sets the axial length of the color sampling volume.

color line density: The number of color scan lines across the color field of view that affects the frame rate.

color map: Assignment of various shades or brightness of color to depict different velocities while maintaining directional information.

color map invert: Control that reverses the colors on the color scale bar as well as the colors in the image where flow is present. This inversion may be applied to preferentially show the vessel or cardiac structure as red or blue.

color M-mode: The presentation of the color Doppler image in conjunction with the M-mode trace. The sampling direction for the M-mode trace is shown on the color Doppler image.

color persistence: Frame averaging in Doppler imaging.

color reject: Doppler imaging control that sets the minimum signal strength for the display of color Doppler signals.

color velocity scale: Incorporated into the color flow display and shown as the color scale bar with the maximum velocity indicated (usually in centimeters per second).

color wall filter: A high-pass filter that eliminates low-frequency Doppler shift frequencies associated with slow-moving structures in the color flow image.

combined Doppler mode: The presentation of the color flow image in conjunction with the time display of the pulsed-wave spectral analysis.

comet tail artifact: An artifact created from small, highly reflective interfaces. Multiple internal reflections are ultimately detected and are mapped in the image extending distally from the reflector.

compound linear array: A linear array transducer that steers the beam via electronic phasing to extend the width of the field of view. Incorporates characteristics from both the linear array and the phased array.

compressibility: The ease with which a medium can be reduced in volume. The velocity of sound in a medium is inversely proportional to the square root of the compressibility of the medium.

compression (wave propagation): A high-pressure region or a region of increased density of particles created by the action of the sound wave.

contrast enhancement: An image processing technique that changes the association between pixel values and gray levels to display pixels with similar signal levels as different shades of gray.

contrast resolution: The ability to resolve two objects with similar reflective properties (signal levels) as separate entities.

curvilinear array: Multiple crystal elements arranged linearly on a curved surface. The width of the field of view extends beyond the physical dimension of the row of crystal elements.

cycle: A sequence of events recurring at regular intervals in time or space. For example, particle density varies from a maximum in the compression zone to a minimum in the rarefaction zone and back to a maximum in the successive compression zone to complete one cycle.

dead zone: The distance from the face of the transducer to the closest identifiable echo.

decibel: Unit expressing relative intensity.

density: A physical parameter that describes the mass per unit volume of a medium.

depth of field: Length of the focal zone for a focused transducer.

derating factor: Fractional reduction in intensity or pressure caused by attenuation in tissue.

diffraction: The spreading out of the beam that results when the beam passes through a small aperture.

diffuse reflection: The reflection of an ultrasound beam in multiple directions from a large rough-surfaced object.

divergence: The spreading out of a beam from a source of small physical dimensions, diffraction, or scattering. Divergence reduces beam intensity.

Doppler angle: The angle between the beam axis and the direction of travel for the moving reflector.

Doppler cursor: Means to denote the sampling direction for Doppler spectral waveform acquisition.

Doppler effect: Relative motion between the sound source and sound receiver causing a change in the observed frequency.

Doppler gain: Doppler control that amplifies the complex Doppler signal.

Doppler imaging: Moving reflectors encoded in color and stationary reflectors encoded in shades of gray are depicted throughout the field of view in real time.

Doppler output power (control): Control that varies the excitation voltage applied to transducer elements to adjust the intensity of the transmitted beam for Doppler acquisition.

Doppler reject: Control that eliminates low-amplitude signals to suppress noise in the spectral display. The threshold for rejection is based on signal level rather than on frequency.

Doppler shift frequency: The change in frequency between the transmitted frequency (f) and received frequency by reflection from an interface moving with velocity (v) at an angle (θ) to sound propagation:

$$\text{Doppler shift} = \frac{2fv \cos \theta}{c}$$

where c is the velocity of sound in the medium.

Doppler spectral waveform: The time display of the velocity distribution present in the Doppler signal.

duty factor: The fraction of the time the transducer is actively producing the ultrasound beam. Duty factor equals pulse duration divided by pulse repetition period.

dwell time: The time required to interrogate one line of sight.

dynamic range: A measure of the spread of signal magnitudes that can be represented or processed by a device.

dynamic receive focusing: An electronic focusing method that uses continuously variable delay lines to sweep the receive focal zone through all depths during the reception of returning echoes.

echo ranging: A technique to determine the distance of an object from the transducer that relies on the measured time delay from pulse transmission to echo detection.

edge enhancement: A filtering technique to make the boundaries of structures more distinct.

elasticity: Property of a medium to return to its original shape after being deformed by a force.

elastography: An imaging modality that depicts the resistance of tissue to a change in shape when force is applied.

electronic focusing: Electronic delay lines connected to individual crystals of multiple-element transducers are adjusted to cause the ultrasonic wavefronts to reach the point of interest in phase (focus) and to reinforce the induced signals on reception of the echo.

endosonography: Specialized real-time imaging with small probes that can be inserted into various body cavities (e.g., endovaginal and endorectal).

enhancement: An image artifact caused by unequal attenuation along scan lines. Reflectors distal to a low-attenuating object appear with a greater signal level than do identical reflectors located in the neighboring region.

epidemiologic studies: Investigations of human populations to identify adverse effects associated with a particular agent.

extended field of view: Imaging method to enlarge the field of view of a real-time transducer. As a transducer is moved across the patient, successive frames are combined to form a panoramic image.

far field: The region beyond the near field for a nonfocused transducer in which the ultrasound beam diverges rapidly. Also called Fraunhofer zone.

fast Fourier transform (FFT): Mathematical algorithm that separates a waveform into its various frequency components. Spectral analysis of the complex Doppler signal identifies the Doppler shift frequencies and their relative importance.

field of view (FOV): The physical region probed by the ultrasound beam that corresponds to the image.

focal length: The distance from the front face of the transducer to the focal point.

focal zone: For a focused transducer, the region defined by the pressure amplitude that is within 3 decibels (dB) of the maximum pressure amplitude of the transmitted beam. The focal zone corresponds to the region of minimal beam width.

focusing: A process whereby the beam width is reduced by mechanical or electronic means.

footprint: The active piezoelectric area of a transducer that transmits ultrasound waves.

fractional bandwidth: The spread of frequency components in a transmitted wave expressed as a fraction of the center frequency.

frame averaging: The process whereby multiple successive frames separated in time are combined to produce an image with lower noise.

frame rate: In B-mode imaging, the number of images acquired per second. Also describes the refresh rate of a display.

free-field conditions: Pressure (intensity) measurements are performed in water without reflectors or other disturbances to the ultrasonic field.

freeze frame: A single image acquired during real-time scanning that is designated for display.

frequency: The number of wave cycles passing a given point in a given increment of time. The unit is cycles per second or hertz. Frequency is the inverse of period.

frequency averaging (frequency compounding): A method whereby frequency components in the echo signal are processed separately and then recombined in a single image to improve penetration, resolution, or tissue texture.

geometric distortion: Deviation from true spatial relationships corresponding to anatomic structures.

ghost image: An artifact whereby an object located distal to refractive structures is replicated multiple times in the image.

grating lobes: Secondary intensity lobes created by the regular spacing of crystal elements.

high-PRF mode: A method to reduce aliasing by increasing the pulse repetition frequency above the constraint imposed by echo ranging but with some ambiguity in depth position.

horizontal distance: Measurement of distance in the direction perpendicular to the central axis of the beam.

hydrophone: A device to measure pressure variations in the ultrasonic field.

intensity: A physical parameter that describes the amount of energy flowing through the cross-sectional area of a beam each second.

interference: The superposition or algebraic summation of waves. Constructive or destructive interference can occur.

lateral resolution: The ability to resolve, as separate entities, two adjacent objects that lie perpendicular to the beam axis. Lateral resolution depends on beam width.

lead zirconate titanate (PZT): A crystalline material with piezoelectric properties.

line of sight: The sampling direction of the sound beam. Multiple lines of sight are necessary to compose a B-mode image.

linear array: A multiple-element transducer in which the crystal elements are positioned next to one another in a row. Selective activation of crystal elements determines the direction of sampling. The image format is rectangular.

longitudinal wave: A wave in which the particle motion is along the same direction as the propagation of the wave energy (direction of travel of the wave).

matching layer: A layer of material placed next to the radiating surface of the crystal in the transducer to facilitate the transmission of sound energy into the patient.

matrix size: The number of rows and columns of pixels that compose the image.

maximum depth of visualization: The maximum depth at which scatterers are perceived.

maximum velocity waveform: The time display of the highest velocity component of the Doppler signal.

mean frequency: The average of all Doppler shift frequencies in the Doppler signal.

mechanical index: A parameter that describes the acoustic output in terms of the likelihood of cavitation, predicted by the ratio of the peak rarefactional pressure to the square root of the frequency.

mirror image artifact: An artifact in which an object is duplicated in the image. The incorrect placement of the object occurs distal to the strong reflector in the image.

M-mode scanning: A scanning technique that depicts the reflector position with respect to time in a two-dimensional display.

near field: For the nonfocused transducer, the region that extends from the front face to the beginning of divergence.

noise: Random variations that do not correspond to reflectivity in measured echo signals.

nonlinear propagation: At high intensity, the sound wave is distorted from the sinusoidal shape with the introduction of additional frequency components (harmonics).

Nyquist limit: The minimal rate at which the Doppler signal can be sampled without aliasing.

output display standard (ODS): The effect of current operating parameters on acoustic output expressed as the thermal index (TI) and the mechanical index (MI).

packet size: The number of transmit pulses used to sample a color line of sight in Doppler imaging. Also called ensemble length.

panning: Translation of the write zoom field of view within the limits of the field of view imposed by the transducer.

partial volume: The assignment of an intermediate signal level when the ultrasonic beam encompasses objects with different reflectivities.

period: The time for one complete wave cycle. Period is the inverse of wave frequency.

phase aberration: Loss of signal coherence during beam formation caused by differences in acoustic velocity in tissue.

phased array: A multiple-element transducer in which the beam is electronically steered and focused by time-delayed excitation of the crystals. The image format is sector.

piezoelectric effect: A pressure wave (sound wave) incident on a material with aligned dipolar molecules that induces an electrical signal. This permits the material to be used as a receiver of sound waves.

position generator: Device to determine the two-dimensional location of the echo origin.

power: A measure of the total energy transmitted per unit time summed over the entire cross-sectional area of the beam (intensity multiplied by area). The unit of power is the watt (joule per second).

power Doppler: Doppler imaging technique in which the signal strength (not velocity) of moving reflectors at each sampling site is encoded by color.

power spectrum: Graphic representation of the spectral analysis in which the magnitude of each frequency is plotted as a function of frequency.

propagation: The transmission of sound energy to regions remote from the sound source.

pulse average: The duration of a single pulse that prescribes the time interval over which the intensity is measured.

pulse duration (temporal pulse length): The time interval during which the transmitted pulse is generated. The pulse duration is calculated by multiplying the number of cycles in the pulse by period.

pulse repetition frequency (PRF): The number transmitted pulsed waves generated each second. The maximum PRF depends on the scan range (R) and the acoustic velocity (c):

$$PRF_{max} = \frac{c}{2R}$$

pulse repetition period (PRP): The time interval between successive transmit pulses. It is equal to the inverse of pulse repetition frequency.

quadrature phase detector: Signal processing to identify the forward and reverse components of the complex Doppler signal.

Q-value: A transducer parameter that characterizes the pulse length and bandwidth of the transducer.

radiation force: Acoustic pressure applied over the surface of an object causing translational or rotational motion.

range ambiguity artifact: The misplacement of a reflector in the B-mode image when the detected echo was not created from the most recent transmitted pulse.

range gate: The selection of a time interval (time delay and time length) after pulsed-wave transmission during which the detected echoes are processed for display. Since distance from the transducer is defined by the elapsed time, analysis is restricted to echoes originating from a specific depth.

rarefaction: A low-pressure region or a region of decreased density in a medium created by the action of the sound wave.

read zoom: A method to magnify the image size on the monitor.

receive beam formation: Echo-induced signals from multiple crystal elements are delayed in time and then

summed to maximize the net signal associated with the reflector.

receive beam former: Executes dynamic receive focusing of the detected echo across several crystal elements.

reflection coefficient: The fraction of incident intensity reflected by an acoustic interface.

reflectivity: The combination of factors—including acoustic impedance mismatch, size, shape, and angle of incidence—that determines the intensity of a reflected echo from an interface.

refraction: A process whereby sound enters one medium from another, resulting in a bending or deviation of a sound beam from the expected straight-line path. Refraction obeys Snell's law, which is based on the ratio of the velocity of sound in the respective media.

registration arm: The scanning mount for the static B-mode transducer, which senses transducer position and orientation.

reverberation: An artifact in B-mode imaging created when repeated reflections occur between two strong reflectors.

sample volume: Defined region within which echoes must originate in order to be processed for display.

scan converter: A device that stores scan data in the form of echo signal strengths with the corresponding locations of the interfaces.

scan line: The sampling direction of the sound beam. Multiple lines of sight are necessary to compose a B-mode image. Also called line of sight.

scan line density: The number of scan lines per unit length or angular degree.

scan range: The maximum depth from which a returning echo can be detected with the correct assignment of reflector depth. The maximum depth of the field of view.

scattering: The redirection of sound energy resulting from the sound beam striking an interface whose physical dimension is less than one wavelength. Also called nonspecular reflection.

sector scanner: A real-time scanner that produces a pie-shaped field of view.

sensitivity: The ability of the scanner to detect weak-reflecting objects at a specific distance from the transducer.

shadowing: The reflectors distal to a highly attenuating object that appear lower in signal strength than adjacent reflectors with similar reflectivities.

signal processing: The manipulation of a received echo signal to enhance the presentation of scan data.

slice thickness: The out-of-plane (elevation) thickness contributing to the echo formation at that location in the image.

smoothing: A spatial filtering technique for reducing noise in the image.

Snell's law: A mathematic description of the principle of refraction that relates the bending of the wave with the ratio of the acoustic velocities for the media.

spatial average intensity: Average of intensity measurements over the cross-sectional area of the beam.

spatial compounding: A real-time imaging method in which scan lines for consecutive frames are steered at different angles and the scan data are combined to form a composite image.

spatial peak intensity: The location in the ultrasonic field where intensity has the highest value.

spatial pulse length: The spatial extent of the transmitted pulse. The spatial pulse length is the product of the number of cycles in the pulse and the wavelength.

speckle: Interference pattern incident on a transducer produced by echoes from multiple scatterers. The signal does not exhibit a one-to-one correspondence with the scatters. The speckle pattern is frequency-dependent.

spectral analysis: The process of determining the individual Doppler shift frequencies that are present in the complex Doppler signal and the relative importance of each.

spectral broadening: The introduction of additional frequency components in the complex Doppler signal caused by limitations in the detection technique.

spectral invert: A control to alter the assigned flow direction of the Doppler spectral waveform with respect to the baseline.

specular reflector: An interface much larger than the wavelength of the sound wave.

stable cavitation: The expansion and contraction of preexisting microbubbles in response to the applied pressure oscillations.

static B-mode: Generation of a single B-mode image by moving the transducer across the patient's surface.

subdicing: The crystal element of an array is divided into several smaller subelements. These subelements are electrically wired together to act conjointly. Subdicing helps to reduce the intensity of grating lobes.

sweep speed: Control to set the temporal resolution in the M-mode or spectral Doppler display.

temporal average intensity: The time average of intensity at a point in space.

temporal peak intensity: The peak value of the intensity at a point in space.

temporal resolution: The ability to depict the movement of structures accurately.

thermal index: The ratio of the in situ acoustic power to the acoustic power required to raise tissue temperature by 1°C.

threshold: The minimal level that the dose of an agent must exceed in order to induce an adverse effect.

tissue harmonic imaging: Imaging mode that detects harmonic frequencies created by the nonlinear propagation of ultrasound through tissue.

tissue-mimicking (TM) phantom: A phantom made of materials that mimic the ultrasonic properties of tissue with respect to velocity, attenuation, and scattering. Small, strong reflectors are placed in well-defined geometric patterns within the phantom to assess axial resolution, lateral resolution, dead zone, and distance accuracy.

transducer: Any device that converts one form of energy into another form. In ultrasound, a piezoelectric crystal converts an electrical stimulus into an ultrasound pulse and the returning echo into an electrical signal.

transient cavitation: A condition in which short-lived bubbles undergo large variation in size before collapsing completely.

transit time broadening: Introduction of frequency components above and below the actual Doppler shift because sampling is performed with a finite beam size.

transmission coefficient: A coefficient that describes the fraction of intensity of a beam transmitted through an acoustic interface.

transmit beam former: Timed sequence of excitation pulses applied to crystal elements across the aperture to enable focusing and/or steering of the ultrasound beam.

transverse wave: The motion of the particles in the medium is perpendicular to the direction of wave propagation.

uniformity: Signals obtained for interfaces with similar reflective properties located at the same depth have the same amplitude.

variance map: Color assignment in Doppler imaging based on the distribution of velocities within the sampling volume.

vector array: A transducer with multiple crystals in a linear format that steers the beam via electronic phasing to extend the width of the field of view. Also called compound linear array.

velocity error: The incorrect assignment of reflector size or position caused by acoustic velocity deviation from 1540 meters per second (m/s) along the beam path. Also called propagation error.

velocity scale: In flow detection, the range of velocities that can be displayed without aliasing.

vertical distance accuracy: Measurement of distance in the direction along the central axis of the beam.

voxel: Volume element is the smallest three-dimensional component of a scanned volume data set.

wall filter: A high-pass filter that eliminates low-frequency Doppler shift frequencies associated with slow-moving structures such as vessel walls.

wavelength: A physical characteristic of a wave that is the distance for one complete wave cycle.

write zoom: Magnification technique applied during data collection to improve spatial detail by mapping the detected echoes within a field of view that has reduced physical dimensions.

zone sonography: A B-mode imaging method in which echo wavetrain data for each channel following a series of broad-beam transmitted pulses are mathematically reconstructed to form the image.

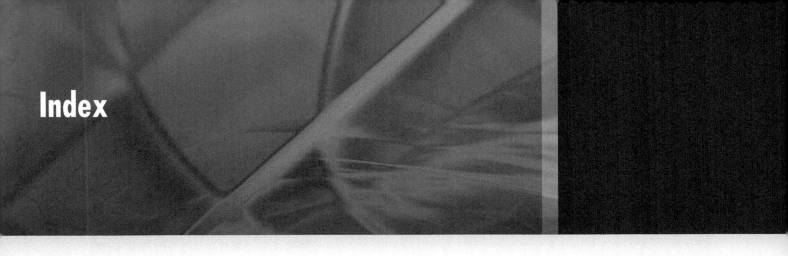

Index

Note: Page numbers followed by *b* indicate boxes, *f* indicate figures and *t* indicate tables.

A

Absorption, 17–18, 18*f*
Acoustic impedance
    of the matching layer, 32–33
    in ultrasound, 10–11, 11*t*
Acoustic intensity, 21
Acoustic lenses, 43
Acoustic noise, 121–122
Acoustic radiation force, 102
Acoustic velocity
    change in intensity and, 21
    in ultrasound physics, 4–5, 5–6, 7*t*
Acoustic velocity equation, 6, 7*t*
Adaptive frame averaging, 112
Adaptive time-gain compensation, 106
AIUM. *See* American Institute of Ultrasound in
        Medicine (AIUM)
Aliasing
    color, 177, 177*f*
    Doppler spectral analysis and, 162–163,
        163*f*
    pulsed-wave Doppler and, 149–150, 149*f*
A-line echo signal, 102
American Institute of Ultrasound in Medicine
        (AIUM), 191, 193–194, 197
A-mode scanner/scanning, 45, 48
    block diagram of, 52*f*
    illustrative, 52–53, 53*f*, 54*f*
    role in current clinical practice, 51–52
Amplification, 46
Amplitude, 3
    peak, 25
    ratio, decibels *vs.*, 25*t*
Analog scan converter, 55, 55*f*
Analog-to-digital conversion, 58–59
    height conversion, 58–59, 59*f*
    serial sampling, 59, 59*f*
Annular phased arrays, 65, 77, 77*f*
Aperture focusing, 70–72, 73*f*
Apodization, 77–78
Applications of color Doppler imaging,
        180–181, 180*f*
Arrays, 118–119, 128. *See also* Phased arrays
    annular phased, 65, 77, 77*f*
    compound linear, 77
    curvilinear, 74–75, 75*f*, 118–119, 128
    linear, 66–68, 67*f*, 68*f*, 118–119, 128
    multielement, 101
    2D, 101

Artifacts, 117–118, 124–125
    attenuation, 177
    color aliasing, 177, 177*f*
    color bleed, 179, 179*f*
    color noise, 179, 179*f*
    flash, 179–180, 180*f*
    high pulse repetition frequency, 177
    image, 127–139
    mirror-image artifact, 178, 179*f*
    misregistration of color, 179–180, 180*f*
    multiple-angle, 178, 178*f*, 179*f*
As low as reasonably achievable,
        principle of, 195
Asynchronous autocorrelation system,
        171–172
Asynchronous linear array, 172*f*
Asynchronous scanner, 168
Attenuation, 9, 24, 27, 177
    artifacts related to, 128–129, 128*f*, 129*f*
    interactions and, 18, 18*t*, 19*f*
Attenuation rate, 26
Autocorrelation, 169–171
    Quadrature detection, 169–170
    signal processing, 170–171, 170*f*, 171*f*
        dwell time, 170
        fixed echo canceller, 171
Autoscanning. *See* Scanned mode
Axial resolution, 30, 39–41, 40*f*, 41*t*, 117–118,
        118*f*, 203, 203*f*, 204*f*, 205*f*, 205*t*
Azimuthal resolution. *See* Axial resolution

B

Backing material, 32
Banding, 129, 129*f*
Bandwidth, 35–37, 36*f*
    broad, 89
    calculation of, 36, 37*f*
    fractional, 36–37
    matching layer effect and, 37
    pulse duration and, 35, 37*f*
    pulsed-wave, 150
BART format. *See* "Blue away, red toward"
        (BART) format
Baseline, 159
Beam formation, 75
Beam steering, 76*f*
Beam width, 39, 44, 44*f*, 62–63, 63*f*
    effective, 73
    and lateral resolution, 41*f*, 45*t*

Beat frequency, 144
Bilinear interpolation, 108
Binary encoding, 93–94, 94*f*
Bioeffects Committee of the AIUM,
        193–194
Black and white inversion, 110
Bladder, reverberation artifacts in, 130*f*
"Blue away, red toward" (BART)
        format, 168
B-mode image, 102*f*, 103*f*, 151
B-mode imaging, M-mode with, 184, 185*f*
B-mode imaging system, lateral resolution of,
        118
B-mode scanner/scanning. *See also* Static
        B-mode scanning
    motion and, 183
    with multiple-element transducer, 84*f*
    operation of, 62
    real-time, 57
Breast with cyst, sonogram of, 27*f*
Broadband techniques, 89
Broad bandwidth, 89
Broad-bandwidth transducers, 118
Bulk modulus, 5–6, 7*t*

C

Capacitive micromachined ultrasonic
        transducers (CMUTs), 80
Cavitation, 188–189, 192
    stable, 188–189
    transient, 189
Center frequency, 34, 36
Channel, 72
Cine loop, real-time instrumentation
        and, 87
CIRS, Inc., 198–199
Clinical applications, of elastography,
        102–103, 102*f*, 103*f*
Clinical efficacy in obstetrics, 194
Clinical image quality, evaluation of, 215–216,
        216*f*
Clinical safety, 187–196
    American Institute of Ultrasound in
        Medicine, 193–194
    clinical efficacy in obstetrics, 194
    display of output indices, 192
    education and training, 195
    epidemiologic studies, 189–190
    Mechanical index, 191, 192

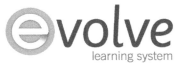
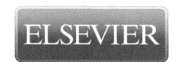
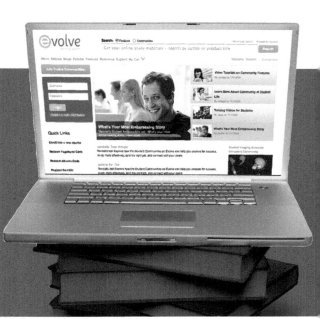

Printed and bound by CPI Group (UK) Ltd, Croydon, CR0 4YY

03/10/2024

01040349-0019